OXFORD MEDICAL PUBLICATIONS

Autoimmune Rheumatic Disease

'The conquerors make war upon themselves, blood
against blood, self against self.'

From King Richard III
William Shakespeare 1592
(Perhaps the first published reference to autoimmunity!)

Autoimmune Rheumatic Disease

Second edition

JOHN MORROW
Senior Lecturer in Immunopathology
St Bartholomew's and The Royal London
School of Medicine and Dentistry
London, UK

J. LEE NELSON
Associate Member, Fred Hutchinson Cancer Research Center,
Seattle; and Associate Professor of Medicine, University of
Washington, USA

RICHARD WATTS
Consultant Rheumatologist, The Ipswich Hospital NHS Trust,
Ipswich; and Honorary Senior Lecturer, University of
East Anglia, UK

DAVID ISENBERG
ARC Diamond Jubilee Professor of Rheumatology
University College London, UK

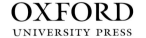

OXFORD

UNIVERSITY PRESS

OXFORD

UNIVERSITY PRESS

Great Clarendon Street, Oxford OX2 6DP

Oxford New York

Athens Auckland Bangkok Bogota Buenos Aires Calcutta
Cape Town Chennai Dar es Salaam Delhi Florence Hong Kong Istanbul
Karachi Kuala Lumpur Madrid Melbourne Mexico City Mumbai
Nairobi Paris São Paulo Singapore Taipei Tokyo Toronto Warsaw

and associated companies in
Berlin Ibadan

Oxford is a trade mark of Oxford University Press

Published in the United States
by Oxford University Press Inc., New York

First edition published 1987

Second edition published 1999

British Library Cataloguing in Publication Data
Data available

Library of Congress Cataloging in Publication Data

1 3 5 7 9 10 8 6 4 2

ISBN 0 19 262883 6

Typeset by
EXPO Holdings, Malaysia
Printed in Hong Kong

Preface

It is a little over 10 years since the first edition of *Autoimmune Rheumatic Disease* appeared. During this time a vast amount of information on virtually every aspect of these diseases, from aetiopathogenesis to treatment has been published. New sets of clinical features have come to be recognized, most notable being the appreciation that the phospholipid syndrome exists as a primary entity separate from systematic lupus erythematosus.

To help assimilate and clarify this information for the second edition the original authors, John Morrow and David Isenberg, have been joined by Lee Nelson and Richard Watts, whose major interests are, respectively, in immunogenetics and new approaches to therapy. By emphasizing these topics, whose rapid growth has been remarkable, we believe that the fresh and timely approach of the first edition is enhanced.

Our major objective in the first edition was to draw clinicians and basic scientists together by providing clear accounts of the clinical expression of the autoimmune rheumatic diseases, a comprehensive review of their immunopathology, a critical analysis of their animal models, and explanations of the laboratory tests used to study them. As we recalled in the preface to the first edition the need for this approach was emphasized by overhearing the comment of a laboratory technician who, after listening to a lecture by one of us on the clinical aspects of SLE, was heard to remark, 'I never realized there was a human model for this animal disease'. This objective remains paramount in the second edition and has been reinforced by a reciprocal anecdote. Not long after the first edition was published one of us struck up a conversation with a junior clinician about experimental therapies for lupus and, in particular, the NZB/W mouse. 'That's fantastic,' he said, 'You mean there is an animal model for lupus?'. This question would not have been so surprising if the individual in question had not just carried out a residency in a department at the National Institutes of Health famous for its work on experimental autoimmunity!

The layout of the chapters broadly follows that of the first edition though with even greater use of original artwork and colour. The section describing the fundamental concepts of immunogenetics has been completely updated. The development of a variety of new animal models is also emphasized and much attention is paid to the potential of monoclonal antibody and other new forms of therapy.

The integrated use of colour throughout the volume with diagrams and illustrations situated close to their text has also been maintained in order to provide logical presentation of clinical features and histopathology (a butterfly rash or histology slide stained with haematoxylin and eosin shown in black and white rather misses the point!).

Drug schedules are continually being revised and new side-effects recognized. Although guidance about the type of drugs used to treat patients with autoimmune rheumatic diseases is discussed, the book is not intended to be a pharmacopoeia. Readers who wish to learn more about precise dosage schedules are advised to consult the pharmaceutical company's printed instructions before administering any of the drugs recommended.

W.J.W.M.
J.L.N.
R.A.W.
D.A.I.

October 1998

Acknowledgements

We would like to acknowledge gratefully the tremendous secretarial and administrative support given to us by Ann Maitland. We also thank those who kindly allowed us to use material from their photograph collections, including Elizabeth Adams, Meryl Griffiths, Lorin Lakasing, Paul Plotz, Michael Snaith and Tom Stoll. Lesley Isenberg, Brendan Murphy, Keith Nye, Elizabeth Ross and Nadeem Sheikh very kindly donated original material. We are especially grateful to Elizabeth Jeffery not only for extensive comments on the pathological mechanisms in rheumatoid arthritis but for providing the immunofluorescence slide used for the cover design. Discussions with Lori Tucker and Pat Woo encouraged us to emphasize the development of autoimmune rheumatic disease during childhood. Ramesh Nayak brought our attention to the Shakesperian quote used at the beginning of the book.

We also wish to thank several pharmaceutical and other companies whose kind support has enabled us to integrate the colour plates throughout the text. We thank Abbott Laboratories, Alpha Laboratories, The Binding Site, Boehringer Ingelheim, ImmunoConcepts, Novartis, Pharmacia, and Searle. We are also indebted to ImmunoConcepts for providing the immunofluorescence slides and photographs of other immunological assays that appear in Chapter 2.

Contents

1 | Introduction: the immune system — order and disorder

Introduction

Since their recognition almost five decades ago, the immune processes underlying autoimmune rheumatic disease have been the subject of intense clinical and laboratory research. These efforts have had several consequences. Most obviously, the diagnosis and management has improved. Although treatment remains less than satisfactory in many cases, certain serious complications such as renal lupus can now be controlled much more effectively. In addition, immunological investigations, aided by the derivation of animal models, have enabled major advances in the understanding of the immunopathological mechanisms involved. These latter findings have provided a greater insight into all autoimmune conditions, including thyroiditis, diabetes mellitus, and myasthenia gravis which are not dealt with in this text.

We do not intend to instruct the reader in basic immunology. Such a task is beyond the scope of this book and there are many excellent primers on this subject available. Rather, the aim of this chapter is to review the immune system in sufficient detail in order that the concepts that are thought to underlie the aetiology and pathophysiology of autoimmune disease may be introduced in a manner that is comprehensible to the relatively inexperienced reader.

The normal immune response

Innate immunity

The immune response can be categorized as either *innate* or *specific*, although there is considerable interaction between these components. Innate immunity comprises elements of the immune system that can mount a non-specific, 'immediate' response. These are directly activated by infectious agents, inflammation, or tumours. The innate response has the advantage of speed, but lacks specificity and may cause host tissue damage and is frequently involved in the inflammation that can follow autoimmune events. The principal components of the innate immune response are as follows.

Neutrophils

The neutrophil (or polymorphonuclear cell) is a specialized phagocyte that is frequently involved in the inflammatory responses found in autoimmune diseases. These cells are released from the bone marrow in large numbers during acute infection or inflammation, and new cells are produced by the action of granulocyte and granulocyte-macrophage colony stimulating factors (G-CSF and GM-CSF) to cause the characteristic neutrophil leucocytosis.

Powerful chemoattractants are released at sites of infection or inflammation. These are principally the complement activation products C5a and C3a and the macrophage-derived leukotriene, B4. These substances cause migration of neutrophils to the inflamed site by: (i) upregulation of adhesion molecules on neutrophils, which increases margination and adhesion of neutrophils to the vascular endothelium; and (ii) stimulating neutrophil chemotaxis. Cells pass between endothelial cells into the tissues by a process known as *diapedesis*.

Phagocytosis occurs by the formation of pseudopodia around the organism or particle to be ingested. Owing to the fluidity of the cell membrane, the tips eventually fuse to form a membrane-bound vesicle. The phagosome fuses with the neutrophil cytoplasmic granules to form a phagolysosome. Within this localized environment, killing occurs. There are two major mechanisms: (i) O_2-dependent response, or respiratory burst, in which there is production of reactive oxygen metabolites, such as hydrogen peroxide, hydroxyl radicals, and singlet oxygen, via the reduction of oxygen by an NADPH oxidase; and (ii) O_2-independent response, owing to the toxic action of preformed cationic proteins and enzymes contained within the neutrophil cytoplasmic granules.

Eosinophils

These cells comprise up to 5% of white blood cells in healthy individuals and appear to be used selectively for fighting parasitic (particularly nematode) infections. Eosinophils also participate in immediate hypersensitivity type inflammatory reactions, although they appear to be involved in autoimmune reactions on rare occasions. They have low-affinity surface receptors for antibodies of the IgE class. They are not phagocytic, but they contain many large granules, which are cytotoxic when released by the binding of IgE (through the cellular Fc receptor) and complexed antigen.

Basophils and mast cells

Mast cells consist of at least two distinct populations, which are distinguished by their enzyme content. The T mast cells contain trypsin alone and were formerly termed 'mucosal mast cells' owing to their location near mucosal surfaces. The TC mast cells contain both trypsin and chymotrypsin and were formerly described as 'connective tissue mast cells', owing to their location. The TC mast cells contain more histamine, which is released following stimulation with basic amines. Conversely, only T mast cells contain cytoplasmic IgE.

Basophils, and the morphologically similar mast cells, make up only a very small proportion of the granulocytic white blood cell population. Basophils are involved in inflammation, although their role is rather obscure. The cytoplasmic granules of basophils and mast cells contain histamine and other vasoactive amines. These cells also bear high-affinity IgE Fc receptors and participate in immediate hypersensitivity reactions.

Complement

Complement is involved in the eradication of organisms and immune complexes, as well as in inflammation and immunoregulation. The complement system comprises a series of at least 20 serum glycoproteins that are activated in a cascade sequence, with proenzymes that undergo sequential proteolytic cleavage, similar to the coagulation pathway.

Two main pathways of activation exist, termed the classical and alternative pathways (Fig. 1.1a). These converge in the activation of C3, both forming individual C3 convertases. This leads into the final common pathway with the assembly of C5–C9 into the membrane attack complex (MAC), which forms a 'doughnut-like' transmembrane channel leading to cell lysis by osmotic shock. A mannose binding lectin pathway which activates C3 has also been recognized.

Activation of the classical pathway
Activation of the classical pathway is calcium- and magnesium-dependent and occurs by the binding of C1q (a subcomponent of the C1 molecule) with either IgG- or IgM-containing antigen–antibody immune complexes (Fig. 1.1b).

Activation of the alternative pathway
The main components of this pathway are, factor B, factor D, and properdin (Fig. 1.1c). In the presence of factor D, factor B is cleaved (to Bb) and combines with C3b to form the alternative pathway C3 convertase, C3bBb. This convertase is stabilized by properdin. The alternative pathway is continually turning over at a low rate. This is markedly accelerated by alternative pathway activators, which provide a 'protected' site for the C3bBb convertase by enhancing the binding of properdin and preventing degradation of the complex. Activators of the alternative pathway include: yeast cell walls, IgA, endotoxin (Gram-negative bacterial cell walls), and C3 nephritic factor (an autoantibody that stabilizes the convertase), found in patients with membrano-proliferative glomerulonephritis.

Regulation of complement activation
Complement activation does not occur in the fluid phase, but is localized on the surface of the organism, cell, or immune complex that triggered the reaction. This is essential, as many of the by-products of complement activation are potent mediators of inflammation, and would cause extensive tissue damage if not controlled. In addition to the activation sequences described, there are regulatory proteins (factors H and I) that suppress the activation.

Effector functions of complement
The most important effects of complement activation are:

(a)

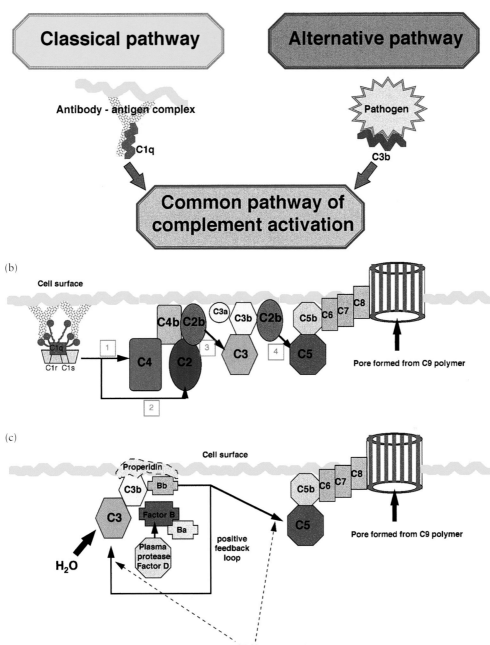

(b)

(c)

Fig. 1.1(a–c). The complement system is made up of a series of serum proteins that interact in a cascade. Most of the early components are serine proteases, which activate each other sequentially. There are initially two main activation pathways, *classical* and *alternative*, which lead to a final common pathway. The classical pathway is activated by antibody–antigen complexes, while the alternative pathway is initiated when a pre-activated complement component (C3b) binds to the surface of a pathogen, where it is protected.

- Destruction of pathogens and tumour cells by the lytic process described above and by opsonizing them for phagocytosis.
- Recruitment of cells and proteins to inflammatory sites, by the chemoattractant activity of the proteolytic products C5a and C3a, and the increase in vascular permeability also produced by these factors (sometimes called anaphylatoxins).
- Removal of immune complexes by opsonization, solubilization (alternative pathway), and prevention of precipitation (classical pathway).
- Immunomodulation, especially of B cell responses.

Acute phase proteins

Acute phase reactants are proteins that are synthesized in response to trauma, infection, necrosis, tumours, or other inflammatory events (Table 1.1). Although of

Table 1.1   Acute phase proteins

- C-reactive protein
- Fibrinogen
- Serum amyloid A
- Serum amyloid P
- Haptoglobin
- Complement components
- Mannan binding protein
- α_1-antitrypsin
- α_2-macroglobulin
- Ceruloplasmin

secondary importance, these substances play a part in non-specific defence mechanisms and also appear to be involved in immunopathological processes. The measurement of C-reactive protein in the serum is particularly useful in monitoring disease activity.

Heat shock proteins

Heat shock proteins are a family of highly conserved proteins that act as immunodominant antigens in many infections (Table 1.2). They act as molecular chaperones (housekeeping proteins within cells), preserving the cell's protein structure. They are similar in configuration to the antigens found on certain microorganisms and may induce autoimmunity through molecular mimicry.

Table 1.2   Major stress or heat shock proteins

Low molecular weight
- HSP27 kDA
- HSP32 kDA (haem oxygenase)
- HSP47 kDA
- HSP56 kDA

High molecular weight
- HSP60 kDA Family
    HSP65
- HSP70 kDA Family
    HSC70 (constitutively expressed form)
    HSP72
    Glucose regulated protein (Grp)75
    Grp78
- HSP kDA90 Family
    HSP90
    Grp94/96

Specific immunity

Specific or adaptive immunity is the hallmark of the immune system. It is achieved by a mechanism involving multiple rearrangements of original (germline) DNA in T and B lymphocytes. The altered DNA codes for proteins with hypervariable regions and creates the specific antigen-binding T cell receptor and antibody molecules. This genetic diversity allows the production, for example, of over 10^8 different antibodies, enough to cover the spectrum of antigens encountered by humans.

Antibody molecules (immunoglobulins)

Antibodies are serum glycoproteins that are produced as a highly specific response to an antigenic challenge. Collectively they are termed immunoglobulins. Briefly, they consist of two heavy chains (each with four domains) and two light chains (termed either κ or λ polypeptides, each with two domains). Hypervariable amino acid sequences occur in certain regions of both chains and it is here that antigen binding occurs (Fig. 1.2). A wealth of data exists regarding the physicochemical and functional characteristics of various antibody classes and subclasses, and these are summarized in Table 1.3. Some important terms, which the reader should be aware are:

Variable 'V' domains. These are regions on the immunoglobulin molecule that have great variation in amino acid and have short segments of hypervariable regions.

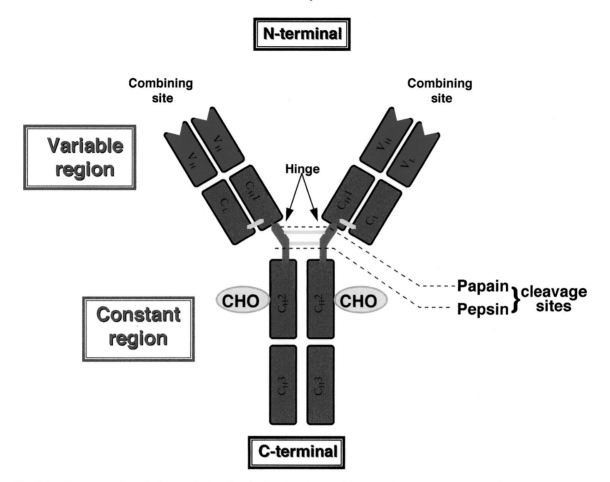

Fig. 1.2. Representation of a human IgG molecule showing the variable (V) and constant (C) regions, heavy (H) and light (L) chains, the location of carbohydrate (CHO) molecules and the carboxy terminal region (COOH). Enzymatic cleavage sites are indicated. The darkly shaded areas represent the hypervariable regions. The idiotypic region is located in the hypervariable section. The isotypic determinants are the heavy-chain constant region structures. Allotypes are antigenic markers located on the heavy chain. In three dimensions the CHO molecules interact 'connecting' the two C_H2 domains.

Idiotype. These structures are specific markers found in the hypervariable region of any given antibody and are associated with the antigen-binding site or *parotope*. The idiotype is also antigenic and can be determined by serological techniques. The smallest definable part of an idiotype is called an *idiotope*.

Fab (fragment antigen binding). Antigen binding occurs where the loops bearing the hypervariable regions of the light and heavy chains come together in space. The conformational structure of the binding site largely determines the 'goodness-of-fit', or affinity/avidity, of any particular antibody for an antigen.

Constant 'C' domains. The constant domains are regions of the molecule in which the amino acid sequences are relatively conserved.

Fc (fragment crystalline). This part of the immunoglobulin is formed from constant domains and regulates the effector functions (including binding to cell surface receptors and complement fixation), leading to elimination of the bound antigen.

The Hinge region. This structure gives flexibility to the antibody molecule, allowing ease of binding to antigen and cell surface receptors.

Table 1.3 Summary of the major biological and physico-chemical characteristics of the immunoglobulins

	IgG	IgM	IgA	IgE	IgD
Principal feature	Dominant class of antibody	Produced first in immune responses	Found in mucous membrane secretions including breast milk	Responsible for the symptoms of allergy. Probably important in defence against nematode parasites	Found almost solely on lympho-cyte cell surface membrane
Molecular weight	150 000	900 000 (pentamer)*	160 000 (dimer)*	180 000	200 000
Sedimentation coeff.	7S	29S	7, 9 or 11S†	8S	7S
Heavy chain	gamma	mu	alpha	epsilon	delta
Light chain	kappa + lambda	kappa + lambda	kappa + lambda	kappa + lambda	kappa + lambda
Carbohydrate content (%)	3	12	8	12	13
Mean adult serum conc. (mg/ml)	13.5	1.5	3.5	5×10^{-1}	0.03
Half-life (days)	21	10	6	2	3
Agglutination ability	+	+++	+	–	–
Precipitin formation	+++	+	+	–	–
Complement fixation:					
Classical	++	+++	–	–	–
Alternative	–	–	+/–	–	–
Binds to mast cells	–	–	–	+	–
Crosses placenta	+	–	–	–	–

*Both IgM and IgA molecules comprise the monometric forms bound by J (joining) chain.
†Depends on whether the molecule is in mono- or dimeric form and if secretory component is attached.

Allotype. Allotypic variation is a phenomenon that describes the occurrence of different alleles of the same immunoglobulin between individuals. Such genetic markers are primarily associated with the constant region of immunoglobulins and include the Gm specificities of IgG (which functionally indicate an interaction with rhesus D antigens) of which over 25 variants have been identified.

Isotype. The isotypic markers are the constant-region, heavy chain structures linked with the various immunoglobulin classes found in an individual. Thus, in practice, the term is a synonym for antibody class.

Genetics of antibody production

Antibody production is unusual in the way the immunoglobulin molecule is encoded within three separate chromosomes: (i) chromosome 14 for the heavy chain; (b) chromosome 2 for the light chain; and (iii) chromosome 22 for the light chain. Furthermore, rearrangement of the multiple elements of germline DNA leads to production of antibodies with many different antigen-binding sites (clonal diversity of Fab, Fig. 1.3).

Successive recombinations of VDJ to different C domains causes progressive switching in the

(a)

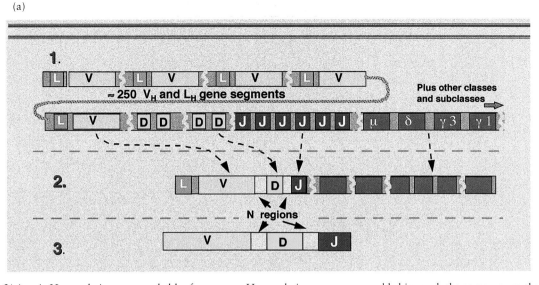

Fig. 1.3(a). 1. Heavy chains are encoded by four exons. Heavy chain genes are assembled in much the same way as the light chain genes with the addition of an $\cong$ 13 bp diversity or D segment between the V_H and J_H segments. 2. During lymphocyte differentiation a single $L_H - V_H$ unit is joined to a D segment and a J_H unit through somatic recombination. During this stage of the process the D segment is flanked by short segments of random sequence known as N regions. 3. The rearranged gene is transcribed in the daughter B cells and finally spliced to join the previously selected $L_H - V_H - N - D - N - J_H$ unit to one of the 8 C_H segments.

isotype of the antibody, but, since the Fab gene is not altered, the same antigen-binding region is maintained.

This explains why the primary immune response is of the IgM isotype, as this is the first to be translocated. Switching to subsequent isotypes requires help from T lymphocytes. IgG and other isotype responses therefore develop later. However, once the switch has occurred, memory B cells remain. These react rapidly to any further challenge and the IgG of the secondary response is produced. The extensive variability of antibody molecules and their predicted ability to combine with more than 10^8 different antigens is explained by the following factors:

- Multiplicity of V (25–100 genes), D (10 genes), and J (5–6 genes) genes within the DNA.
- Combinational freedom of VJ and VDJ genes and light and heavy chain genes, i.e. any of the multiple genes above can join each other.
- Junctional diversity: splicing of the genes together is frequently inaccurate and 'frame-shift' in base

pairs leads to misreading and production of the 'wrong' amino acid.
- Somatic mutation in V genes.

T cell receptor complex

Antigen recognition at the T cell level is accomplished by a mechanism quite similar to that employed by immunoglobulin (and immunoglobulin genes). Essentially, a limited set of gene segments can recombine to encode a highly diverse set of receptor specificities. The T cell antigen receptor is a structure on the surface of all thymus-derived lymphocytes. It comprises two transmembrane glycoprotein chains, termed α and β (although analogous structures named γ and δ can be found on some immature T cells). As with antibody, the polypetide chains have both a variable (V) and a constant region (C) of amino acid residues (Fig. 1.4). In the β chain the variable region is encoded by V-, D-, and J-like elements. The α chain is made up of V- and J-like elements. The polypeptide chains of the receptor are linked by disulfide bridges. Furthermore, the whole

(b)

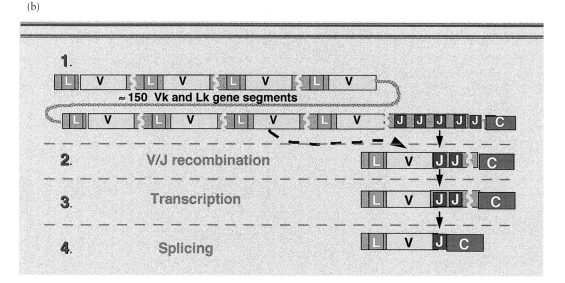

Fig. 1.3(b). 1. κ light chains are encoded by four exons (i) A leader or L_κ segment which encodes a 17–20 residue hydrophobic signal peptide. This directs *de novo* κ chains to the endoplasmic reticulum where it is removed. (ii) A V_κ segment which encodes the first 95 of the κ chain's 108-residue variable region. (iii) A joining or J_κ segment which encodes the 13 remaining residues of the variable region. (iv) The C_κ segment encodes the κ chain constant region. 2. During lymphocyte differentiation a single $L_\kappa - V_\kappa$ unit is joined to a J_κ unit through somatic recombination. 3. The rearranged gene is transcribed in the daughter B cells. 4. Finally splicing to join the previously selected L_κ, V_κ, J_κ exons with the C_κ exon.

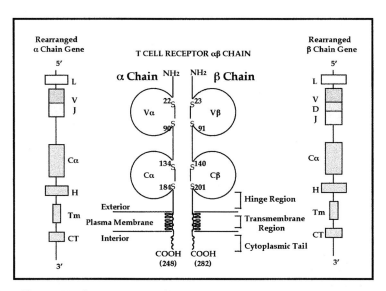

Fig. 1.4. Organization of human T cell receptor genes. The α and γ TCR genes are arranged in a single complex which spans over one million base pairs on chromosome 14. The $D\delta$, $J\delta$ and $C\delta$ genes are sandwiched between the interspersed $V\alpha/V\delta$ and $J\alpha$ genes such that the δ genes are deleted with rearrangement of the α gene. The β and γ TCR genes span approximately 600 and 150 kb respectively and are located at opposite ends of chromosome 7 with D, J and C genes downstream of the V genes. Abbreviations: V variable; D diversity; J joining; C constant.

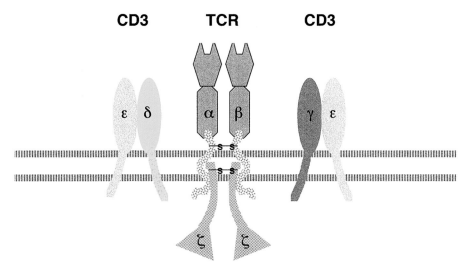

Fig. 1.5. Association of T cell receptor and CD3 molecules in the cell membrane.

molecule is arranged on the T cell membrane as a complex with another structure known as CD3 (Fig. 1.5). It is thought that this association is necessary for the antigen receptor to be expressed at the cell surface. The receptor also has a transmembrane tail. When an antigenic peptide is received by the receptor, a signal, manifesting as a series of enzyme phosphorylation reactions, is transmitted to the nucleus and the cell the responds accordingly by becoming activated, releasing cytokines, etc.

Organization of the lymphoid system

The immune system comprises several masses of lymphoid tissue or organs located throughout the body, as well as circulating leucocytes. The circulating cells originate from the bone marrow, which is the primary site of haematopoeisis in mammals. They subsequently differentiate and are programmed to fulfil certain roles by certain lymphoid organs. For example, the thymus processes 'virgin' lymphocytes into T cells, whereas B lymphocytes arise from the tonsils and gut-associated lymphoid tissue.

The cells of the immune system

Circulating leucocytes can be subdivided into several groups that are characterized by morphology, cell surface markers, and biological function. There are two families of molecular structures on the cell surface, called clusters of differentiation (CD; Table 1.4) and adhesion molecules (Table 1.5). The biological function of many of the CD molecules is now known and knowledge of their presence is very useful in identifying specific leucocyte subpopulations. Adhesion molecules facilitate many biological activities, particularly those involved in cell–cell recognition. Their functions include cellular activation, cytokine release, capture and 'rolling' of leucocytes along the endothelial cell lining of blood vessels, and extravasation. There is an overlap between these two families and certain adhesion molecules have also been assigned CD numbers.

An important function of cells of the immune system is the production and release of biologically active chemical messengers termed *cytokines*. The substances have a diverse range of functions and are summarized in Table 1.6. Cytokines are associated with inflammatory responses as well as specific types of immune response (see below). Quite recently an additional group of chemical messengers known as *chemokines* has been identified. These substances are of low molecular weight and categorized according to the presence of paired cysteine amino acid motif. Chemokines are primarily associated with the recruitment of mononuclear cells. The principal chemokines identified to date are summarized in Table 1.7.

Lymphocytes

Lymphocytes are spherical cells, approximately 10 μm in diameter, with a prominent nucleus of densely

Table 1.4 Major CD antigens and their cellular distribution

Cluster designation	Tissue distribution	Function
CD1	Cortical thymocytes	
CD2	All T cells and NK cells	Ligand for CD58; forms an adhesion pair, e.g. between T cell and antigen-presenting cell
CD3	Found on all mature T cells; intimately associated with the T cell receptor	Signal transduction following antigen presentation
CD4	T helper/inducer lymphocytes; comprise 2–3 circulating T cells	Ligand for class II MHC molecules associated with processed antigen fragments
CD5	T cells, also B cells	Ligand for CD72
CD8	Cytotoxic/suppessor T cells	Ligand for class I MHC molecules associated with processed antigen fragments
CD11a	Lymphocytes (especially memory T cells), granulocytes, monocytes, and macrophages	Part of adhesion molecule LFA-1
CD14	Macrophages	Receptor for bacterial lipopolysaccharide
CD16	Natural killer cells and macrophages	CD16 is a low-affinity Fc receptor involved in signal transduction
CD19	All mature B cells	Signal transduction
CD20	All mature B cells	Involved in cell activation; may be a calcium channel
CD21	Mature B cells, follicular dendritic cells, pharyngeal, and cervical epithelial cells	Complement C3d receptor
CD28	Activated T cells and some B cells	Activation of naive T cells
CD45	All cells of haematopoietic origin; also called *leucocyte common antigen*	Two isoforms, Ro and RA. Ro is associated with memory. Functions by cell signalling through the T cell receptor
CD56	NK cell marker	Mediates cell adhesion
CD72	All mature B cells	Ligand for CD5; involved in signalling
CD80/86	Antigen-presenting cells	Co-stimulatory ligands for CD28

Note: This list is far from exhaustative and has been confined to the CD types most commonly encountered in a clinical immunology setting.

packed nuclear chromatin. There are two main populations, the T and B lymphocytes.

T cells

T cells have two principal functions, and are divided into two groups.

Helper (CD4⁺) cells

T helper cells can be distinguished by the presence of the CD4 protein on their surface. These cells enhance certain immune responses. They receive antigen from specialized presenting cells and initiate or reinforce antibody production, natural killer cells, and cytotoxic responses, mainly by the production of certain cyto-

Table 1.5   Adhesion molecules

Adhesion molecule	Tissue distribution	Ligand
Immunoglobulin superfamily		
ICAM-1	Endothelial cells, monocytes, T and B cells, dendritic cells, keratinocytes, chondrocytes, epithelial cells	LFA-1
ICAM-2	Endothelial cells, monocytes, dendritic cells, subpopulations of lymphocytes	LFA-1
ICAM-3	Lymphocytes	LFA-1, Mac-1
VCAM-1	Endothelial cells, kidney epithelium, macrophages, dendritic cells, myoblasts, bone marrow fibroblasts	VLA-4
PECAM-1	Platelets, T cells, endothelial cells, monocytes, granulocytes	?
MAdCAM-1	Endothelial venules in mucosal lymph nodes	$\alpha 4\beta 7$ integrin and L-selectin
Selectin family		
E-Selectin/ELAM-1	Endothelial cells	?
L-Selectin	Lymphocytes, neutrophils,	?
P-Selectin	Megakaryocytes, platelets, and endothelial cells	?
Integrin family		
VLA subfamily		
VLA-1 to VLA-4	Endothelial cells, resting T cells, monocytes, platelets, and epithelial cells	Various molecules, including laminin, fibronectin, collagen, and VCAM-1
VLA-5 (fibronectin receptor)	Endothelial cells, monocytes, and platelets	Laminin
VLA-6 (laminin receptor)	Endothelial cells, monocytes, and platelets	Laminin
$\beta 1\alpha 7$	Endothelial cells, ?	Laminin
$\beta 1\alpha 8$	Endothelial cells, ?	?
$\beta 1\alpha_v$	Platelets and megakaryocytes	Fibronectin
$\beta 2$	Widely distributed	Collagen, laminin, vitronectin
Leucam subfamily		
LFA-1	Leucocytes	ICAM-1 to -3
Mac-1	Endothelial cells, ?	ICAM-1, fibrinogen, C3bi
Cytoadhesin subfamily		
Vitronectin receptor	Platelets and megakaryocytes	Vitronectin, fibrinogen, laminin, fibronectin, von Willebrand factor, thrombospondin
$\beta 4\alpha 6$	Endothelial cells, thymocytes, and platelets	Laminin
$\beta 5\alpha_v$	Platelets and megakaryocytes, ?	Vitronectin, fibronectin
$\beta 6\alpha_v$	Platelets and megakaryocytes, ?	Fibronectin
$\beta 7\alpha 4$/LPAM-1	Endothelial cells, thymocytes, monocytes	Fibronectin, VCAM-1
$\beta 8\alpha_v$	Platelets and megakaryocytes, ?	?

Abbreviations are as follows: intercellular adhesion molecule, ICAM; vascular cell adhesion molecule, VCAM; endothelial leucocyte adhesion molecule, E-selectin or ELAM; lymphocyte Peyer's patch adhesion molecule, LPAM; platelet/endothelial cell adhesion molecule, PECAM; very late antigen, VLA; leukocyte function-associated antigen, LFA; mucosal addressin, MAdCAM

Adapted from Table 2.15, Clinical Medicine (4th edition) eds P. Kumar and M. Clark. W.B. Saunders, Edinburgh, 1999.

Table 1.6 Cytokines: origin and biological function

Cytokine	Source	Mode of action
IL-1	Macrophages	Immune activation: induces an inflamatory response
IL-2	Primarily T cells	Activates T (and NK) cells and supports their growth. Formerly called *T cell growth factor*
IL-3	T cells	Primarily promotes growth of haematopoietic cells
IL-4	T helper cells	Lymphocyte growth factor; involved in IgE responses
IL-5	T helper cells	Promotes growth of B cells and eosinophils
IL-6	Fibroblasts	Promotes B cell growth and antibody production
IL-7	Stromal cells	Lymphocyte growth factor, important in the development of immature cells
IL-8	Primarily macrophages	Chemoattractant
IL-10	CD4 cells, activated monocytes	Inhibits the production of IFN-γ, IL-1, IL-6, TNF-α, and antigen presentation
IL-12	Monocyte/macrophages	Augments Th1 responses and induces IFN-γ
IL-13	Activated T cells	Stimulates B cells
G-CSF	Primarily monocytes	Promotes growth of myeloid cells
M-CSF	Primarily monocytes	Promotes growth of macrophages
GM-CSF	Primarily T cells	Promotes growth of monomyelocytic cells
IFN-α	Leucocytes	Immune activation and modulation
IFN-β	Fibroblasts	Immune activation and modulation
IFN-γ	T cells and NK cells	Immune activation and modulation
TNF-α	Macrophages	Stimulates generalized immune activation as well as tumour necrosis. Also known as *cacechtin*
TNF-β	T cells	Stimulates immune activation and generalized vascular effects. Also known as *lymphotoxin*
TGF-β	Platelets	Immunoinhibitory but stimulates connective tissue growth and collagen formation

Abbreviations: tumour necrosis factor, TNF; transforming growth factor, TGF; interleukin, IL; interferon, IFN; granulocyte-macrophage colony stimulating factor, GM-CSF; granulocyte colony stimulating factor, G-CSF; monocyte colony stimulating factor, M-CSF.

kines. In the last few years two types of T helper cell have been categorized into two major subpopulations based on their ability to produce certain cytokines. T cells of the T helper 1 (Th1) class produce IL-2, IL-3, and interferon-γ. These cytokines will promote immune responses that are primarily cell mediated or inflammatory. Lymphocytes of the T helper 2 (Th2) category produce cytokines that favour antibody

Table 1.7 Chemokines and associated function

Chemokine	Class	Site of production	Biological activity
MCP-1	-CC-	Monocytes, macrophages, fibroblasts, keratinocytes	Attracts monocytes and memory T cells to inflammatory sites
MIP-1α	-CC-	Macrophages	Attracts monocytes and T cells
MIP-1β	-CC-	Monocytes, macrophages, endothelial cells, T and B cells	Attracts monocytes and CD8+ T cells
RANTES	-CC-	Platelets and T cells	Attracts monocytes, T cell and eosinophils
IL-8	-CXC-	Macrophages	Attracts neutrophils, naive T cells
SDF-1α	-CXC-	Stromal cells	Attracts hemopoietic progenitor cells

Abbreviations: macrophage chemoattractant protein, MCP; macrophage inflammatory protein, MIP; regulated on activation, normal T-cell expressed and secreted, RANTES; stromal-derived factor, SDF.

responses, i.e. IL-4, IL-5, IL-10. Cells termed Th0 are CD4-positive T cells that have yet to differentiate into a Th1 or Th2 type. Recently, a third type of T helper cell has been described; this population has been termed Th3 and is associated with immunosuppressive effects mediated by TGF-β (Table 1.6).

Cytotoxic (CD8+) cells

The cytotoxic lymphocyte can be recognized by the presence of the CD8 cell surface molecule and has the ability to kill other cells in an MHC-restricted (major histocompatibility complex) manner. This kind of response is used in dealing with virus infections and cancer cells. The cytotoxic cell can down-regulate immune responses at an appropriate time. It may function by releasing soluble factors or messenger molecules, which act on the B lymphocytes to reduce their output of antibodies, although the suppressive function of these cells is still controversial.

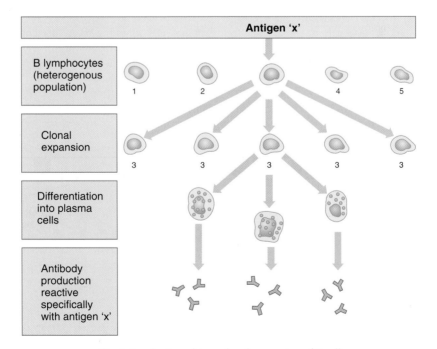

Fig. 1.6. Antigen-driven clonal expansion of B cells.

B cells

These cells produce antibody and comprise approximately 25% of the lymphocyte population. B lymphocytes capable of producing a specific antibody to a given antigen are rapidly encouraged to multiply by a mechanism called clonal expansion (Fig. 1.6). In this process, once a B cell has been exposed to a specific antigen (which it recognizes through immunoglobulin molecules located in the cell membrane), and in the presence of cytokines (interleukins 1–6 and B cell growth factors), it is activated and divides. Following this expansion step, B lymphocytes differentiate to become plasma cells which produce large amounts of antibody. Morphologically, plasma cells are distinguished by a cytoplasm containing large amounts of endoplasmic reticulum. The plasma cell has a relatively short half-life and is 'terminally differentiated', i.e. after it has fulfilled its antibody-producing function it dies. Following the death of these cells, the expanded B cell population shrinks back to its original size, although some remain as memory cells. As well as surface immunoglobulin, B lymphocytes can be distinguished by the presence of the CD19 and CD20 molecules.

HLA genes and molecules

As mentioned above, a unique feature of the immune response is its ability to react specifically to a given antigen. Because the term antigen is not restricted to microbial pathogens and toxins, but includes such materials as foreign organs (i.e. following transplantation) and certain tumour-associated structures, it can be said that the immune system has the ability to discriminate between 'self' and 'non-self' antigens. This process is facilitated by a recognition system called the *major histocompatibility complex* (MHC), which dictates the way antigen is processed and recognized as foreign.

The major histocompatibility complex

The human MHC is located on the short arm of chromosome number six. As the name implies, genes in the MHC in significant part determine the distinction between self and non-self, thus determining the compatibility or incompatibility of transplanted tissue. Numerous genes in the MHC complex encode for products that are critical determinants in the generation of immune responses. Although HLA-typing techniques have been developed so that genes in the MHC can be studied directly, other HLA-typing techniques detect the molecules encoded by these genes. The term HLA (human leucocyte antigen) derives from initial descriptions of HLA molecules in which the typing technique utilized antibodies that react with HLA molecules expressed on the surface of leucocytes isolated from peripheral blood samples. HLA molecules, however, are widely expressed on numerous cell types (*vida infra*).

The MHC complex includes class I, class II, and class III genes (Fig. 1.7). The class I region includes HLA-A, -B, and -C loci (gene regions) that encode for molecules that are referred to as classical class I antigens, and HLA-G, -F, and -E that are referred to as non-classical, class Ib, HLA antigens. Whereas there is extensive polymorphism (variability) at the HLA-A, -B, and -C loci, much less polymorphism is found in HLA-G, -F, and -E.

The class III region contains a number of genes, some of which are also important in immune

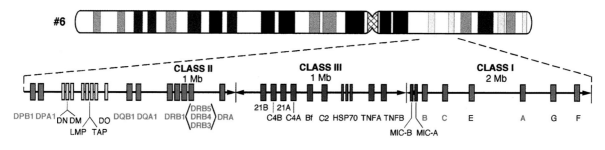

Fig. 1.7. Simplified schematic of the human major histocompatibility complex. DRB3, DRB4, and DRB5 are present only on some haplotypes and are further illustrated in Figure 1.8. Distances are not drawn to scale and genes that are not known to be expressed and pseudogenes are not shown.

responses. Noteworthy are the genes for the complement proteins C4A, C4B, and C2, the gene for heat shock protein 70, and genes for tumour necrosis factors (TNF) α and β.

HLA class II genes and molecules

The most frequent description of MHC gene associations with autoimmune diseases have been with HLA class II genes. The HLA class II region includes genes that encode for three distinct families of molecules: HLA-DR, -DQ, and -DP. An individual inherits genes that encode for one HLA-DQ, one HLA-DP, and at least one HLA-DR molecule from each parent. The 'block' of genes inherited from one parent can be referred to as a *haplotype*.

The class II molecules HLA-DR, -DQ, and -DP each consist of two chains that are non-covalently associated on the cell surface. The two chains are referred to as the α and β chains and the genes that encode them are

referred to as A and B, respectively; for example, the DQA1 gene encodes the DQα1 chain, DQB1 encodes the DQβ1 chain, etc. Thus at least six HLA class II genes are inherited on each parental haplotype.

An interesting aspect of the class II region is that some haplotypes, but not others, will have an additional gene. This phenomenon is illustrated in Fig. 1.8. Whereas all individuals will have a DRB1 gene, only some will also have a DRB3, DRB4 or DRB5 gene. Each of the DRB genes encodes for a DRβ chain that pairs with a DRα chain on the cell surface; thus, individuals with a DRB3, DRB4, or DRB5 gene will also express an additional molecule on the cell surface. These molecules are referred to as the DR52, DR53, and DR51 families, respectively. DR1 to DR18 are the families of molecules encoded for by the DRB1 gene. There is almost no variability in the DRA gene (thus none in the corresponding DRα chain) so that the polymorphism of DR molecules is almost entirely determined by the DRβ chain. The DQA1 and DQB1 genes are both polymorphic so that variability of DQ

The HLA Class II Loci DRB3, DRB4 and DRB5

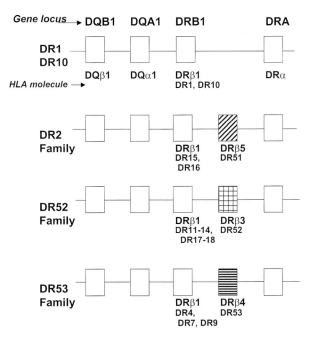

Fig. 1.8. The HLA class II DRB gene loci. All haplotypes have a DRB1 gene. If the DRB1 gene has an allele from the DR1 or DR10 family there is no DRB3, DRB4 or DRB5 gene on the haplotype. If the DRB1 locus has an allele from the DR15 or DR16 family a DRB5 gene is also present on the haplotype. If the DRB1 locus has an allele of the DR11-DR14 or DR17-DR18 families, a DRB3 gene is also present on the haplotype. If the DRB1 allele is from the DR4, DR7 or DR9 families, the haplotype will also have a DRB4 gene.

Table 1.8   Polymorphism in HLA genes

HLA-A	B	C						
87 (83)	187 (173)	45 (39)						
DRA	DRB1	DRB3	DRB4	DRB5	DQA1	DQB1	DPA1	DPB1
2 (2)	197 (178)	17 (14)	7 (7)	14 (13)	19 (15)	35 (30)	13 (10)	83 (77)

The number of alleles that have been identified at each HLA locus is given as of 1998. Some nucleotide differences do not result in amino acid differences. The number of alleles that encode for different amino acids is given in parenthesis.

molecules is expressed on both chains of the molecule. The same is true for DPA1 and DPB1 and for the DP molecule.

Polymorphism, a hallmark feature of HLA genes and molecules

A hallmark feature of HLA genes (both class I and class II) is extensive polymorphism. The alternative forms of a gene at a given locus are called alleles; for example HLA-A*0101 is one of 86 alleles that have been identified at the HLA-A locus. The number of recognized alleles at each HLA locus has increased markedly over the years. A summary of the number of recognized alleles at each of the class II and class I loci, as of 1998 (see Table 1.8).

The techniques that are used to identify polymorphism in HLA class II genes and the molecules they encode include serology, cellular, and DNA-based typing methods. These methods are described in Chapter 2. Although HLA terminology can seem confusing at first, the concept behind the terminology is simple. The concept is simply that of 'splitting', which became increasingly more extensive with the application of better techniques. For example, the molecule that was first called 'HLA-DR4' using serological typing techniques, with the application of DNA-typing techniques, is now known to consist of a family of at least 27 molecules.

Linkage disequilibrium in the MHC complex

In the MHC complex there is a tendency for genes to be inherited *en bloc* and this is referred to as linkage disequilibrium (Fig. 1.9). The linkage disequilibrium between DR and DQ genes is particularly strong (Tsjui *et al.* 1991). As discussed above, another interesting aspect of linkage disequilibrium in the HLA class II region is the predictability with which DRB3, DRB4, and DRB5 genes are present only on some haplotypes

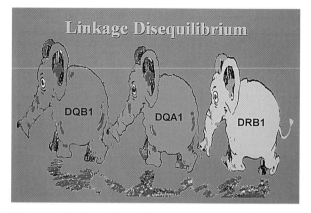

Fig. 1.9. Linkage disequilibrium. HLA genes often travel 'en bloc'. Linkage disequilibrium is particularly strong in the HLA class II region between the DRB and DQ loci. (Picture by Neal Branfield.)

dependent on the specific allele at the DRB1 locus. It is particularly important in view of the strong linkage disequilibrium in the class II region to consider all of the class II molecules that an individual expresses when seeking to understand the role of HLA genes and molecules in autoimmunity.

Structure of the HLA molecule

The crystallographic three-dimensional structure of the class II molecule HLA-DR1 has been described and in most respects the structure is similar to that of the HLA class I molecule. The α and β chains contribute to the formation of a platform of β-pleated sheets and each forms an α helix, creating the antigen-binding site and ligand for the T cell antigen receptor. The mouth of the antigen binding cleft is thought to be more open in class II molecules and longer peptides can be bound by class II than by class I molecules. Knowledge of the three-dimensional structure of the class II molecule, and of the sequence of a particular HLA allele, allows

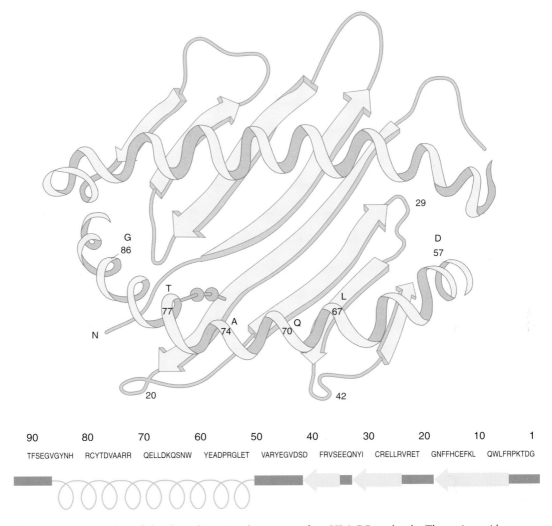

Fig. 1.10. Schematic representation of the three dimensional structure of an HLA-DR molecule. The amino acid sequence encoded by the DRB1*0101 allele is given as an example and some of the locations of various polymorphic residues on the three-dimensional DR1 molecule are shown. The schematic below the figure follows the amino acid sequence and indicates where the α-helix is (loops), β pleated sheets (line with arrow) and turns in the β pleated sheets (line without arrow).

prediction of where specific amino acid residues would be located on the class II molecule. A schematic representation for one of the alleles of the DR1 family (DRB1*0101) is shown in Fig. 1.10. Polymorphism in HLA molecules and the locations at which they occur are important since it is predicted that amino acid differences at particular locations of the HLA molecule will influence the repertoire of peptide antigens that can be bound by a specific HLA molecule and/or interactions with the T cell receptor.

Distribution of HLA molecules

There are important differences in the distribution and function of HLA class I and class II molecules. HLA class I molecules are expressed on platelets and nearly all nucleated cells. HLA class II molecules have a much more limited distribution. Class II molecules are constitutively expressed primarily on monocytes, macrophages, B lymphocytes dendritic cells, and certain marrow-derived precursor cells. Expression of class II molecules can be induced on T cells by activation and can be increased on monocytes, endothelial cells, and fibroblasts by certain cytokines such as γ-interferon. There are also differences between class I and class II molecules in antigen processing and in antigen presentation.

Antigen processing

The current view of antigen processing is that HLA class I molecules predominantly bind peptides from cytosolic antigens and class II molecules from endosomal antigens. The intracellular pathways for antigen processing and transport also differ for class I and class II molecules. A basic principle common to both, however, is the importance of protein fragmentation in the generation of epitopes or profiles for T and B cell recognition. Intracellular proteases such as endopeptidases, which cleave from the centre, and exopeptidases, which cleave from the end, are involved in antigen breakdown.

HLA class I molecules are synthesized in the endoplasmic reticulum where they bind peptides mainly from proteins that have been endogenously synthesized in the cytosol. Genes that encode subunits of the protease which is a large catalytic protein, are also located in the MHC complex. The transporter protein associated with antigen processing (TAP), also located in the MHC complex, encode for products that transport peptides from the cytosol to the endoplasmic reticulum. The peptide–HLA class I complexes travel to the cell membrane, where they become available for recognition by the T cell receptor of $CD8^+$ T cells.

Similar to HLA class I molecules, HLA class II molecules are also synthesized in the endoplasmic reticulum. However, unlike class I molecules, the peptide-binding cleft of class II molecules is prevented from binding ligands in the endoplasmic reticulum by invariant chain, a non-polymorphic polypeptide. Subsequent to travel of the invariant chain–HLA complex to endosomes, a heterodimer encoded by other genes in the MHC complex (DMA and DMB) assists in the exchange of invariant chain (a portion called 'CLIP') for a peptide. In contrast to class I, where peptides are usually 8–9 amino acids long, peptides binding to class II molecules are usually 12–25 amino acids long. The peptide–HLA class II complexes then travel to the cell membrane, where they become available for recognition by the T cell receptor of $CD4^+$ T cells.

Antigen presentation

HLA class I and class II molecules present antigen fragments to T cells. In general, antigens that are presented by class II molecules are recognized by $CD4^+$ T helper cells. Antigens that are presented by class I molecules are presented to $CD8^+$ T cells and a cytotoxic response results. The responding population of T cells thus recognizes the combined shape and other features (such as the charge of specific amino acids) of the antigen and the HLA molecule. The combination of T cell receptor, HLA molecule, and antigen fragment is known as the trimolecular complex. Because of genetic variation in HLA molecules, given a particular HLA molecule, some antigens may be more effective than others in inducing immune responses. For example, an antigen might present an optimum shape or conformation to the T cells in the context of the particular MHC molecule or might bind or not bind to particular MHC molecules. Immune responses that only occur with certain antigen–HLA combinations are called HLA restricted.

Antigen-presenting cells

Several cell types, sometimes termed *accessory cells*, facilitate the antigen-presenting process.

Macrophages and monocytes (mononuclear phagocytes)

These cells are distributed throughout the body, in the tissues (as macrophages) and in the blood (as monocytes). Macrophages are equipped with various features that make them particularly effective at removing foreign antigens that are ready for presentation. They are phagocytic and have, on their surface, receptors that recognize the Fc region of antibody molecules, as well as biologically active fragments of complement (C3b). The presence of these structures on cells in the macrophage–monocyte family makes it easy for them to intercept and dispose of antigen–antibody complexes.

Follicular dendritic cells

Follicular dendritic cells are non-phagocytic and are located in the germinal centres of lymph nodes (follicles). They are surrounded by B lymphocytes to which they present antigen, usually complexed with antibody, on the surface of their dendrites. Their surfaces are rich in Fc and C3b receptors to facilitate antigen trapping.

Langerhans' cells and dendritic cells

The Langerhans' cell is found primarily in the skin. The dendritic (or veiled) cell is present in the blood (and is different to the follicular dendritic cell described above). They are of macrophage/monocyte lineage.

From HLA molecules to autoimmunity

A striking feature of the autoimmune diseases as a group (both rheumatological and non-rheumatological) is the finding of particular HLA class II molecules in association with increased risk of disease. HLA class II associations are described for each of the autoimmune rheumatic diseases in the ensuing chapters, and, when relevant, other genes in the MHC complex are included. Prodigious work over the past 20 years has contributed to a substantial knowledge base describing particular HLA genes that are increased in patients with autoimmune rheumatic diseases. Genetic contributions outside of the MHC complex are also likely; however, in contrast to MHC associations, these studies are in their infancy (and no attempt is made to cover this subject in the current context).

The mechanisms by which HLA molecules contribute to the pathogenesis of autoimmune diseases remain unknown. Explanations that have been proposed include molecular mimicry, in which a particular HLA molecule shares an amino acid sequence stretch with an invading microorganism so that the HLA molecule becomes the target of a cross-reactive immune response. Another explanation that has been proposed is that the influence of particular HLA molecules is exerted at the level of thymic selection. Particular HLA molecules might select a population of potentially autoreactive T cells that become expanded and pathogenic at a later time in life when the individual is exposed to an appropriate trigger (e.g. a particular microorganism). It has also been proposed that the peptide binding repertoire of a particular HLA molecule might contribute directly to autoimmunity. Others propose that the association of HLA molecules with autoimmune diseases is not due to the molecules themselves, but rather to genes that are in linkage disequilibrium with them. Numerous recent studies have shown that, in addition to presenting foreign antigens, HLA molecules also present peptides derived from other HLA molecules and still another possibility is that

HLA molecules contribute to autoimmunity because they themselves are presented as self-peptides in other HLA molecules. An example of this model is the hypothesis that implicates a peptide derived from the DRβ1 chain presented by a DQ molecule in the pathogenesis of rheumatoid arthritis (see Chapter 5). Finally, in another recently described hypothesis, it has been proposed that persistent microchimerism (non-host cells) may contribute to the pathogenesis of some autoimmune diseases (see Chapters 4 and 8). Clearly, the mechanisms by which HLA molecules contribute to autoimmunity are likely to be complex and may differ for different autoimmune diseases. Another important consideration in the pathogenesis of autoimmune diseases is tolerance, and factors that could affect the breakdown of the normal mechanisms of tolerance, and these are discussed further below.

Immune tolerance

Tolerance is a state in which the immune system fails to respond to a given antigen. This mechanism evolved from a need for the body to prevent its tissues being attacked by its own defence network. On occasions when tolerance fails or is incomplete, autoimmunity can result.

Positive and negative selection

During the early stages of the development of the immune system in the life of an individual, lymphocytes are made tolerant to self-antigens. Several types of tolerance can occur, although the most important process occurs in the thymus by means of a complicated, multistep selection mechanism. In the first stage of this process, immature T cells, which do not bear either of the CD4 and CD8 molecules (double-negative cells) enter the subcapsular region of the thymus, divide, and proliferate. T cell receptors and CD4 and CD8 molecules are then co-expressed simultaneously; these cells are termed 'double-positive'. Maturing cells migrate towards the cortex of the thymus where the selection process occurs. T cells that encounter and can engage with MHC class I or II molecules on the epithelium of the thymic cortex are said to be 'positively selected' and they undergo further processing. Cells that do not interact with the MHC die as a result of mechanism termed programmed cell death, or apoptosis. They will also lose either the CD4 or

CD8 co-receptor, depending on which particular MHC molecule they engage. For example, CD8 cells bind to MHC class I molecules, and CD4 to class II. Thus, after positive selection, only cells that can recognize MHC molecules (and thus antigenic peptides presented in association with these structures) remain.

However, another step is necessary to remove cells that can react with self-peptides and this occurs through negative selection. This part of the selection process occurs in the cortico-medullary junction, which is rich in dendritic cells and macrophages. If either CD4 or CD8 cells engage with cells bearing MHC class I or II molecules containing self-peptide (i.e. autoreactive T cells) they undergo apoptosis and are clonally deleted. Cells that do not interact with MHC–peptide complexes pass through the thymus and become part of the mature T cell pool. Negative selection is generally regarded as the most important aspect of tolerance induction. During these early stages of development it is evident that a lot of apoptosis-induced cell death occurs in the thymus. Both positive and negative selection occur through a similar binding mechanism (CD4/8 to MHC–self-peptide complex); however, the different outcomes are thought to be due to the differences in binding affinities. Positive selection is a result of a weak binding affinity, whereas negative selection is favoured by a high binding affinity. It has been postulated that some cells of intermediate binding affinity may escape negative selection and pass into the periphery, where they are potentially autoreactive.

Peripheral tolerance

Self-reactive cells can, on occasion, escape the elimination process in the thymus and become part of the circulating pool of T cells. While these lymphocytes may become autoaggressive there are several other forms of tolerance that occur outside the thymus. Again, these mechanisms are rather complicated, not particularly well understood, and a full description is outside the scope of this chapter. Nevertheless, it will suffice to say that processes exist to eliminate or inactivate (anergize) both self-reactive T and B lymphocytes. The so called 'veto' effect can occur when self-peptides are presented to the autoreactive lymphocyte. Specialized cytotoxic T cells may kill the autoreactive cell if the self-peptide is presented in association with an MHC class I molecule. Self-reactive, antibody-producing B cells may be deleted, in certain circumstances, when they encounter autoantigen. Alternatively, it is thought that they may be regulated by anti-idiotypic antibodies that bind to the idiotype marker on the B cell in question.

Breakdown of tolerance

Clearly the ability of the immune system to recognize and discriminate self from non-self is an essential factor in host survival. If this ability is challenged autoimmunity may result. The exact mechanisms that maintain the tolerant state are not fully understood but are thought to include the following factors:

Defective immunoregulation

If the inherent control mechanisms built into the immune system are dysfunctional, aberrant responses may occur. This may occur through deletion (such as viral infection e.g. HIV) or immunophysiological effects such as cytokine imbalances. For example, if a Th1 response, which is generally thought to be inflammatory, is sustained and does not switch to a Th2 type response, autoimmunity may result. Furthermore, reduced numbers of CD8 cell have been observed in many autoimmune disease. The suppressive role of these cells has long been established and should they been functionally impaired due to quantitative or qualitative defects, there is a high likelihood that the immune system will be in a state of imbalance. Defective immunoregulation is closely related to cytokine imbalances (see below).

Cytokine imbalances

Inappropriate production of cytokines can cause a large number of immune abnormalities. In particular they may upregulate MHC class II molecules and thus cause immune activation and increased antigen presentation. It has also been speculated that sustained production of the pro-inflammatory cytokines TNFα, IFNγ and IL-2 may disrupt peripheral tolerance although the precise mechanisms remain to be elucidated.

T cell by-pass

Immune responses are regulated by T helper cell populations which generally function in an antigen specific manner. T helper cells for autoantigens are functionally deleted in ontogeny and thus a state of self tolerance occurs. However, in certain circumstances, new sets of T helper cells can be recruited which do drive immune responses to self antigens. For example if an autoantigen becomes slightly modified due to infection or an environmental influence such as UV light, chemicals or a drug reaction it may be recognized in a very different way and solicit help from novel T cell clones. Alternatively the need for T cell help may be circumvented entirely if B lymphocytes are activated by an infection such as Epstein Barr virus which has a highly specific tropism for these cells.

Molecular mimicry

Molecular mimicry generally refers to a condition in which micro-organism-derived antigens resemble an autoantigen and inadvertently provoke a cross reacting immune response to host tissues. A well-known example is the autoimmune attack that sometimes occurs against heart muscle (myosin) following infection with group A streptococci (rheumatic fever).

Release of hidden antigens

Tissue injury following mechanical trauma or infection may release antigens that have been previously hidden from the immune system thus provoking anti-self responses. For example, autoimmune uveitis can be induced in laboratory animals following induced mechanical damage to the eye.

The immune system in concert

Following an antigenic stimulus, the components of the immune system co-operate to meet and eliminate the challenge. The foreign antigen is picked up by a cell of the monocyte/macrophage series and the antigen is degraded or processed and presented to both the B and T lymphocytes. T helper cells are generated, which enhance the antibody response made by B cells. Some of this augmentation is due to secreted lymphokines or cytokines from the T helper population. It should be noted that cytotoxic T cells may be generated if foreign antigens, typically viruses, are presented directly to this cell population. Bacteria are most likely to be processed through the MHC class II pathway and thus generate, primarily, antibody responses. The B cells, once triggered, will differentiate into plasma cells producing specific antibody, which binds to the antigen and further triggers the complement system. The complement system, in turn, recruits neutrophils which together eliminate the antigen, perhaps with additional help from lymphokine-activated macrophages. Once

the immune system has detected 'foreign antigens' it can communicate this information to other systems, particularly to the brain and neuroendocrine systems. For example, following infection, there is an increase in both pituitary and adrenal gland secretion. Figure 1.12 indicates the complex nature of these relationships.

Immunopathology of autoimmune disease

Formation of autoantibodies may be a normal physiological process. However, excessive production of such antibodies can be harmful. The ways in which autoantibodies cause structural damage to the body's tissues are varied. Antibodies may react directly with a specific tissue, resulting in inflammation and tissue damage, such as anti-glomerular basement membrane antibodies in Goodpasture's syndrome, or they may affect function directly, for example acetylcholine receptor antibodies in myasthenia gravis (type II hypersensitivity).

Alternatively, circulating immune complexes may be formed. Immune complexes are biologically active entities that, in themselves, have certain characteristics. These properties determine whether immune complexes become harmful and cause extensive tissue damage. Inflammation or autoimmune conditions resulting from the formation of immune complexes are classified as type III hypersensitivity reactions. The complexes are often deposited in the kidney, skin, joint, and nervous system. This results in complement activation, accumulation, and activation of neutrophils, with the release of proteolytic enzymes and further damage. It should also be noted that mononuclear cells are also implicated in tissue destruction. Both CD4+ and CD8+ lymphocytes are observed routinely as infiltrates in inflammatory lesions. While there is little doubt that these cells contribute to tissue destruction, their precise role in the pathological processes is uncertain. The complexity of the autoimmune diseases is quite formidable, largely because there is so much variation in the interplay of the different factors that can influence the reactivity of the immune system to the body's tissues.

Summary

The immune system is a complex defence system essential for the health and survival of the host. It comprises organs and tissues which 'train' highly specialized lym-

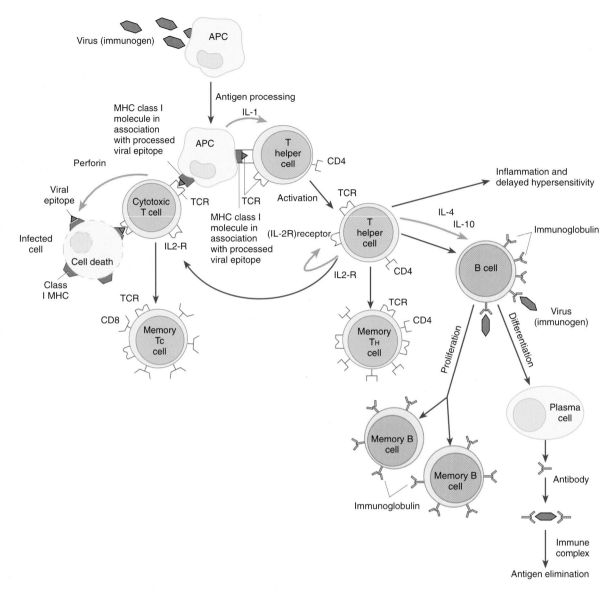

Fig. 1.12.   The immune system in concert.

phocyte sub-populations. These cells have a range of effector functions including direct cytotoxic effects and the production of antibodies as well as a diverse array of communications molecules (cytokines and chemokines). The hallmark of the immune system is its ability to react with foreign antigens in a highly specific manner and to discriminate between self and non-self targets. When this capability fails and the state of self tolerance is challenged, inflammation and autoimmunity may result.

References

General Reading

Callard RE, Gearing AJH. *The cytokine facts book*. Academic Press, London. 1997.

Barclay AN *et al. The leucocyte antigen facts book*. Academic Press, London. 1997.

Janeway CA, Travers P. *Immunobiology: the immune system in health and disease*, 3rd Edition. Current Biology, London. 1997.

Isenberg DA, Morrow WJW. *Friendly fire*. Oxford University Press, Oxford. 1995.

Maddison PJ, Isenberg DA, Woo P, Glass DN. *Oxford Textbook of Rheumatology*. 2nd Edition. Oxford University Press, Oxford. 1998.

Peakman M, Vergani D. *Basic and clinical immunology*. Churchill Livingstone, Edinburgh. 1997.

Pigott R, Power C. *The adhesion molecule facts book*. Academic Press, London. 1997.

2 | *Immunological methodology*

Introduction

The autoimmune rheumatic diseases may present in many different ways and thus be problematic to diagnose. The enormous clinical diversity can also make treatment unsatisfactory. Thus the immunological tests available are used to help establish the diagnosis and, in some cases, to monitor the disease.

At present these rheumatic diseases are treated according to end-organ function, specific details of which will be given in the relevant chapters, and not according to results obtained from any one laboratory test. The clinical rheumatologist may be bewildered by the apparently large number of assays that are described in the literature and wonder not only which can be reasonably requested for his patients but moreover at the clinical relevance of the result.

The aim of this chapter is to acquaint the reader with some basic principles of practical immunology, as well as the most important laboratory tests that may be used to evaluate and research these diseases. Critical comments are provided as to the usefulness and practicality of these assays as both diagnostic tools and prognostic indicators. Advice as to the value of different combinations of tests in the different diseases is given in the relevant chapters.

Fundamentals of practical immunology

Antigen-antibody interactions

When antigens and their complimentary antibodies meet they combine, an *immune complex* is formed, and several outcomes are possible. If the antigen is a large soluble macromolecule the complex may *precipitate* from the solution. Alternatively, *agglutination* may occur in the case of insoluble antigens such as bacteria. These reactions form the basis of several assays used in immunological investigations and may be encountered in studies of the autoimmune rheumatic diseases.

Precipitation tests

The formation of a precipitate in an antigen–antibody reaction is dependent on the ratio of the reactants. In 1935, Heidelberger and Kendall demonstrated that peak precipitation occurs at the point of *equivalence*, when antigen and antibody are in optimal proportions. Prior to reaching this point antibody is present in excess quantities and afterwards antigen is the dominant reactant (Fig. 2.1). This phenomenon is probably a consequence of lattice formation, which would explain the variable solubility of antigen–antibody complexes (Fig. 2.2). Based on these theoretical considerations, two tests are of particular note.

Double diffusion assay

This procedure was first described by Ouchterlony in 1954. Solutions of antigen and antibody are placed in adjacent wells cut in an agar plate and are allowed to diffuse. A precipitin line will form if the antibody is specific for the antigen. The appearance of the line is dependent on several factors including the relative concentrations of the reactants (Fig. 2.3). The test is very simple to perform and is a general purpose immunological tool; its limitation is that it is qualitative rather than quantitative.

Single radial immunodiffusion

Described by Mancini and colleagues in 1954, this test is a modification of the Ouchterlony method can be used for the quantification of antigens. In this case antibody specific for the antigen to be quantified is first incorporated into the agar plate. A precipitin line will form at the equivalence point (Fig. 2.4). The concentra-

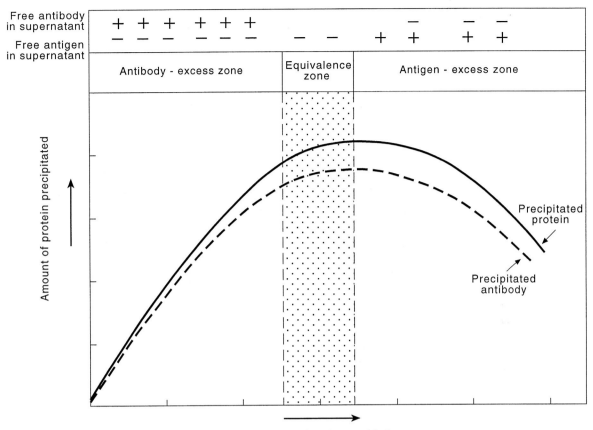

Free antibody in supernatant + + + + + + − − − −

Free antigen in supernatant − − − − − − − − + + + +

Antibody - excess zone | Equivalence zone | Antigen - excess zone

Amount of protein precipitated

Precipitated protein

Precipitated antibody

Amount of antigen added

Fig. 2.1. The classical precipitin curve as described by Heidelberger and Kendall in 1935. At the point of equivalence the antigen binding sites of the antibody are largely saturated and maximum precipitation occurs, leaving virtually no free antigen or antibody in the supernatant.

tion of antigen is calculated by measuring the diameter of the precipitin ring and relating it to a standard curve. This procedure is simple, inexpensive, and versatile and can be used to quantify any antigen provided the investigator has access to a suitable supply of antiserum. The lower limit for the detection of antigen is 5–10 μg/ml.

Probably the most common agglutination assay used in studies of the rheumatic diseases is the latex bead test for rheumatoid factor. As described previously, antibody will macroscopically agglutinate or clump antigen; the kinetics of this reaction are similar to precipitin formation. In the rheumatoid factor agglutination test, latex beads are precoated with human gammaglobulin (usually purchased in this form from a commercial source). A small aliquot of the beads is incubated for a few minutes with test serum on a dark glass slide. If antiglobulin autoantibodies (of the IgM class: IgM is a particularly efficient agglutinator because of its high valency) are formed, then the beads will be seen to agglutinate within a minute or so (Fig. 2.5).

Labelled antibodies

A range of important test procedures have been developed from antibodies labelled with markers (such as enzymes, fluorochromes, or radioisotopes) which can then be used in sensitive detection systems. The most important applications of labelled antibodies are detailed below.

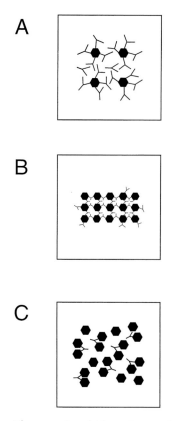

A

B

C

Fig. 2.2. The ways in which antigen and antibody may combine to form complexes: antibody excess is depicted in (**a**) the zone of equivalence in (**b**) and antigen excess in (**c**).

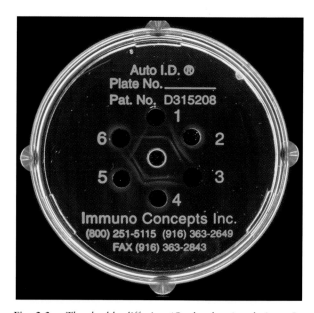

Fig. 2.3. The double diffusion (Ouchterlony) technique. In this diagram antiserum placed in the central well has reacted with four different antigen preparations in the peripheral wells. Non-identity and partial identity of antigens are shown respectively by crossing over and spur formation between precipitin lines.

Immunofluorescence

This technique is based on the principle that antibodies conjugated with a fluorochrome such as fluorescein or rhodamine can be detected by irradiating them with light of a specific wavelength (usually ultraviolet). The light will excite the fluorochromes and cause them to emit light of a different wavelength. In the case of fluorescein, maximum absorption of the exciting radiation occurs at 490–495 nm, and the characteristic green fluorescence is emitted at 517 nm. The technique is very powerful as it is sensitive, specific, and adaptable; it can be used to detect almost any antigen including aetiological agents, cellular determinants, and even antibodies themselves.

Thus, such conjugated antibodies can be used to detect specific antigens in a variety of substrates, including tissue specimens, cell monolayers (fixed on the surface of microscope slides), or in suspension. There are two major staining techniques used in

immunofluorescence procedures: the *direct* method in which labelled antibody is incubated directly to the sample, and the *indirect* method in which an unconjugated antibody is used as well as the labelled species. These approaches are summarized in Fig. 2.6. There are two major uses of immunofluorescence

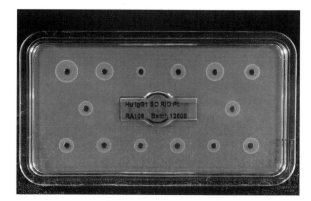

Fig. 2.4. The single radial immunodiffusion (Mancini) assay. The diameter of the precipitin ring is directly proportional to the quantity of antigen that has been placed in the wells. The ring size is related to a calibration curve in which known amounts of antigen are used.

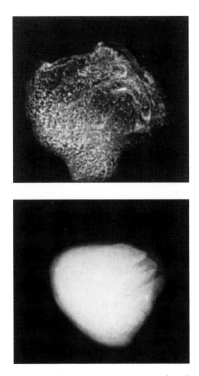

Fig. 2.5. Latex agglutination test. Latex beads sensitized with a single component protein antigen rapidly agglutinate in the presence of a specific antiserum. The top slide shows strong agglutination, indicating a positive test. The lower slide shows a negative control.

techniques and these are immunohistology and cell sorting/flow cytometry.

Immunohistology

The conjugated antibodies are applied either directly or indirectly to the tissue specimens under investigation and then examined using a microscope fitted with a suitable light source (usually a mercury vapour lamp) which will excite the fluorochromes. By using filters, the wavelength of the light can be altered and double staining with different conjugates, e.g. fluorescein and rhodamine (which give green and red fluorescence, respectively), can be carried out. The results of double staining can be visualized simultaneously using double-exposure photography and appear most elegant.

Cell sorting/flow cytometry

The fluorescence-activated cell sorter (FACS) was devised as a method of separating subpopulations of cells. The cells to be sorted are first incubated with fluorescent-labelled antibody(ies) of the desired specificity. The suspension is then passed through a vibrating nozzle which has the effect of forming liquid droplets, each containing a single cell. Laser beams illuminate the suspension and those cells identified by a labelled antibody are detected by their excitation energy as they pass through a high voltage field and are sorted and collected aseptically. A schematic depiction of a FACS is shown in Fig. 2.7.

Flow cytometry is a modification of FACS. It operates on a similar principle but does not separate cell populations but father simply counts them. As such the technique has become very popular for analysing lymphocyte populations since it automates the tedious, labour-intensive counting procedures that were necessary previously with conventional microscopy, and also because of the universal availability of monoclonal antibodies that identify these cell populations. As with the FACS, flow cytometry can determine dual-labelled populations such as $CD4^+$, $CD3^+$ T helper cells. A *dot plot* of such an analysis is shown in Fig. 2.8.

Radioimmunoassay

Another very powerful procedure of great use in investigating autoimmune rheumatic diseases is radioimmunoassay. Originally developed by Berson and Yalow in 1960 (the latter received the Nobel Prize for this work), radioimmunoassay is in many ways similar to immunofluorescence in that a *labelled* antibody, in this case conjugated with a radioisotope, is used to detect a specific antigen. The technique is very sensitive and can detect antigens in the picogram range. Numerous variations of radioimmunoassay exist: the methods for labelling antisera (or in some cases, antigens) with a radioisotope are very straightforward and thus assays can easily be customized to suit the needs of individual investigators. For practical reasons it is often convenient to have the principle reactants adsorbed on to the wall of the 'test tube' (more commonly the wells of a microtitration plate are used). Such a technique is called a *solid phase assay*. When the reaction is carried out entirely in solution it is called a *liquid phase assay*.

ELISA

One inherent drawback of radioimmunoassays is the requirement for radioisotopes. This characteristic can be disadvantageous from the point of view of safety or, more realistically, because of the need for expensive equipment to measure radioactive emissions. This latter

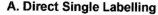

A. Direct Single Labelling

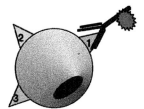

B. Indirect Single Labelling

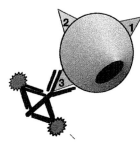

C. Direct Double Labelling

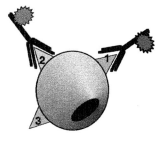

D. Combined Direct and Indirect Labelling

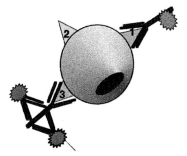

Fig. 2.6. Diagrammatic representation of immunofluorescence. In the direct method (a) antigen-1 in the substrate is detected with a labelled (i.e. FITC) fluorescent antibody. The indirect single labelling method (b) requires that an unlabelled antibody binds to the antigen-3 which is then in turn visualized with a flurochrome-conjugated antiglobulin reagent, typically F(ab')$_2$ fragments. In practice, the indirect technique is the most useful as it may be it is less prone to background fluorescence and is more sensitive because of the increased number of binding sites that are available for the labelled antibody to attach. Variations in these methods include direct double labelling to detect multiple antigens (antigen-1 and antigen-2) (c). Each antibody would be conjugated with different flurochromes, typically fluorescein isothiocyanate (FITC) and rhodamine or phycoerythrin (PE). Finally a combination of direct and indirect double labelling can be carried out (d). Unlabelled antibody specific fro antigen-3 is visualized with isotype-specific, FITC labelled F(ab')$_2$ fragments in combination with directly conjugated, phycoerythrin labelled antibody to antigen-1.

requirement can be particularly problematic in 'field' situations. For these reasons the *enzyme-linked immunosorbent assay* (ELISA) was devised. Instead of antibodies being attached to a radiochemical they are coupled to an enzyme such as a horseradish peroxidase or alkaline phosphatase. Assays are carried out, usually in flat-bottom 96-well plates, in a similar way to radioimmunoassay except that at the final stage detection of the antibody (and thus the antigen) is facilitated by the addition of a substrate and a developer that will generate a colour reaction if the enzyme-linked anti-body is present. The end-point colour, which gives a quantitative estimation of the reactant to be measured, can theoretically be read in any spectrophotometer but more usually the plate is scanned in an ELISA reader. The particular advantage of this method is the speed at which the reading takes place: usually less than one minute for a 96-well plate.

Although not by any means limited to this type of test, the *avidin-biotin* system has proved to be particularly useful when applied to ELISA assays. Biotin is a vitamin and avidin is a glycoprotein that may play a

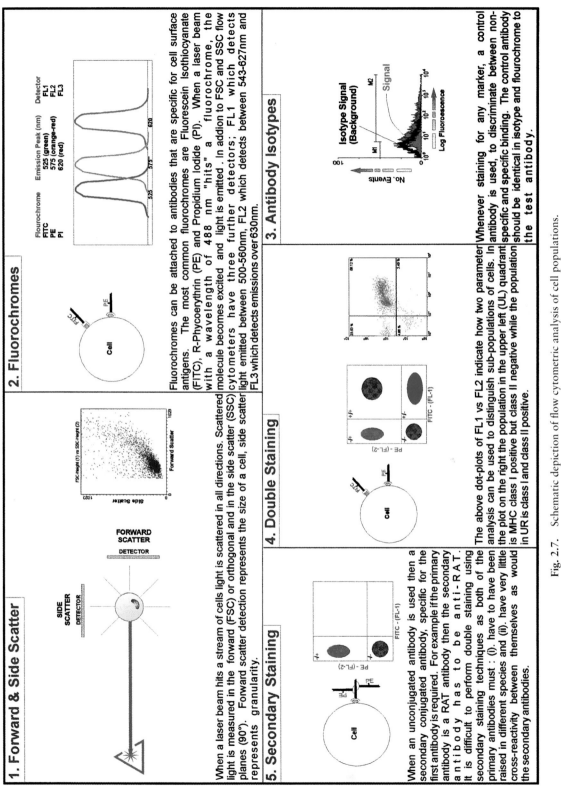
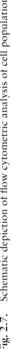

Fig. 2.7. Schematic depiction of flow cytometric analysis of cell populations.

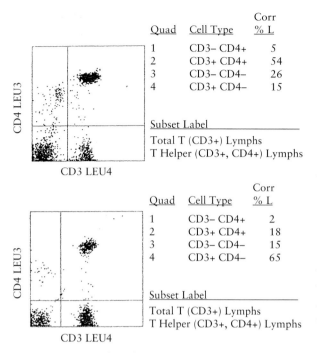

Quad	Cell Type	Corr % L
1	CD3– CD4+	5
2	CD3+ CD4+	54
3	CD3– CD4–	26
4	CD3+ CD4–	15

Subset Label

Total T (CD3+) Lymphs
T Helper (CD3+, CD4+) Lymphs

Quad	Cell Type	Corr % L
1	CD3– CD4+	2
2	CD3+ CD4+	18
3	CD3– CD4–	15
4	CD3+ CD4–	65

Subset Label

Total T (CD3+) Lymphs
T Helper (CD3+, CD4+) Lymphs

Fig. 2.8. *Dot plot* showing simultaneous two-colour fluorescence analysis of human CD3+, CD4+ T cells. Each dot represents an individual labelled cell. The top panel is representative of cells from a normal individual whereas the lower panel shows cells from a patient with AIDS.

role in embryonic development, as well as having antimicrobial properties. The major significance of these two apparently unrelated substances is that they will bind together most tenaciously. The avidin molecule has four sites that will bind biotin with a very high affinity; the biological significance of this interaction is unknown but it has been employed at a practical level to amplify the sensitivity of immunoassays. There are many permutations of the avidin–biotin system in use in ELISA as well as in radioimmunoassays, immunocytochemistry, flow cytometry, electrophoresis, and many other techniques.

Electrophoresis

Electrophoretic techniques, the separation of macromolecules in an electric field according to their charge, are numerous in biomedical research and it is beyond the scope of this text to attempt to describe them, even in limited detail. Instead, we will discuss two procedures that are of particular use in immunological research.

Immunoelectrophoresis

In this technique, proteins are placed in a small well cut in an agar plate, an electrical potential is then applied to the plate, and the protein macromolecules separate according to their charge. When the electrophoresis has been completed the proteins are both fixed and visualized by the application of a suitable antiserum to a well that runs the length of the plate. Antigens and antibodies will diffuse towards each other and will be seen to appear as a series of precipitin arcs. The technique is a moderately sensitive qualitative assay, useful for detecting serological abnormalities (paraproteinaemias etc.) as well as the performance of separation techniques, although the technique has now been largely superseded by Western blotting (see below). Numerous ingenious variants of the basic technique have been described; one in particular, termed countercurrent immunoelectrophoresis, is used routinely in immunology laboratories to screen for autoantibodies to extractable nuclear antigens (see below).

Immuno (Western)-blotting

This technique has gained great popularity since its description in 1979. Basically, it adds an additional step to the polyacrylamide gel procedure, making it a highly sensitive, and thus very powerful, analytical tool. Proteins are separated on a polyacrylamide gel, the pore size of which is 'tailored' to suit the molecular weight of the protein/ antigens being studied. When the electrophoresis has been completed the separated macromolecules are transferred electrophoretically to a nitrocellulose sheet that is a replica of the original gel. Thus, with immunoblotting there is the option not only of visualizing the separation of the material by conventional staining of the gel (the limitation of which is that the identification of separated molecules is limited by guessing their molecular weights), but also of using antibodies to identify specific antigens that have been transferred to the nitrocellulose sheet. The nitrocellulose sheet can be probed with either enzyme conjugated antibodies, usually in combination with the biotin-avidin system, or radiolabelled antibodies (Fig. 2.9).

Polymerase chain reaction

The polymerase chain reaction (PCR) technique has rapidly become established as one of the most powerful

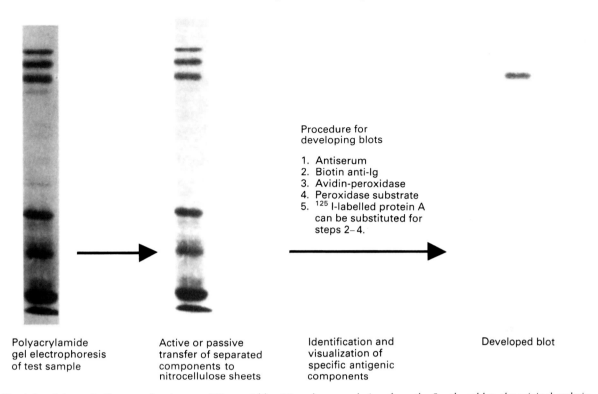

| Polyacrylamide gel electrophoresis of test sample | Active or passive transfer of separated components to nitrocellulose sheets | Procedure for developing blots

1. Antiserum
2. Biotin anti-Ig
3. Avidin-peroxidase
4. Peroxidase substrate
5. ^{125}I-labelled protein A can be substituted for steps 2–4.

Identification and visualization of specific antigenic components | Developed blot |

Fig. 2.9. Schematic diagram of an immuno(Western) blot. Note the name derives from the *Southern* blot, the original and virtually identical method used to visualize DNA fragments and named after its inventor. This method subsequently gave rise to the *Northern* blot which is used for studying RNA, and the Western blot described here.

techniques available in molecular biology and has been applied widely to the field of diagnostics. It was conceived (supposedly while driving up the California coast) and developed by Dr Kary Mullis just over 10 years ago and has subsequently found utility in a diverse range of applications, including diagnosis of slow-growing microorganisms such as mycobacteria and HIV, forensic studies, evolutionary biology, and phylogenetics, as well as a central role in the human genome project. In immunology PCR is now used routinely for HLA typing and has numerous research applications, such as determining cytokine production at the intracellular level. In recognition of the importance of his discovery, Dr Mullis was awarded the Nobel prize for Chemistry in 1993.

PCR analysis is based on the principle that nucleic acids representing the analyte in question can be amplified logarithmically and identified. The technique can be carried out using very small starting quantities of DNA or RNA (theoretically only one molecule is necessary) and be configured to give either qualitative or quantitative read-outs. Oligonucleotide primers representing the analyte in question (e.g. a specific HLA type or cytokine) are incubated with the DNA starting material (if RNA is used as a starting point it is first reverse transcribed into DNA) and a DNA polymerase enzyme (most commonly Taq polymerase derived from the bacterium *Thermophilus aquaticus*). In a repetitive heat cycling process, the primers are extended using the original DNA as a template. The DNA product accumulates exponentially and as much as 1 μg may result from a 30-cycle PCR reaction. This process is summarized in Fig. 2.10. There are now numerous variants of PCR and it is outside the scope of this chapter to do anything but describe the technique in its basic form: for further reference see McPherson *et al.* (1995).

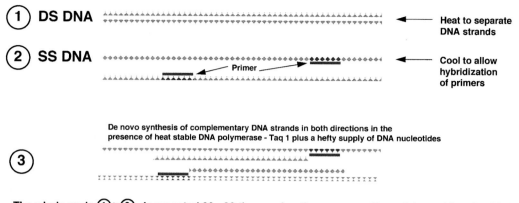

Fig. 2.10. Scheme depicting the amplification of a specific DNA sequence using the *polymerase chain reaction*. PCR allows the amplification of a chosen DNA fragment without the need for restriction enzymes, vectors or host cells. As can be seen from the diagram, at each round of thermal cycling the DNA is increased by the Taq polymerase enzyme (an excess of nucleotides is present).

Immunological tests used for evaluation of the autoimmune rheumatic diseases

Serology

Immunoglobulin levels

Although a very non-specific test of immunological function, estimates of serum immunoglobulin concentrations, IgG and IgM, are the most useful, straightforward, and simple to carry out. Small laboratories may utilize either home-made or commercially available radial immunodiffusion kits. Larger service laboratories may employ semi-automated nephelometric techniques.

Autoantibodies

Rheumatoid factor

The rheumatoid factor (Rf) test is of great importance in this group of diseases and plays a central role in differential diagnosis. As all of the disorders considered in this text have, by definition, a rheumatic element, this test is carried out on virtually every patient presenting in a rheumatology clinic. Rf is, primarily, in IgM antibody that is directed against the patient's own IgG molecules; thus it is sometimes termed *antiglobulin*. This antibody is usually detected using gelatin particles coated with denatured IgG, although in the past fixed animal erythrocytes were used. In the presence of rheumatoid factor a gross macroscopic agglutination of the particles (see Fig. 2.5) will be seen within a minute or so. This effect can be titred and thus the levels of antibody can be quantified. The assay method is based on a modification (Heller's modification) of the Waaler–Rose test. The test is sometimes known as RAPA (rheumatoid arthritis particle agglutination assay), although the term RAHA (rheumatoid arthritis haemagglutination assay) is (incorrectly) in quite common usage and stems from the days when the test used fixed erythrocytes. Latex beads coated with IgG can also be used in a similar way: this latter test is considered to be more sensitive than RAPA, although the RAPA test is more specific.

The advantages of this test are its speed and simplicity; it can be carried out in the most basic of facilities, and is commercially available. Its shortcomings are that it is qualitative rather than quantitative (titrating out the end-point agglutination can provide a semi-quantitative result) and that it measures, primarily, rheumatoid factors of the IgM class. Antiglobulins of other isotypes can be measured, by solid phase radio or ELISA immunoassays, and can be used to show that the patient with so called 'seronegative' rheumatoid arthritis does in fact have circulating rheumatoid factor.

Anti-nuclear antibodies (ANA)

In 1958, George Friou and colleagues, in a series of articles, described and partially characterized the phenomenon by which serum from patients with SLE (systemic lupus erythematosus) binds to nuclear antigens in fresh-frozen tissue. Using fluorochrome-labelled antisera, it was shown that the component binding to the nucleus was in fact antibody from the patient. This finding clearly demonstrated that an autoimmnue pathology was underlying the disease and heralded a new era of research in SLE.

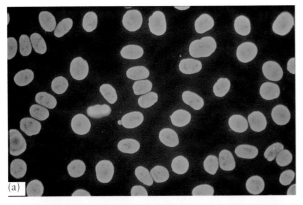
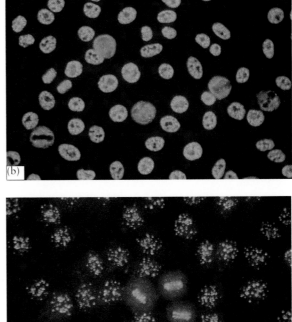
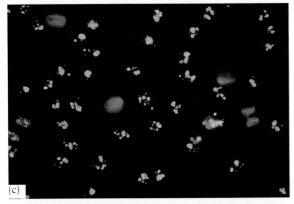
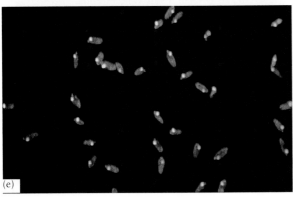
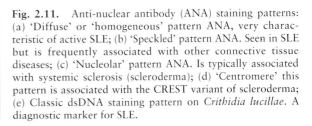

Fig. 2.11. Anti-nuclear antibody (ANA) staining patterns: (a) 'Diffuse' or 'homogeneous' pattern ANA, very characteristic of active SLE; (b) 'Speckled' pattern ANA. Seen in SLE but is frequently associated with other connective tissue diseases; (c) 'Nucleolar' pattern ANA. Is typically associated with systemic sclerosis (scleroderma); (d) 'Centromere' this pattern is associated with the CREST variant of scleroderma; (e) Classic dsDNA staining pattern on *Crithidia lucillae*. A diagnostic marker for SLE.

Screening for anti-nuclear antibodies (ANA), or anti-nuclear factor (ANF) as it is sometimes called, is an important primary step in the diagnosis of lupus, although, to some extent, this test has been superseded by the DNA-binding assay. The test is usually performed in fresh-frozen sections of rodent liver or kidney, or both together, or cell lines such as Hep-2. Several fluorescent staining patterns occur, reflecting the different antigenic specificity of the autoantibodies that are associated with the clinical conditions.

Testing for ANA by immunofluorescence provides a very useful screening method for the clinical immunologist/rheumatologist. The test requires an experienced technician to 'read' and interpret the slides and thus the results are prone to some subjective bias. However, the different staining patterns that are obtained with various connective tissue diseases (Fig. 2.11) yield valuable diagnostic information and more than compensate for this shortcoming.

Anti-DNA autoantibodies

Coincident with Friou's remarkable observations on ANA, reports from other laboratories in Europe and America appeared describing antibodies in the sera of lupus patients that would bind to native DNA. The detection of antibodies binding to double-stranded (ds) DNA is central to the diagnosis of SLE. Antibodies binding to single-stranded (ss) DNA are much less disease specific and are found in a wide variety of autoimmune and infectious diseases. Many versions of this test exist and their advantages and disadvantages are summarized in Table 2.1; currently the *Crithidia lucillae* assay is thought to be the 'gold standard' (Fig. 2.11).

Antibodies to extractable nuclear antigens (ENA)

The extractable nuclear antigen (ENA) test measures antibodies to a number of non-DNA proteins and nucleic acids. Antibodies to ENA seem to be par-

Table 2.1 Methods of detecting and measuring anti-DNA antibodies

Test	Comments
Precipitation assay	Performed by double diffusion in dilute agarose gel or counter immunoelectrophoresis. The former method is insensitive and not quantitative, the latter is sensitive but the results seem to differ from those obtained using other assays.
Passive haemagglutination	DNA is adsorbed on to tanned or formalinized erythrocytes. The method is sensitive but requires fresh preparations of coated cells and there is much interassay variability.
Complement fixation	Potentially important since complement-fixing antibodies in serum may correlate with the development of lupus nephritis. However, not all anti-DNA antibodies fix complement.
Radioimmunoassays (RIA)	Cultured cells can be internally labelled with ^{3}H-thymidine or ^{125}I-iodocytidine and thus act as a source of radioactive DNA. In the Farr assay, bound and free DNA are separated by precipitating immunoglobulins with 50% saturated ammonium sulfate. Bound, radioactive DNA precipitates with the immunoglobulins, whereas free DNA remains in the supernatant. This method is reproducible, but may miss low avidity anti-DNA antibodies. In contrast, the nitrocellulose filter method allows free DNA to pass through the filter but dsDNA protein complexes do not. Retained radioactivity on the filter is proportional to the serum anti-DNA antibody concentration. Polyethylene glycol may also be used to precipitate complexes of DNA–anti-DNA antibodies. Finally, another variant is a solid phase RIA in which non-radioactive DNA is bound to a Sephadex column and radiolabelled anti-IgG/IgM is added after serum incubation.
ELISA	A simple, rapid quantitative, and reproducible technique in which DNA is applied to the wells of polystyrene plates and the amount of anti-DNA antibodies in the serum is measured colorimetrically by adding an enzyme-labelled, affinity-purified anti-immunoglobulin antiserum, and, subsequently, an appropriate substrate.
Immunofluorescent assays	The haemoflagellate *Crithidiae lucillae* has a kinetoplast containing circular dsDNA. The parasite is fixed to a microscope slide, incubated with test serum, and fluorescent anti-immunoglobulin added. The test has good specificity; quantitation is expressed by titre. Another fluorescence method employs human metaphase chromosomes as a substrate.

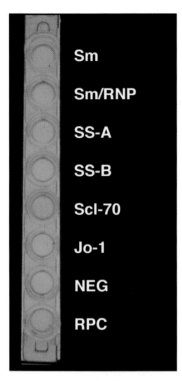

Fig. 2.12. ELISA colour reaction. In this case the assay has been set up to measure extractable nuclear antigens (ENA) although they can also be detected with the Ouchterlony immunodiffusion technique.

ticularly useful in diagnosing patients with auto-immune rheumatic disease. Antibodies may be detected to nuclear components extracted from calf thymus cells and commonly induce a speckled fluorescent staining pattern (Fig. 2.11). Most laboratories use the immunodiffusion technique to detect antibodies to these antigens, although, more recently, radioimmunoassay and ELISA (Fig. 2.12) have been utilized.

Enzyme digestion studies have revealed that these antigens are sensitive to RNase and trypsin and are composed of ribonucleoprotein (RNP). Another closely related antigen, designated Sm (so named because it was first found in the serum of a patient named **Sm**ith), has been found to be resistant to RNase and trypsin.

Many studies have been undertaken to purify and characterize the RNP and Sm antigens. In 1979, Lerner and Steitz demonstrated that both of these antigens contain a small series of nuclear RNA species (U1, U2, and U4–6) which were associated with eight proteins (called bands A–G according to their electrophoresis pattern on polyacrylamide gels). Subsequently, the RNP antigenic determinants were found on protein bands A and C in association with U1 RNA, whereas Sm determinants were present on the other six proteins in association with U1, U2, and U4–6 RNA.

Other important nuclear antigens include the Sjögren's syndrome A and B (SS-A and SS-B) antigens. Originally termed 'Ro' and 'La', they have since been found to be antigenically identical to two entities named SS-A and SS-B, respectively, by Alspaugh and Tan in 1975 who were studying patients with Sjögren's syndrome. They are thought to be cellular ribonuclear proteins although they remain to be fully characterized. SS-A (Ro) is usually extracted from human spleen and SS-B(La) from calf thymus.

Anti-neutrophil antibodies (ANCA)

Over the past decade, intense interest has been focused on the measurement of anti-neutrophil cytoplasmic antibodies (ANCA) and this test is now arguably one of the most useful immunopathology assays for diagnosing a clinical condition, specifically *Wegener's granulomatosis*. ANCA are specific for granule proteins of neutrophils and monocytes and in immunofluorescence assays induce two primary staining patterns (Fig. 2.13), namely *cytoplasmic staining* (cANCA) and *perinuclear staining* (pANCA). A further staining pattern, which does not have a clear-cut association with a distinct granule protein, is sometimes seen in chronic inflammatory bowel diseases.

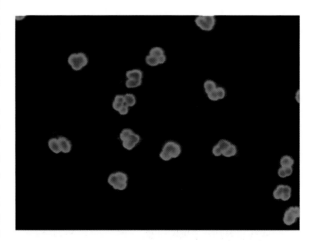

Fig. 2.13. Anti-neutrophil cytoplasmic antibody (ANCA) staining patterns: (a) cytoplasmic staining (cANCA) classically associated with Wegener's granulomatosis; (b) perinuclear staining (pANCA) associated with various vasculitides and general autoimmune rheumatic disease. This pattern is much less disease specific than cANCA.

cANCA is strongly associated with *Wegener's granulomatosis* (a necrotizing vasculitis, probably immune complex-mediated, of the small arteries and veins occurring particularly in the lungs and kidneys; see Chapter 11). This staining pattern is induced by antibodies directed against proteinase 3 (PR3; PR3-ANCA) in about 90% of all ANCA-positive sera. Anti-PR3 ELISAS are carried out in some laboratories but are not yet standardized or in common usage.

The pANCA staining pattern is, in most cases, induced by antibodies against myeloperoxidase (MPO; MPO–ANCA) but may depend upon antibodies against other antigens in the cytoplasm. Perinuclear-type staining may also be seen in patients who are ANA-positive. PANCA appears to be less specific than cANCA but these antibodies have been described in certain subtypes of primary vasculitides, including polyarteritis and glomerulonephritis and Churg Strauss vasculitis.

It is equivocal whether the ANCA titre reflects disease activity (but given the association between disease and a positive test result it is always prudent to recommend careful follow-up of the patient). The role of the ANCA antibody/antigen in the pathology of the above diseases is uncertain.

Anti-cardiolipin antibodies

Anti-phospholipid antibodies bind to phospholipids, particularly cardiolipin. They are associated with blood clotting disorders, particularly in patients with autoimmune rheumatic disease, as well as strokes, thrombosis, and recurrent fetal loss. They are usually detected by anti-cardiolipin ELISAS which are commercially available. Quite recently it has been recognized that a large portion of antibodies directed against cardiolpin are in fact binding an associated co-factor known as β_2 glycoprotein (β_2GP-1). Currently, many laboratories are measuring anti-β_2GP-1 antibodies as well as anti-phospholipid *per se*. The clinical and pathological significance of these antibodies is discussed in Chapter 9.

Other autoantibodies

Numerous tests for other antibodies binding to a wide spectrum of autoantigens exist in the autoimmune rheumatic diseases: these are discussed in the appropriate chapters. In this section we have described antibodies that the physician and scientist will most commonly encounter when studying these disorders. In Fig. 2.14 we have outlined a decision tree which may aid in the choice of serological tests that should be conducted in order to diagnose patients with rheumatic diseases.

Circulating immune complexes

In the 1970s and early 1980s there was intense interest in the measurement of immune complexes in patients with autoimmune rheumatic diseases. The rationale for measuring these entities was that complexes of antigen and (auto) antibody may be formed during the course of the disease and be deposited in tissues such as the kidney, brain, joints, or blood vessels, from which point they initiate a sequence of inflammatory events that perpetuate or even exacerbate the disease process. This viewpoint catalysed the development and introduction of numerous types of tests. Some of these proved to be fairly reliable and would give more-or-less reproducible results from one laboratory to another, while others could at best be described as unpredictable. Yet even the best of these assays produced results that frequently did not correlate with one another; a discrepancy that can be attributed to the fact that the tests selected for different physicochemical characteristics of the complexes (such as size, affinity of the bound antibody, and its ability to bind complement components). Although immune complex measurement has not found its way into the panel of tests used for the routine monitoring of autoimmune rheumatic diseases, on occasion it may be considered useful. In these circumstances several assays are available commercially. These are based on the polyethylene glycol precipitation method (PEG) or C1q binding. The PEG test is the simplest and most economical of immune complex assays and is based on the principle that this reagent excludes macromolecules from the liquidphase. PEG-precipitated material, including immunoglobulins of all classes and sub-classes, as well as complement components and acute phase proteins, can be measured by radial immunodiffusion or nephelometry. The disadvantage of this technique is that it takes some time to complete (up to three days if the Mancini radial diffusion assay is used) and it has been criticized for its lack of specificity.

C1q-based systems are based on the principle that immune complexes fix complement by binding to this molecule, its first component. Although numerous variations of this test have been described, the most practical is the C1q–IgG ELISA system. This assay is a 'two-site' or 'sandwich' system designed to detect immune complexes in human serum that contain two antigens; C1q and IgG. ELISA microtitre plates are

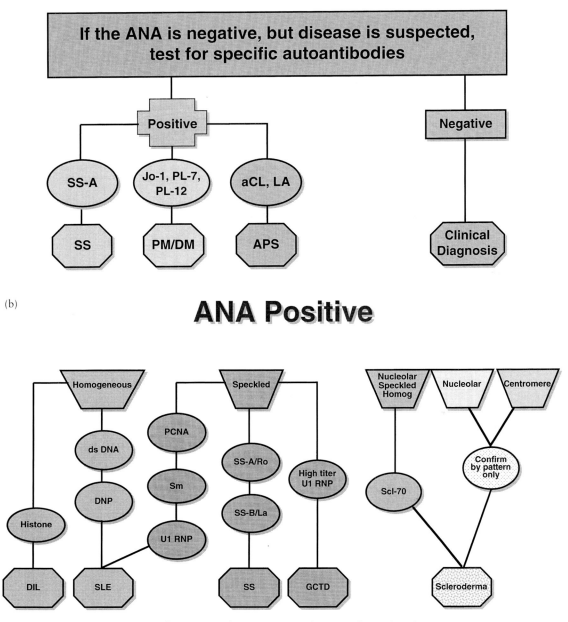

(a)

ANA Negative

If the ANA is negative, but disease is suspected, test for specific autoantibodies

Positive

Negative

SS-A

Jo-1, PL-7, PL-12

aCL, LA

SS

PM/DM

APS

Clinical Diagnosis

(b)

ANA Positive

Homogeneous

Speckled

Nucleolar Speckled Homog

Nucleolar

Centromere

PCNA

ds DNA

SS-A/Ro

High titer U1 RNP

Confirm by pattern only

Sm

DNP

Scl-70

Histone

SS-B/La

U1 RNP

DIL

SLE

SS

GCTD

Scleroderma

Fig. 2.14. Diagnostic 'decision tree' for autoimmune rheumatic disease based on ANA positivity.

coated with a monoclonal anti-C1q antibody which is capable of capturing immune complexes containing C1q. The bound complexes are quantitated with a murine monoclonal anti-IgG antibody conjugated to horse-radish peroxidase. After suitable colour development the plates are scanned in an ELISA reader.

Complement and acute phase proteins

Measurement of these serum components can be extremely useful in the management of autoimmune rheumatic diseases. For example, low complement levels in a patient with SLE can indicate increased consumption and an active disease process. In addition, levels of C-reactive protein can serve as an indicator for differential diagnosis between SLE and RA.

Complement components

Serum concentrations of complement components, primarily C3 and C4, can be measured quite easily by radial immunodiffusion or nephelometry. Activation products of C3, such as C3d, which may act as a more reliable indicator of inflammation, are present at lower levels and although they can be assayed by radial immunodiffusion, more sensitive techniques such as nephelometry are to be preferred.

Functional haemolytic complement

As an alternative to estimations of antigenic complement, functional tests such as the CH_{50} assay can be performed. This test estimates overall levels of serum complement by its ability to cause haemolysis in an indicator system of sheep erythrocytes previously coated with anti-red blood cell antibodies. Although this system has proved to be one of the most accurate indicators of clinical activity, it is highly labour intensive and is not available as a standard procedure in many laboratories.

Cellular assays

In general, cellular immunological techniques are harder to perform on a routine basis than serological tests. In most cases preparations of mononuclear cells, usually isolated by centrifugation on Ficoll density gradients, are necessary. In addition, cell culture facilities and expertise are required, as well as the use of specialized and often expensive reagents, such as radio-isotopes and monoclonal antibodies. Finally, because cellular assays are 'biological' systems, they are prone to giving 'noisy' results. Thus, because of these problems, it is probably fair to say that most clinicians consider tests of cellular immune function to be in an esoteric realm of 'research'. This conclusion is unfortunate as even a modest evaluation of the cellular arm of a patient's immune system can substantially reinforce findings from humoral studies. Some of the more commonly performed investigations are given below.

Proliferation assays

Certain antigens and plant lectins can induce, differentially, subpopulations of lymphocytes to undergo mitogenesis and to proliferate *in vitro*. For example, phytohaemagglutinin and concanavalin A stimulate T cells, whereas bacterial lipopolysaccharide (LPS) selectively affects B cells. The degree of stimulation is determined by the uptake of a pulse of tritiated [^{3}H] thymidine into the DNA of the cell. The degree of responsiveness of the cells is generally thought to correlate with their functionality. Although this test is considered somewhat dated, it remains a good overall test of cellular immune function and is relatively simple and economical to perform. It takes 2–4 days to carry out.

Lectins, however, are non-specific. They bind and activate most receptors on the T cell surface, not only the T cell-specific ones, which is an undesirable property of these substances. More recently, stimulatory anti-CD3 and anti-CD28 antibodies have been used to measure proliferation by activating the T cells in the same way as the lectins mentioned above. The difference lies in the fact that CD3 and CD28 are T cell-specific receptor. CD3 is a complex associated with the T cell receptor, which is necessary for a functional T cell response. CD28 is a cell surface-bound receptor that provides an important co-stimulatory signal without which the T cell would enter a state of non-responsiveness or anergy. Ligation of these two receptors activates, within the T cell-specific signal transduction, pathways that lead to T cell proliferation, which can be used as a measure of T cell responsiveness.

Cytokine assays

Information about cytokines can be most valuable in characterizing the immunopathological features of a given disease. Measurement can be undertaken by a variety of techniques that have various pros and cons. These include the following.

Bioassays

Originally, bioassays that gauged the functionality of the particular cytokine being measured were used. For example, TNF levels were measured by killing of the tumour cell line L929, and IL-2 levels were assessed by its ability to maintain an IL-2-dependent cell line such as HT-2 or CLL. The main disadvantages of bioassays are the availability and maintenance (checking that they are free of mycoplasma infection and that they do not develop a tendency towards cytokine independence) of target cell lines, as well as the relative time and labour involved. In addition, it is hard to quantify the precise amount of cytokine present.

ELISA and ELISPOT

ELISA provides a relatively cheap, rapid, and effective means of measuring the amounts of cytokine in samples from various sources. Briefly, cytokine ELISA utilize monoclonal antibodies bound to the wells of microtitre plates to capture the cytokine of interest. Any other unbound protein is then washed away, a second antibody is then added (usually a polyclonal sera against the cytokine), and, finally, after an incubation period, a third antibody that has specificity against the polyclonal sera is added. This final antibody has an enzyme conjugated to it such alkaline phosphatase or horseradish peroxidase, which, as described previously, will catalyse a colour reaction in the presence of a suitable substrate. The amount of colour can be correlated with the quantity of cytokine present. One requirement of these assays is that the monoclonal antibody used to capture the cytokine must be raised against the fully functional, bioactive, molecule: if it is not then non-functional cytokine will be measured. There have been a number of adaptations of this assay; for instance, whole cell ELISA has been developed which relies on cytokine-producing cells being added to the antibody-coated wells. It is thus possible to measure actively secreted cytokine and thus even quantify the number of cells secreting a specific cytokine: such assays are known as ELISPOT. A further variation of this technique is that anti-cytokine antibody may be directly conjugated with an enzyme thus allowing tissue sections to be stained for cytokine expression.

Reverse transcriptase polymerase chain reaction (RT-PCR)

In many cases the amount of cytokine produced is either very low or its turnover is too rapid to be measured by ELISA-based techniques. In such cases, PCR can be used to detect and amplify just one double-stranded piece of mRNA to an amount that can be subsequently quantified. The technique utilizes enzymatic conversion of cytokine mRNA by reverse transcriptase to cDNA, which is then amplified millions of times. This technique relies on the availability of cytokine mRNA-specific primers to mark out the mRNA for the reverse transcriptase. There are a number of disadvantages with this technique including relative expense, operator specialization, and, finally, long assay time.

Intracellular staining

Flow cytometry, has been used for the last decade to assess the number and status of a wide range of cell types. Using this technique, cytokine quantification can be achieved by first permeabilizing cells with a mild detergent in order to allow the conjugated antibody entry into the cell. The advantage of the technique is that distinct cytokine-producing cells can be visualized and identified in a mixed population. In addition, the technique is rapid, typically only requiring one to two hours, although there is a requirement for operator training. The disadvantage of the procedure is that it can be unreliable: once a cell is permeabilized to allow antibody molecules into the cell, cytokine can pass out of the membrane.

Apoptosis

Apoptosis (programmed cell death; PCD) is the process by which cells undergo a series of structural changes leading to death and phagocytosis without the generation of an inflammatory response. Under normal circumstances apoptosis is initiated by limited injury or physiological stimuli and is quite distinct from cell death by necrosis. Abnormalities in the apoptotic process have been implicated in the pathogenesis of autoimmune disease and the measurement of levels of apoptosis may be useful in the investigation of these disorders.

There are several methods available to investigate apoptosis and these include morphological methods using nuclear dyes, methods to demonstrate DNA fragmentation, and those that demonstrate the disruption of membrane asymmetry, an early manifestation of programmed cell death.

DNA fragmentation, as demonstrated by a typical laddering pattern on an agarose electrophoresis gel, is regarded by some researchers as the definitive standard test of apoptosis. However, this technique is relatively slow and other methods have been developed. The use of nuclear stains (May–Grunwald Giemsa/acridine orange) is a simple way to visualize nuclear condensation in apoptotic cells by light or fluorescent microscopy, although flow cytometry is, in most cases, the technique of preference. Intensity of nuclear staining using propidium iodide (PI) can also be used, the nuclei of cells lysed and stained with PI take up stain in different ways. Apoptotic cells will take up less dye owing to nuclear condensation and this can be visualized using flow cytometry.

Another technique useful in the measurement of apoptosis is TUNEL (terminal dUTP nick end labelling). In this procedure the ends of DNA strand breaks or nicks in cells undergoing apoptosis are labelled and quantified in a colour reaction. TUNEL is quite versatile and colour quantification can be carried out by flow cytometry or visually on tissue sections. If the assay is carried out by flow cytometry, individual cells undergoing apoptosis can be quantitated. Because the end-labelling is performed within cells, the technique is by far the most direct method for analysing populations undergoing DNA fragmentation. In addition, because DNA fragmentation is one of the earliest processes in PCD cells can be detected at an early phase. The main disadvantage with TUNEL is the cost of the dUTP and TdT reagents.

Recently, a rapid, sensitive, and relatively inexpensive procedure has been described utilizing annexin V. An early change to cells undergoing apoptosis is the loss of membrane asymmetry leading to the abnormal exposure of phosphotidylserine (PS) on the outer membrane. Annexin V is a phospholipid-binding protein that will bind PS in the presence of calcium. When labelled with a fluorescent dye, annexin V can be used to detect PS on the membranes of cells undergoing apoptosis; again, flow cytometry is the preferred method to quantify the labelled cells.

Cell surface markers

The derivation and general availability of monoclonal antibodies specific for CD or adhesion molecules, labelled with a variety of fluorochromes, as well as the general availability of relatively inexpensive flow cytometers, have revolutionized the quantification of lymphocyte subpopulations. The ever increasing repertoire of cell-specific antibodies allows almost infinite numbers of questions to be asked on a semi-routine basis regarding types and numbers of leucocytes in circulation. The possibilities are almost limitless and because of the general lack of knowledge regarding changes in cell populations in these diseases, basic quantification studies may lead to improved understanding of the immunological basis of these disorders.

The only drawbacks to such analyses are that they are not especially cheap to conduct, they require a flow cytometer, and, from a biological point of view, the correlation between cell phenotype and functional ability may not be absolute.

HLA typing techniques

Methods for studying variation in HLA genes and molecules

The techniques that are used to define HLA genes and the molecules they encode include serological, cellular,

and DNA-based typing methods. The HLA terminology that is used reflects the typing method that is used. Serology utilizes antibodies that detect HLA molecules expressed on the surface of cells. Cellular techniques are functional assays used to subdivide members of a serologically defined family. DNA-typing techniques detect the allele that encodes the corresponding HLA molecule. Much greater discriminatory power is achieved with DNA-based typing techniques.

Serological and cellular typing techniques

HLA antigens were first detected with the use of alloantisera, i.e. sera containing antibodies that react with the HLA molecules. Although some HLA-typing is still done by serology, DNA-typing techniques have largely replaced serological methods. Serological techniques utilize a standardized complement-dependent microcytotoxicity assay. Typing for class I HLA-A, -B, and -C antigens is usually performed on peripheral blood lymphocytes or T cells, with typing for class II HLA-DR and -DQ antigens requiring purification of B lymphocytes (which express DR and DQ antigens).

HLA polymorphism can also be detected by T cell recognition using homozygous typing cells (HTC). The method employs a modified mixed lymphocyte culture in which the homozygous typing cell is cultured with the responder cell of interest. The homozygous typing cell is irradiated so as to function as a stimulator cell only and if the responder cell is not stimulated to proliferate by a HTC, but does react to a standard control, it is presumed to share that specificity. The specificities defined by HTC are termed 'HLA-Dw'. Prior to the advent of DNA-typing techniques, HTC-typing provided a method by which serologically defined specificities could be further subdivided. For example, the serologically defined specificity DR4, when studied further using HTC methods, was found to consist of at least six members and these were designated Dw4, Dw10, Dw13, Dw14, Dw15, and DwKT2 (Table 2.2).

T cell clones have also been used to analyse class I and class II HLA antigens. T cell clones are generated by co-culturing responder cells with irradiated stimulator cells with the specificity of interest. After 7–10 days of culture responding cells are plated at limiting dilution. Positive wells are selected for expansion and then tested against a panel of stimulating cells to determine the specificity of the clone. These clones can then be used as HLA-typing reagents and, similar to the use of HTC techniques, are often able to recognize epitopes within serological typing specificities.

Serological	Cellular	DNA-based
DR4	Dw4	DRB1*0401
	Dw10	DRB1*0402
	Dw13	DRB1*0403
		DRB1*0407
	Dw14	DRB1*0404
		DRB1*0408
	Dw15	DRB1*0405
	DwKT2	DRB1*0406
	No cellular equivalent	DRB1*0409-27

Table 2.2. Serological techniques identified a single DR4 specificity. When cellular techniques were used it was discovered that DR4 is a family of at least 6 HLA molecules. Subsequent application of DNA-based typing techniques indicated that there are at least 27 members of the DR4 family.

DNA-typing techniques

Techniques used to study the DNA that encodes for HLA molecules include restriction fragment length polymorphism (RFLP) analysis, polymerase chain reaction with oligonucleotide probe typing or with sequence-specific primers, and direct gene sequencing.

In RFLP-typing, DNA is isolated from nucleated cells and digested with restriction enzymes. The sample is electrophoresed in an agarose gel, transferred to a nylon membrane by the Southern blotting technique, and then probed with labelled genomic or cDNA probes. RFLP patterns are visualized in different ways depending on the method used for labelling the probes. Polymorphism revealed by RFLP depends upon the restriction enzymes and probes that are used.

The most powerful methods to define variability with HLA genes are those that utilize PCR. PCR-based typing has recently replaced other techniques for HLA typing in most immunogenetics laboratories. PCR is used to amplify a segment of DNA between two regions of known sequence. Two oligonucleotide primers are used and a series of synthetic reactions are catalysed by a DNA polymerase. The primer sequences are selected so as to be complementary to sequences that lie on opposite strands of the template DNA and flank the segment of DNA that is to be amplified. In addition to the primers, the reaction mixture includes template DNA that is denatured by heating, and the four dNTPs, (dATP, dCTP, dGTP, dTTP). The reaction mixture is subsequently cooled, allowing the oligonucleotide primers to anneal to their target sequences, followed by extension of the annealed

primers with DNA polymerase. The cycles of denaturation, annealing, and DNA synthesis are repeated many times. Because the products on one round of amplification serve as templates for the next, successive cycles exponentially increase the amount of the desired DNA product. The initial polymerase utilized to catalyse the PCR reaction was inactivated by the temperatures needed to denature DNA, however, this problem was solved when the thermostable Taq DNA polymerase was introduced.

In HLA-typing the PCR reaction is applied using either group-specific primers or sequence-specific primers. In the latter method a multitude of primer pairs are synthesized, each of which specifically amplifies known alleles at the various HLA loci. In the former technique, group-specific primers are used; for example, a primer pair might be used that amplifies all DR4 alleles. The amplified sample is then blotted on to multiple membranes and hybridized to specific labelled oligonucleotide probes. The pattern of hybridization to these probes allows determination of the specific allele of the sample.

In addition to specificity, PCR-based methods are very sensitive and can be successfully employed to study very small amounts of DNA. To obtain further sensitivity a 'nested' PCR reaction can be employed. Two sequential cycles are used in nested PCR wherein the product of the first amplification is subjected to a second amplification using primers that are internal to the primers used in the first set.

The application of DNA-typing techniques to the study of HLA has essentially revolutionized our understanding of HLA genes and the molecules they encode. A good example of the power of DNA-typing is its application to the study of HLA-DQ (and also DP) molecules, where polymorphism is present on both the α and the β chain. Serological techniques, at best, were able to distinguish nine different DQ molecules. However, we now know that there are DQA1 and DQB1 alleles that encode at least 15 different DQα chains and 30 different DQβ chains. Moreover, what had previously been recognized by serology as a single molecule actually encodes very different molecules, as

Serological		DQ7	DQ7	DQ2	DQ2
DNA typing	DQA1*	0301	0501	0501	0201
	DQB1*	0301	0301	0201	0201

Table 2.3 DNA typing has revealed that what was called DQ7 and DQ2 when serological techniques were used consists of different HLA molecules.

illustrated in Table 2.3. In the example provided, serological methods identify two different molecules as
'DQ7', and another two different molecules as 'DQ2',
whereas the DQα chains differ within each group
and are the same between one member from each group.

Nomenclature

The HLA terminology used reflects the HLA-typing
technique that is used. For example, serological
reagents are capable of distinguishing 18 different molecules that are the product of the DRB1 gene, and these
are called DR1–DR18. However, each of these serologically defined specificities, rather than being a single
molecule, actually represents a family of molecules.
Using cellular typing techniques with homozygous
typing cells, the DR4 family, for example, is further
divided into at least six different members and these
are designated as Dw4, Dw10, Dw13, Dw14, Dw15
and DwKT2. The 'Dw' designation should not be confused with 'DRw', which was previously used for serologically defined specificities when they were only
provisionally recognized by HLA workshop consensus.
With the advent of sequencing and DNA-typing
methods it is now evident that there are far more
members of serologically and cellularly defined families
than were previously appreciated. When DNA-typing
techniques are used to define the specific allele the terminology used indicates the locus and a * sign followed by the number of the allele. Thus, for example,
27 alleles in the DR4 family encode DRB1*0401 to
DRB1*0427 (Table 2.2).

To provide for uniform nomenclature, the World
Health Organization (WHO) established a HLA nomenclature committee. Reports that summarize newly
identified HLA alleles are published periodically, with
updates provided in between summaries. Full sequences
of HLA class I and II alleles are also published
periodically (Marsh *et al.* 1998; Mason and Parham
1998).

Summary

Despite some complex underlying theoretical considerations, clinical immunology is essentially a practical
science. In this chapter we have outlined the most
useful and commonly performed immunological techniques and then described some standard serological
and cellular tests that utilize these procedures and are
used regularly to investigate these diseases at both the
clinical and experimental level. The relative merits of
the tests are also described (although recommendations
for specific assays in the various disorders can be found
in the appropriate chapters for the disorders).

References

Bodmer W, Marsh GE, Albert D *et al.* Nomenclature of the
HLA system, 1996. *Tissue Antigens* 1997; **49**: 297–321.
McPherson MJ, Quirke P, Taylor GR. *PCR: a practical
approach*. IRL Press, Oxford. 1995.
Marsh SGE. HLA class II region sequences, 1998. *Tissue
Antigens* 1998; **51**: 467–507.
Mason PM, Parham P. HLA class I region sequences, 1998.
Tissue Antigens 1998; **51**: 417–66.

General reading

Coligan JE *et al. Current protocols in immunology*. John
Wiley and Sons, New York. 1994.

Introduction

Current, non-selective immunosuppressive therapies for the autoimmune rheumatic diseases, while helping to ameliorate symptoms, contribute both to the mortality and the morbidity. Considerable research effort is aimed at developing new therapeutic modalities. In this chapter the agents used to manipulate the immune system therapeutically will be described. Their use in individual diseases will be described in detail in subsequent chapters.

The functioning of the immune system in the autoimmune rheumatic diseases has been described in Chapter 1. Current ideas about the development of autoimmune diseases such as rheumatoid arthritis (RA) or systemic lupus erythematosus (SLE) are based on the notion that, in genetically predisposed individuals (i.e. those carrying specific HLA class II genes or other genetic factors), an unknown triggering event results in activation of autoreactive lymphocytes which, in the absence of regulation, results in autoimmune disease. Key players in this process are the pathogenic T cell, the autoantigen (usually unknown) that is presented to the T cell in complex with the HLA molecule, and the regulatory T cells (Panayi *et al.* 1992; Feldmann *et al.* 1996), together with the B cells responsible for

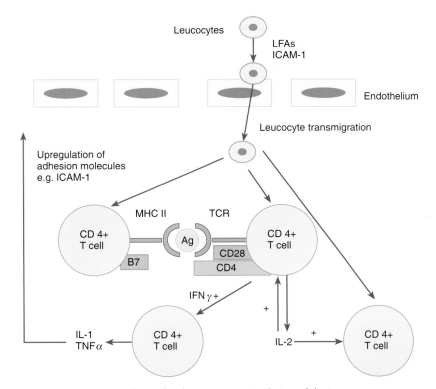

Fig. 3.1. Potential sites for therapeutic manipulation of the immune system.

production of, at least in some cases, pathogenic auto-antibodies. There are a number of points where this immunological process might be blocked or modulated (Fig. 3.1). Modulation can be achieved either non-selectively (using conventional immunosuppressive agents) or selectively (using a variety of biological approaches).

Established non-selective immunotherapy

The use of non-selective immunosuppressive agents forms the mainstay of conventional treatment of chronic immune-mediated rheumatic diseases. Several agents are in use (Table 3.1), including corticosteroids, methotrexate, cyclosporin (Neoral), azathioprine (Imuran), and cyclophosphamide, and these have several potential sites of action (Fig. 3.2).

Methotrexate

Methotrexate inhibits dihydrofolate reductase, interrupting synthesis of purines, and thymidilic and inosinic acids. Other anti-inflammatory effects include reduction in IgM rheumatoid factor production, decrease in chemotaxis, and decrease in IL-2, IL-1, and IL-6 production. Which of these effects is most important in RA is unclear (Cronstein 1996).

Methotrexate is effective in placebo-controlled trials in RA (Weinblatt *et al.* 1994) and is increasingly used in other conditions, either as sole therapy or in combination with corticosteroids. Methotrexate can cause bone marrow suppression, pulmonary toxicity (hypersensitivity), and hepatic fibrosis, and therefore requires careful monitoring in clinical practice.

Azathioprine

Azathioprine is the 1-methyl-4-nitro-5-imidazolyl derivative of 6-mercaptopurine, which is a purine analogue and inhibitor of DNA synthesis. Its active metabolites are 6-thioinosinic acid and 6-thioguanylic acid. Metabolism occurs mainly in erythrocytes and the liver, excretion is predominately renal. The precise mechanism of action is uncertain but cell division rate is decreased with an effect predominately on the S phase of the cell cycle (Spina 1984). Azathioprine inhibits the function of both B and T cells (Yu *et al.* 1974) without altering the ratio of T to B cells. It inhibits immunoglobulin production by B cells (Levy *et al.* 1972) as well as B cell proliferation (Abdou *et al.* 1973). Its effects on T cell function are uncertain, but natural killer cell function and number are reduced (Spina 1984).

Azathioprine is often used in combination with corticosteroids as a 'steroid sparing' agent. Bone marrow suppression may require reduction of dosage. Long-term side-effects include induction of lymphoid tumours. Azathioprine can be used safely in pregnancy despite being able to cross the placental barrier and it is also secreted in breast milk.

Table 3.1   Mechanism of action immunosuppressants

Drug	Mechanism of action
Conventional	
Methotrexate	Inhibits dihyrofolate reductase and purine synthesis
Azathioprine	Inhibits purine synthesis
Corticosteroids	Blocks cytokine gene expression
Cyclosporin	Blocks calcium-dependent T cell activation pathway by binding to calcineurin
Cyclophosphamide	Cross-links DNA, preventing replication
Chlorambucil	Cross-links DNA, preventing replication
Experimental	
Brequinar sodium	Inhibits dihydroorotate dehydrogenase and blocks pyrimidine synthesis
FK506 (Tacrolimus)	Blocks calcium-dependent T cell activation pathway by binding to calcineurin
Leflunamide	Inhibits pyrimidine synthesis; inhibits growth factor receptor-associated tyrosine kinases
Mizoribine	Inhibits purine synthesis
Mycophenolate mofetil	Inhibits inosine monophosphate dehydrogenase and prevents *de novo* guanosine and deoxyguanosine synthesis in lymphocytes
Rapamycin (Serolimus)	Blocks IL-2 and other growth factor signal transduction; blocks CD28-mediated co-stimulatory agents

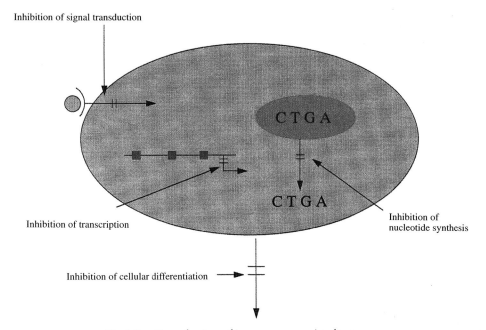

Inhibition of signal transduction

CTGA

CTGA

Inhibition of transcription

Inhibition of nucleotide synthesis

Inhibition of cellular differentiation

Fig. 3.2.   Sites of action of immunosuppressive drugs.

Cyclophosphamide

Cyclophosphamide is derived from nitrogen mustard and the main active metabolite is phosphoramide mustard, which cross-links DNA, preventing replication. Cyclophosphamide has both immunostimulatory and immunosuppressive effects (Turk and Parker 1979) and is toxic to both dividing and resting lymphocytes. Low doses are most toxic to B cells. With increasing doses CD8+ T cells are affected, and CD4+ T cells are most resistant to cyclophosphamide (Bast *et al.* 1983). It acts on the premitotic (G$_2$) phase of the cell cycle. Cyclophosphamide suppresses many cell-mediated responses such as delayed hypersensitivity, cell-mediated cytotoxicity, and antigen- or mitogen-induced blastogenesis.

Cyclophosphamide has a number of toxic effects. Acrolein, the main renal metabolite, has no active role but is responsible for the bladder toxicity, including haemorrhagic cystitis, bladder fibrosis, and bladder carcinoma. Infertility in both females and males occurs according to a dose-dependent relationship (Boumpas *et al.* 1993a). Atypical infections (pneumocystis or fungi) are well recognized (Bradley *et al.* 1989). Malignancy occurs according to a dose-dependent relationship (Baker *et al.* 1987). Because of its toxicity, the clinical use of cyclophosphamide is restricted to severe SLE (typically nephritis) and systemic vasculitis

where it has significantly improved mortality (Fauci *et al.* 1983).

Chlorambucil

Chlorambucil probably has a similar mode of action to cyclophosphamide, through cross-linking of DNA and proteins and preventing cell replication. Chlorambucil itself is not cytotoxic but is rapidly and almost completely metabolized to phenylacetic acid mustard, its most active metabolite. Chlorambucil is established treatment for amyloidosis complicating juvenile chronic arthritis but is rarely used to treat uncomplicated autoimmune disease. The major toxicity of chlorambucil is haematological, together with induction of malignancy.

Corticosteroids

Corticosteroids bind to a cytoplasmic receptor protein, dislodging a complex set of 'chaperon' proteins including heat shock protein 90 (hsp90). The complex of steroid and receptor then moves to the nucleus where it binds to chromatin and induces increased production of mRNA for proteins such as lipocortin. Lipocortin inhibits production of pro-inflammatory cytokines (IL-1, IL-2, IL-2R, IFN-γ, and TNF-α) (Boumpas *et al.*

Table 3.2   Adverse effects of corticosteroid therapy

Metabolic	Truncal obesity
	Electrolyte imbalance
	Glucose/protein metabolism
	Enzyme induction
Infection	
Musculoskeletal	Osteoporosis
	Myopathy
	Tendon rupture
	Osteonecrosis
	Withdrawal syndrome
Gastrointestinal	Peptic ulceration
	Pancreatitis
Ophthalmic	Cataract
	Glaucoma
Cutaneous	Acne
	Striae
	Alopecia
	Bruising
	Skin Atrophy
Central nervous system	Psychosis
	Depression
	Benign intracranial hypertension
Growth retardation	
Suppression of hypothalamic-pituitary-adrenal axis	

1993*b*). At low doses, corticosteroids inhibit the synthesis of pro-inflammatory enzymes such as the metallo-proteinases collagenase and elastase. Other effects of corticosteroids include stabilization of lysosomes, inhibition of macrophage function, and reduction in adhesion molecule expression on cell surfaces. The side-effects of corticosteroids are dose and duration dependent (Table 3.2).

High dose steroids are immunosuppressive and are used to induce remission in vasculitis, SLE, and myositis. Lower doses are used for maintenance therapy, often in combination with other immunosuppressive drugs.

Cyclosporin (Neoral), FK506 (Tacrolimus) and rapamycin

Cyclosporin, FK506 (Tacrolimus), and rapamycin are fungal cyclic peptides which share a number of properties and are potent immunosuppressive agents. Their immunosuppressive effects are secondary to relatively selective T cell inhibition. FK506 and rapamycin are structurally related, but suppress T cell activation at different levels. Cyclosporin and FK506, although structurally dissimilar, share a similar action on the T cell. All three drugs bind to cytoplasmic binding proteins known as immunophilins. FK506 and rapamycin share a common binding protein distinct from the cyclosporin-binding protein (cyclophilin). The drug–immunophilin complex binds to a serine/threonine phosphatase, calcineurin.

Cyclosporin and FK506 inhibit gene transcription of T cell cytokines, including IL-2, IL-3, IL-4, granulocyte-macrophage stimulating factor, TNF-α, and IFN-γ (Herold *et al.* 1986; Sigal and Dumont 1992). Rapamycin, by contrast, has little or no effect on lymphokine transcription or secretion, acting by inhibiting cytokine and growth factor dependent stimulation of T helper cells (Sigal and Dumont 1992).

Cyclosporin has been used to treat many autoimmune conditions, high doses (10 mg/kg/day) were associated with hypertension, angio-oedema, and nephrotoxicity (Isenberg *et al.* 1981). The renal side-effects have been overcome by use of lower doses (< 5.0 mg/kg/day) without loss of therapeutic efficacy (Panayi and Tugwell 1993). Analysis of renal biopsies from patients with RA receiving long-term cyclosporin has shown no increase in structural nephropathy compared with the underlying disease (Rodriguez *et al.* 1996). Cyclosporin is effective in the treatment of RA (Tugwell *et al.* 1990) and has been used in SLE (Caccavo *et al.* 1997). Cyclosporin has also been used in combination with methotrexate in the treatment of severe RA (Tugwell *et al.* 1995).

Tacrolimus and rapamycin have predominately only been used in animal models. Tacrolimus is 10–100 times more potent in suppressing collagen-induced arthritis in rats than cyclosporin (Miyahara *et al.* 1991). Rapamycin can inhibit induction of streptococcal cell wall-induced arthritis but has no effect on established disease. Rapamycin prolongs survival in the MRL/*lpr* mouse (Warner *et al.* 1994). Tacrolimus has recently been reported to be useful in SLE as an alternative to cyclosporin (Duddridge and Powell 1998) and also in Behçet's disease (Suzuki *et al.* 1997).

Non-selective therapies under investigation

Mycophenolate mofetil

Mycophenolate mofetil is the semi-synthetic ethyl ester derivative of mycophenolic acid and is converted into its active metabolite, mycophenolic acid, which is a reversible inhibitor of inosine monophosphate dehydrogenase. T and B cells are more dependent on the *de novo* than the salvage pathways for purine nucleotide biosynthesis, and mycophenolic acid is a relatively specific inhibitor of T and B cell proliferation. It does not inhibit synthesis of IL-2 or expression of IL-2R on mitogen-activated T cells. Mycophenolate mofetil is effective in adjuvant-induced arthritis and has been studied in humans in an open-label study of refractory RA with benefit (Goldblum 1993) and large double-blind trials are underway.

Leflunomide

Leflunomide is an isoxazole drug that exerts part of its action by inhibiting *de novo* pyrimidine biosynthesis through its active metabolite, A77 1726. It has immunosuppressive and antiproliferative effects and has shown therapeutic effects in animal models of autoimmune disease (Bartlett *et al.* 1993). Leflunomide was effective in a placebo-controlled trial in RA and further studies are underway (Mladenovic *et al.* 1995).

Plasmapheresis

Plasmapheresis, or plasma exchange, is the modern version of blood letting and washing. Blood is withdrawn from the patient, plasma is separated off and the cellular components are returned with replacement colloid to the patient. Immune function is affected in many ways including improvement of bacterial killing by monocytes, decrease in anti-T suppressor cell antibodies, alteration in CD4+/CD8+ T cell ratios, and idiotype–anti-idiotype relationships (reviewed in McClure and Isenberg 1997).

Side-effects are common, but severe (1%) or fatal reactions are much less so (0.05–2%). Complications include transient hypotension, problems related to vascular access, and reactions to citrate anticoagulation. The last is a result of a fall in the level of ionized calcium as a result of chelation and usually causes parasthesiae. Infection, air embolism, bleeding, or clotting are much less common. Plasma exchange has been combined with cyclophosphamide (stimulation-depletion) (Schroeder *et al.* 1987) or with immuno-adsorbent columns (Schreider *et al.* 1990).

In conditions where it is thought that immune complexes or autoantibodies in serum are pathogenic (e.g. SLE) then their removal should be beneficial. Plasma exchange has been used in many conditions but proof of its efficacy has remained elusive in most diseases. In most conditions it should be reserved for the severely ill patient.

Intravenous immunoglobulin

Intravenous immunoglobulin (IVIg) has been used extensively to treat autoimmune disease since the first report of its use in a child with thrombocytopaenia and hypogammaglobulinaemia (Imbach *et al.* 1981; Dwyer 1992). In many cases there is little controlled data to support the use of IVIg. IVIg has a clearly defined role in the treatment of immune thrombocytopaenia (ITP) and in Kawasaki disease (Leung 1996).

The mechanism of action of IVIg is uncertain and many different modes of action have been proposed (Table 3.3) (reviewed in Mouthon *et al.* 1996). In ITP there is reduction in antibody production, binding of autoantibody to platelets, and reduced efficacy of the reticuloendothelial system of antibody-sensitized platelets (Clarkson *et al.* 1986).

Table 3.3 Possible mechanisms of action of intravenous immunoglobulin

Modulation of Fc receptor function
Protection of cell surface membranes
Clearance of persistent infectious agents
Suppression of antibody synthesis
Direct inhibition of cytokines by naturally occurring anticytokine autoantibodies
Inhibition of cytokine production/release (IL-1, TNF, IL-6)
Inhibition of superantigen T cell activation
Reduction of adhesion molecule expression (ICAM-1, ELAM)
Upregulation of naturally occurring IL-1 receptor antagonist
Alteration of autoreactive repertoires by V-region-dependent interactions with autoantibodies
Cellular regulation of B and T cell function by administration of anti-idiotypic antibodies
Anti-idiotypic antibody neutralization of autoantibodies
Inhibition of complement binding and activation

Non-steroidal anti-inflammatory drugs

The non-steroidal anti-inflammatory drugs (NSAIDs) are a group of agents widely used in the treatment of autoimmune rheumatic disease to control symptoms (e.g. arthralgia, myalgia) while not being directly immunosuppressive. They share common properties and adverse effects. The major action of NSAIDs is on prostaglandin production with inhibition of cyclo-oxygenase production (COX) activity (reviewed in Vane 1996). Recently, interest has developed in the two isoenzymes of COX: the inducible COX II is predominately expressed in inflamed tissue and brain, whereas the constitutive COX I is normally present in many organs including the kidney and gastrointestinal tract. Selective COX II inhibitors have been reported to reduce gastrointestinal and renal side-effects of NSAID therapy while maintaining anti-inflammatory efficacy (Wojtulewski *et al.* 1996).

Selective immunotherapy

T cell-directed therapy

The T cell is one of the key players in autoimmune disease and a number of different techniques have been applied to modulate its function (Fig. 3.1) (Table 3.4).

Monoclonal antibodies (Mabs) against several T cell targets, including CD4, CD8, CD5, TcR, MHC class

Table 3.4 Strategies for selective manipulation of the immune system

T cells
Antibodies against
- Antigen receptors
- Surface molecules involved in activation
- Surface activation molecules

Vaccination
Inhibition of antigen presentation by MHC class II
- Antibodies
- Peptides

Inhibiting cell traffic

B cells
Manipulate the idiotype network
B cell-specific antibodies
Intravenous immunoglobulin

Cytokines
Cytokine inhibition/stimulation
- Antibodies
- Inhibitors

Administration

II, and IL-2R, have been tried in animal models of autoimmune rheumatic disease, including RA (Wofsy and Seaman 1987; Quagliata *et al.* 1993). Monoclonal antibodies against CD4 (Levitt *et al.* 1992), TCR (Chiocchia *et al.* 1990; Yoshino *et al.* 1991), and CD5, (Larsson *et al.* 1989) but not CD8 (Larsson *et al.* 1989; Levitt *et al.* 1992), were effective in preventing the development of arthritis and reducing severity of established disease.

Anti-lymphocyte monoclonal antibodies have potent immunosuppressive properties and are capable of inducing antigen-specific tolerance (Waldmann 1989); however, a broad spectrum of specificities may be required to induce disease control (Cobbold *et al.* 1992). Anti-CD4 Mabs are able to make activated T cells tolerant, and skin grafts can be achieved across a complete MHC incompatibility (Cobbold *et al.* 1992). Anti-CD4 Mabs alone are capable of inducing tolerance where there are small numbers of autoreactive T cells, but anti-CD8 Mabs are required in addition when there is a greater number of autoreactive T cells. Early experiments used depleting Mabs; however, it is possible that non-depleting agents may be more effective. The precise mechanism of tolerance induction by Mabs is unknown. So far these impressive effects have not been successfully translated into the clinic, suggesting that the objective of inducing immunological tolerance has not yet been achieved (see below). It is not clear why this is so. Studies on synovial fluid and tissue during anti-CD4 Mab treatment have shown a dose-dependent reduction in the number of synovial T cells (Tak *et al.* 1995) suggesting that a better clinical response might have been obtained had higher doses of Mab been used. However, in mice, tolerance can be induced with non-depleting $F(ab')_2$ fragments of anti-CD4 Mab and, furthermore, anti-CD4- Mab-induced tolerance in murine diabetes could be broken by lymphocyte depletion using cyclophosphamide (Parish *et al.* 1993). Thus, higher doses of non-depleting antibodies may be more effective.

The ability of a Mab to deplete depends on a number of factors, including the Mab isotype and the antigen and epitope bound (Bruggeman *et al.* 1987; Bindon *et al.* 1988). The chimeric anti-CD4, Mab cM-T412, has a human IgG1 isotype and this agent produces prolonged CD4 lymphopaenia, whereas a humanized IgG1 anti-CD4 Mab is minimally depleting: this difference must relate to antigen factors such as epitope specificity or affinity (Isaacs *et al.* 1997). It is not possible to predict *in vivo* activity from *in vitro* properties in humans or animals since a human IgG4

Mab had significant depleting activity *in vivo*, which was not predicted by standard *in vitro* tests (Isaacs *et al.* 1996).

The early Mabs used in autoimmune disease were all of rodent origin. However, these generally proved to be immunogenic, with development of human anti-rodent antibodies (Isaacs and Waldmann 1994). This does not necessarily prevent repeated infusions but these may be less effective and potentially dangerous. To reduce immunogenicity, chimeric, primatized, and humanized antibodies have been constructed. Chimeric (rodent variable region in association with a human constant region), primatized (macaque variable and human constant region), or fully humanized antibodies, in which the complementarity-determining regions are all that remain of the 'parent' rodent Mab are shown in Fig. 3.3. The aim of these manipulations is to reduce immunogenicity by minimizing the non-human component of the antibody and also to improve the effector function (Riechmann *et al.* 1988). While anti-allotype and anti-idiotype responses are still possible, chimeric and humanized antibodies as predicted, appear, to be less immunogenic than either rodent or chimeric antibodies, probably through reducing the probability of T cell epitopes within the Mab framework (Isaacs and Waldmann 1994).

Depletion of circulating T cells with both chimeric and humanized Mabs can be profound and prolonged, lasting for several years. A single intravenous infusion of CAMPATH-1H (a humanized Mab directed against the glycoprotein CD52) results in a rapid fall in peripheral blood lymphocytes in all patients, with a nadir occurring within a few hours. The suppression of circu-lating lymphocytes lasts for at least 32 months after multiple intravenous infusions (Watts *et al.* 1994). CD8+ T cells appear to return to the peripheral circulation more quickly than do CD4+ T cells. Peripheral blood B cell (CD19+) numbers approach baseline values by 60 days after treatment.

The mechanism for this depletion of circulating lymphocytes is unknown but suggested explanations include trapping of antibody-coated cells in the phagocytic mononuclear system. Of note is that even with long-lasting lymphocyte depletion, there does not appear to be a significant increase in infections or, at present, malignancy. Clinical trial of non-depleting Mabs, which induce blockade or cellular stasis, may be of value.

Several Mabs cause a first dose reaction with fever, rigors, and rash. First dose reactions reflect the systemic release of cytokines (TNF-α, IL-6, and IFN-γ) (Moreau *et al.* 1996). This is likely to be due to cross-linking of target and effector cells via a-Mab/Fc receptor rather than via complement activation. First dose responses still occur with a humanized antibody of IgG4 isotype (Isaacs *et al.* 1996). It may prove possible to alleviate some of these symptoms by the use of TNF-α antagonists.

Manipulation via T cell receptor and MHC

T cell vaccination

Vaccination against autoimmunity is the holy grail of immunotherapy. To date several forms of vaccination have been attempted in both animal models and

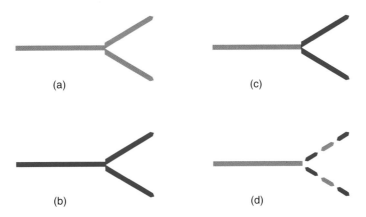

Fig. 3.3. Construction of humanized and chimeric monoclonal antibodies: (a) human antibody; (b) rodent antibody; (c) chimeric antibody — human Fc with rodent variable region; (d) humanized antibody — human Fc and variable framework region, rodent variable region.

clinical trials. T cells that induce adjuvant arthritis on transfer to naive recipients, can be chemically modified and used as a vaccine to prevent or treat adjuvant arthritis. The therapeutic benefit is thought mainly to be due to generation of regulatory T cells that recognize the unique protein sequence of the T cell receptor on disease-causing T cells. Vaccination with activated T cells also leads to generation of regulatory T cells that recognize and suppress activated T cells.

Autologous T cell vaccination using attenuated lymphocytes has been used by three groups in RA. The assumption is that pathogenic T cells being activated have a survival advantage when expanded *in vitro*. This approach has not so far produced significant clinical improvements (Lohse *et al.* 1993; van Laar *et al.* 1993).

Receptors on T cells specific for inducing autoantigen express a conserved number of variable region determinants. The majority of T cells express the α/β form of the TCR on their surface. TCR vaccination may induce tolerance, depletion, suppression, or inactivation of autoreactive TCR. In both collagen- and adjuvant-induced arthritis in animals, vaccination against antigen-specific T cells is effective in preventing arthritis. Unfortunately, in humans, specific disease-associated autoreactive T cells have not yet been identified.

The TCR has been investigated extensively in human autoimmune disease. Several groups have reported specific patterns of TCR Vα or Vβ usage in synovial fluid or tissue. So far no consensus has been reached, although there is some evidence in RA of restriction to Vβ14 and Vβ17 (Howell *et al.* 1991; Zagon *et al.* 1994).

Despite the fact that no clear disease-associated target on T cells has been identified, TCR peptide vaccination in RA has been studied in phase 1 trials using recombinant Vβ14 and Vβ17 in Freund's incomplete adjuvant, the trial of Vβ17 showed some evidence of clinical improvement (Moreland *et al.* 1996). A placebo-controlled trial of a combination of Vβ3, Vβ14, and Vβ17 is underway.

Mucosal tolerance

Oral tolerance is the reduction in systemic immune response following oral administration of antigen. Disease-inducing T cells are of the Th1 phenotype secreting IL-2 and IFN-γ, and these promote immune-mediated tissue damage. A shift from the Th1 to the Th2 phenotype, with production of IL-4 and IL-10, can result in protection from disease. The target antigen of an autoimmune disease can be used to induce such a shift (Weiner *et al.* 1994; Wraith 1996). Protection from disease was associated with emergence of Th2 clones with the same antigen receptor as the pathogenic clones. Antigen presentation in mucosal tissue induces a T cell response that recognizes autoantigen at sites of inflammation. Oral collagen is effective at preventing induction of arthritis and suppressing established disease in collagen-induced arthritis (Nalger-Anderson *et al.* 1986) and rat adjuvant-induced arthritis (Zhang *et al.* 1990). In the collagen-induced model of arthritis, nasal administration of collagen induces a switch from Th1 to Th2 T cells and suppresses induction of arthritis (Staines *et al.* 1996). Disease could also be suppressed using the immmunodominant peptide.

Type II collagen has been chosen for use in humans because it is localized to hyaline cartilage, anti-collagen antibodies can be detected in some RA patients, and oral collagen modulates disease in animal models. In a randomized placebo-controlled trial of type II chicken collagen in 60 RA patients there was a reduction in disease activity in the treated group, but this was only of short duration (Trentham *et al.* 1993). A second study using bovine type II collagen showed no difference between placebo and the treated group (Sieper *et al.* 1996).

MHC antagonists

Modulation of class II MHC alleles has been tried in RA. Induction of autoimmune disease models can be prevented by administration of a competitor peptide for the relevant antigen, resulting in interference of the formation of the trimolecular complex of antigen–MHC–TCR (Adorini and Nagy 1990). Antibodies to MHC molecules will also block the trimolecular complex. Placenta-eluted gammaglobulins containing anti-MHC activity were used in an open study in 80 patients with RA, with some benefit (Combe *et al.* 1985). A murine anti-idiotypic antibody to HLA-DR4 caused clinical improvement in seven of nine RA patients treated (Quagliata *et al.* 1993). An HLA DR4/DR1 peptide vaccine has recently been tried in RA. This combination was chosen because of the strong association between RA and DR4 or DR1 in different ethnic groups (Pratt *et al.* 1995). The desired antibody response was mounted to a single intramuscular injection of the vaccine.

Adhesion molecules

Intracellular adhesion molecule-1 (ICAM-1, CD54) is expressed on many cell types, including monocytes and lymphocytes. Inhibition of ICAM-1 is attractive since this may block leucocytes migrating into inflammatory sites and also prevent T cell activation. In an open study, a murine anti-ICAM-1 Mab resulted in modest improvement in clinical status (Kavanaugh *et al.* 1997). During treatment a CD3+ and CD4+ lymphocytosis developed, together with a peripheral mononuclear cell increase in mRNA for IFN-γ (Schulze-Koops *et al.* 1995).

Monoclonal anti-CD18 (β_2-integrin) administered at the same as intra-articular antigen injection in rabbits reduces inflammatory exudate and synovitis (Jasin *et al.* 1992). Collagen-induced arthritis can be delayed by anti-CD44 Mab (Verdengh *et al.* 1995).

The interaction of B7 molecules on antigen presenting cells with CD28 or CTLA-4 antigens on T cells provides a second signal for T cell activation. Selective inhibition of the B7–CD28 or B7–CTLA4 interaction produces antigen-specific T cell unresponsiveness *in vitro* and suppresses immune function *in vivo*. In lupus prone mice (NZB/W$_{F1}$), treatment with a B7-binding protein, CTLA4–Ig, resulted in marked improvement, with prolongation of life and decreased autoantibody production (Finck *et al.* 1994).

Cytokines

The function of cytokines can be manipulated in several ways: (i) Mab directed against the cytokine itself, where binding inhibits interaction of cytokine with its receptor; (ii) soluble cytokine receptors bind to free cytokine and also inhibit interaction between cytokine and membrane-bound receptor; (iii) cytokine receptor antagonists, which compete with cytokine for binding to receptor but fail to activate it; and (iv) administration of cytokines antagonistic to target cytokines. These approaches have been used in animals and in clinical trials, mainly in RA.

Interleukin-1 receptor antagonist

Interleukin-1 receptor antagonist (IL-1Ra) is a naturally occurring inhibitor of IL-1; it blocks binding of IL-1 to its receptor but does not possess agonist activity. A large excess of IL-1Ra over IL-1 is required to block cell function. Recombinant IL-1Ra has been used in a double-blind, placebo-controlled trial in RA with encouraging results; there was a significant reduction in disease activity and a reduction in the rate of erosion (Bresnihan *et al.* 1996).

Soluble interleukin-I receptor

The extracellular part of the IL-1 receptor is shed to form soluble IL-1 receptor (sIL-1R). sIL-1R binds specifically to IL-1 and prevents binding of IL-1 to the cell surface receptor. Administration of sIL-1R in RA has not so far shown any significant clinical benefit.

Monoclonal antibodies against TNF-α

Chimeric and humanized Mabs against TNF-α have been used in both open and controlled trials in RA with encouraging results. Retreatment may be effective but development of antibodies against the rodent component may limit the length of the response. Encouraging results have also been obtained with a TNF-α Mab plus methotrexate combination (Maini *et al.* 1998). Several patients developed autoantibodies against cell nuclei and DNA (Elliot *et al.* 1994; Rankin *et al.* 1995). In addition, at least one patient has subsequently developed clinical features typical of SLE (M. Feldmann, personal communication). It is tempting to speculate that this form of Mab therapy may, through some unknown mechanism, be upregulating IL-10, a potent inducer of anti-DNA antibodies.

Immunoadhesins

The use of monoclonal antibodies to treat human autoimmune disease is limited by a number of factors, including immunogenicity, despite the use of humanized Mab. One approach to these difficulties is the construction of immunoadhesins. Immunoadhesins are fusion proteins between the extracellular portions of cell surface molecules and the immunoglobulin constant region. The extracellular component provides for binding to the natural ligand, while the Fc prolongs half-life, permits dimerization, increases avidity, and provides for other effector functions. Immunoadhesins are relatively easy to design and construct providing the DNA sequence of the receptor is known.

In humans TNFR–Ig has shown clinical benefit in a double-blind, placebo-controlled trial (Baumgartner *et al.* 1996; Moreland *et al.* 1997). The efficacy was dose related and antibodies to the agent were not detected. Combinations of p75TNFR–Ig and anti-CD4 Mab have been successfully tried in collagen-induced arthritis (Williams *et al.* 1995) and are being tried in humans.

Manipulation of the idiotypic network

Manipulation of the idiotypic network has been proposed as a novel method of therapy for autoimmune disease (for review see Zouali *et al.* 1996). There are several possible methods by which the idiotype network might be manipulated: (i) direct injection of a common idiotype, with formation of anti-idiotype and downregulation of pathogenic (e.g. DNA) antibodies); (ii) injection of anti-idiotype, with the anti-idiotype directly downregulating anti-DNA antibodies; (iii) injection of anti-idiotype conjugated to a cytotoxic agent whereby the anti-idiotype targets antibody-producing cells and the toxin destroys them; and (iv) passage of plasma over an anti-idiotype column which removes antibodies bearing the common idiotype. In lupus-prone mice, anti-idiotype administration suppresses both anti-DNA antibody production and nephritis. The effect was transient and antibodies appeared that did not bear the idiotype (Hahn and Ebling 1983). Conjugation to a cytotoxic agent eliminates anti-DNA-producing cells *in vivo* (Sasaki *et al.* 1986). In humans, removal of specific idiotype-bearing DNA antibodies using an anti-idiotype immunoadsorbent column has been possible without significant toxicity (Macleod *et al.* 1988).

Gene therapy

Gene therapy refers to any technique that regulates a genetic product that may be involved in a disease process. More specifically this can mean the replacement or missing or defective genes or the introduction of regulatory gene sequences. Numerous techniques may be employed to achieve these outcomes including antisense and ribozyme-based strategies, retroviral delivery systems, *ex vivo* cellular manipulation and naked DNA and genetic immunization. This aspect of molecular medicine is a fast moving and very exciting growth area and full review of these technologies is beyond the scope of this chapter and we refer readers to some of the excellent synoptic overviews currently available (Anderson 1998; Mathiesen and Tuohy 1998; Romano *et al.* 1998; Yanez and Porter 1998). The autoimmune rheumatic diseases are a group of disorders which may benefit greatly from this technology and several novel therapeutic strategies have been suggested (Chernajovsky *et al.* 1998; Evans *et al.* 1998) and experimental and clinical outcomes are awaited with much interest. In several animal models *ex vivo* gene transfer has been used to obtain local sustained production of human IL-1Rα in the knee. In collagen-induced arthritis not only the injected knee, but also the contralateral knee also improved (Bakker *et al.* 1997).

Stem cell transplantation

Autologous haemopoietic stem cell transplantation (AHSCT) following bone marrow ablation has been used to treat isolated cases of severe treatment resistant autoimmune disease. Allogenic bone marrow transplantation can cure a variety of autoimmune diseases in experimental animal models (reviewed in Marmont 1997) and interest is developing for clinical trials, particularly in RA (Wicks *et al.* 1997) and systemic sclerosis (Tyndall *et al.* 1997).

Summary

The development of novel therapies for autoimmune disease is rapid and several diverse technologies have been introduced. It is to be hoped that some of these new treatments will prove successful in the clinic, but there is still a long way to go before curative treatments are routinely available.

References

Abdou NI, Zweimann B, Casella SR. The effects of azathioprine therapy on bone marrow dependent and thymus dependent cells in man. *Clin Exp Immunol* 1973; **13**: 55–64.

Adorini L, Nagy ZA. Peptide competition for antigen presentation. *Immunol Today* 1990; **11**: 21–4.

Anderson WF. Human gene theapy. *Nature* 1998; **392**(Suppl): 25–30.

Baker GL, Kahl LE, Zee BC *et al.* Malignancy following the treatment of rheumatoid arthritis with cyclophosphamide. Long term case control study. *Am J Med* 1987; **83**: 1–9.

Bakker AC, Joosten LAB, Arntz OJ *et al.* Prevention of murine collagen induced arthritis in the knee and ipsilateral paw by local expression of human interleukin-1 receptor antagonist protein in the knee. *Arthritis Rheum* 1997; **40**: 893–900.

Bartlett RR, Anagnosopulos H, Zielinski T *et al.* Effects of leflunamide on immune responses and models of inflammation. *Springer Semin Immunopathol* 1993; **14**: 381–94.

Bast RC Jr, Reinerz EL, Maver *et al.* Contrasting effects of cyclophosphamide and prednisolone on the phenotype of human peripheral blood lymphocytes. *Clin Immunol Immunopathol* 1983; **28**: 101–14.

Baumgartner S, Moreland LW, Schiff H *et al*. Double-blind, placebo-controlled trial of tumour necrosis factor receptor (p80) fusion protein (TNFR:Fc) in active rheumatoid arthritis. *Arthritis Rheum* 1996; **39**: 574–9.

Bindon CI, Hale G, Waldmann H. Importance of antigen specificity for complement mediated lysis by monoclonal antibodies. *Eur J Immunol* 1988; **18**: 1507–14.

Boumpas DT, Austin HA, Vaughan EM *et al*. Risk of sustained amenorrhoea in patients with SLE receiving intermittent pulse cyclophosphamide. *Ann Intern Med* 1993a; **119**: 366–9.

Boumpas DT, Chrousos GP, Wilder RL *et al*. Glucocorticoid therapy in immune mediated diseases — basic and clinical correlates. *Ann Intern Med* 1993b; **119**: 1198–208.

Bradley JD, Brandt KD, Katz BP. Infectious complications of cyclophosphamide therapy for vasculitis. *Arthritis Rheum* 1989; **32**: 45–53.

Bresnihan B, on behalf of the collaborating investigators, *et al*. Treatment with recombinant human interleukin-1 receptor antagonist (rhu-1ra) in rheumatoid arthritis: results of a randomised double blind placebo controlled multicenter trial. *Arthritis Rheum* 1996; **39**(Suppl.); S73.

Bruggeman M, Williams GT, Bindon CI *et al*. Comparison of the effector functions human immunoglobulins using a matched set of chimeric antibodies. *J Exp Med* 1987; **166**: 1351–6.

Caccavo D, Lagana B, Mitterhofer AP *et al*. Long-term treatment of systemic lupus erythematosus with cyclosporin A. *Arthritis Rheum* 1997; **40**: 27–35.

Chernajovsky Y, Annenkov A, Herman C, *et al*. Gene therapy for rheumatoid arthritis. Theoretical considerations. *Drugs Aging* 1998; **12**: 29–41.

Chiocchia G, Boissier MC and Fournier C. Therapy against murine collagen induced arthritis with T cell V beta-specific antibodies. *Eur J Immunol* 1990; **21**: 2899–905.

Clarkson SB, Bussel JB, Kimberly RP *et al*. Treatment of refractory immune thrombocytopaenia with an anti-Fc-gamma receptor antibody. *N Eng J Med* 1986; **314**: 1236–42.

Cobbold SP, Qin S, Leong LYW, Martin G, Waldmann H. Reprogramming the immune system for peripheral tolerance with CD4 and CD8 monoclonal antibodies. *Immunol Rev* 1992; **129**: 165–201.

Combe B, Cosso B, Bonneau M *et al*. Human placenta-eluted gammaglobulins in immunomodulating treatment of rheumatoid arthritis. *Am J Med* 1985; **78**: 920–8.

Cronstein BN. Methotrexate and its mechanism of action. *Arthritis Rheum* 1996; **39**: 1951–60.

Duddridge M, Powell RJ. The treatment of severe and difficult cases of systemic lupus erythematosus with tacrolimus — a report of three cases. *Ann Rheum Dis* 1997; **56**: 690–2.

Dwyer JM. Manipulating the immune system with immune globulin. *N Eng J Med* 1992; **326**: 107–16.

Elliot MJ, Maini RN, Feldmann M *et al*. Randomised double blind comparison of chimeric monoclonal antibody to tumour necrosis factor α (cA2) versus placebo in rheumatoid arthritis. *Lancet* 1994; **344**: 1104–10.

Evans CH, Whalen JD, Ghivizzani SC, Robbins PD. Gene therapy in autoimmune diseases. *Ann Rheum Dis* 1998; **57**: 125–7.

Fauci AS, Haynes BF, Katz P, Wolff SM. Wegener's granulomatosis: prospective clinical and therapeutic experience with 85 patients for 21 years. *Ann Intern Med* 1983; **98**: 76–85.

Feldmann M, Brennan FM, Maini RN. Rheumatoid arthritis. *Cell* 1996; **85**: 307–10.

Finck BK, Linsley PS, Wofsy D. Treatment of murine lupus with CTL4Ig. *Science* 1994; **265**: 1225–7.

Goldblum R. Therapy of rheumatoid arthritis with mycophenolate mofetil. *Clin Exp Rheum* 1993; **11**(Suppl. 8): S117–19.

Hahn B, Ebling F. Suppression of NZB/NZW murine nephritis by administration of a syngeneic monoclonal antibody to DNA: possible role of anti-idiotypic antibodies. *J Clin Invest* 1983; **71**: 728–36.

Herold KC, Lancki DW, Moldwin RL *et al*. Immunosuppressive effects of cyclosporin A on cloned T cells. *J Immunol* 1986; **136**: 1315–21.

Howell MD, Diveley JP, Lundeen KA *et al*. Limited T cell receptor β-chain heterogeneity among interleukin 2 receptor-positive synovial T cells suggests a role for superantigen in rheumatoid arthritis. *Proc Natl Acad Sci USA* 1991; **88**: 10921–5.

Imbach P, Barandun S, d'Apuzzo V *et al*. High dose intravenous immunoglobulin for idiopathic thrombocytopaenia in childhood. *Lancet* 1981; **ii**: 1228–32.

Isaacs JD, Waldmann H. Helplessness as a strategy for avoiding antiglobulin responses to therapeutic antibodies. *Ther Immunol* 1994; **1**: 303–12.

Isaacs JD, Wing M, Greenwood JD *et al*. A therapeutic human IgG4 monoclonal antibody that depletes target cells in humans. *Clin Exp Immunol* 1996; **106**: 427–33.

Isaacs JD, Burrows N, Wing M *et al*. Humanised anti-CD4 monoclonal antibody therapy of autoimmune and inflammatory disease. *Clin Exp Immunol* 1997; **110**: 158–66.

Isenberg DA, Snaith ML, Morrow WJW *et al*. Cyclosporin A for the treatment of systemic lupus erythematosus. *Int J Immunopharmacol* 1981; **3**: 163–5.

Jasin HE, Lightfoot E, Davis LS *et al*. Amelioration of antigen induced arthritis in rabbits treated with monoclonal antibodies to leucocyte adhesion molecules. *Arthritis Rheum* 1992; **35**: 541–9.

Kavanaugh AF, Schulze-Koops H, Davis LS *et al*. Repeat treatment of rheumatoid arthritis patients with a murine anti-intracellular adhesion molecule-1 monoclonal antibody. *Arthritis Rheum* 1997; **40**: 849–53.

Larsson P, Holmdahl, R, Klareskog L. In vivo treatment with anti-CD8 and anti CD5 monoclonal antibodies alters induced tolerance in adjuvant induced arthritis. *J Cell Biochem* 1989; **40**: 49–56.

Leung DYM. Kawasaki syndrome: immunomodulatory benefit and potential toxin neutralisation by intravenous immuno globulin. *Clin Exp Immunol* 1996; **104**(Suppl. 1): 49–54.

Levitt NG, Fernandez-Madrid F, Wooley PH. Pristane induced arthritis in mice. IV. Immunotherapy with monoclonal antibodies against lymphocyte subsets. *J Rheumatol* 1992; **19**: 1342–7.

Levy J, Barnett EV, MacDonald NS *et al*. The effect of azathioprine on gammaglobulin synthesis in man. *J Clin Invest* 1972; **51**: 2233–8.

Lohse AW, Bakker NPM, Hermann E *et al*. Induction of an anti-vaccine response by T cell vaccination in non-human primates and humans. *J Autoimmun* 1993; **6**: 121–30.

Macleod B, Lewis E, Schnitzer T *et al*. Therapeutic immuno-adsorbtion of anti-native DNA in SLE, clinical studies with a device utilising monoclonal anti-idiotypic antibody. *Arthritis Rheum* 1988; **31**(Suppl.): 15.

McClure CE, Isenberg DA. Does plasma exchange have any part to play in the management of SLE? *Controversies in Rheumatology*, eds Isenberg DA, Tucker LB, Martin Dunitz, London 1997; 78–85.

Maini RN, Breeolveld FC, Kalden JR *et al*. Therapeutic efficacy of multiple intravenous infusion of anti-tumour necrosis factor *α* monoclonal antibody combined with low dose weekly methotrexate in rheumatoid arthritis. *Arthritis Rheum* 1998; **41**: 1552–63.

Marmont AM. Stem cell transplantation for severe auto-immune disorders, with special reference to rheumatic diseases. *J Rheum* 1997; **24**(Suppl. 48): 13–18.

Mathisen PM, Tuohy VK. Gene therapy in the treatment of autoimmune disease. *Immunol Today*; 1998; **19**: 103–5.

Miyahara H, Hotokebachi T, Arita C *et al*. Comparative studies of the effects of FK506 and cyclosporin A on passively transferred collagen induced arthritis in rats. *Clin Immunol Immunopathol* 1991; **60**: 278–88.

Mladenovic V, Domlijan Z, Rozman B *et al*. Safety and effect-iveness of leflunamide in the treatment of patients with active rheumatoid arthritis. *Arthritis Rheum* 1995; **38**: 1595–603.

Moreau T, Coles A, Wing M, *et al*. Transient increase in symptoms associated with cytokine release in patients with multiple sclerosis. *Brain* 1996; **119**: 225–37.

Moreland LW, Heck LW, Koopman WJ *et al*. V*β*17 T cell receptor peptide vaccination in rheumatoid arthritis: results of phase I dose escalation study. *J Rheumatol* 1996; **23**: 1353–62.

Moreland LW, Baumgartner SW, Schiff MH *et al*. Treatment of rheumatoid arthritis with a recombinant human tumour necrosis factor receptor (p75)-Fc fusion protein. *N Eng J Med* 1997; **337**: 141–7.

Mouthon L, Kaveri SV, Spalter SH *et al*. Mechanisms of action of intravenous immunoglobulin in immune-mediated diseases. *Clin Exp Immunol* 1996; **104**(Suppl. 1): 3–9.

Nalger-Anderson C, Bober LA, Robinson ME *et al*. Sup-pression of type II collagen induced arthritis by intragastric administration of soluble type II collagen. *Proc Natl Acad Sci USA* 1986; **83**: 7443–6.

Panayi GS, Tugwell P. An international consensus report: the use of cyclosporin A in rheumatoid arthritis. *Br J Rheumatol* 1993; **32**(Suppl. 1): 1–3.

Panayi GS, Lanchbury JS, Kingsley GH. The importance of the T cell in initiating and maintaining the chronic synovitis of rheumatoid arthritis. *Arthritis Rheum* 1992; **35**: 729–35.

Parish NM, Hutchings PR, Waldmann H *et al*. Tolerance to IDDM induced by CD4 antibodies in nonobese diabetic mice is reversed by cyclophosphamide. *Diabetes* 1993; **42**: 1601–5.

Pratt W, Heck L, Moreland LW *et al*. Safety and immuno-genicity of a single intramuscular injection of a synthetic HLA-DR4/1 peptide vaccine with alum adjuvant in rheuma-toid arthritis patients. *Arthritis Rheum* 1995; **38**(Suppl.); S281.

Quagliata F, Schenkelaars EJ, Ferrone S. Immunotherapeutic approach to rheumatoid arthritis with anti-idiotypic antibodies to HLA-DR4. *Israel J Med Sci* 1993; **29**: 154–9.

Rankin ECC, Choy EHS, Kassimos D *et al*. The therapeutic effects of an engineered human anti-tumour necrosis factor *α* antibody CDP571 in rheumatoid arthritis. *Br J Rheumatol* 1995; **34**: 334–42.

Riechmann L, Clark M, Waldmann H *et al*. Reshaping human antibodies for therapy. *Nature* 1988; **332**: 323–7.

Rodriguez F, Krayenbuhl JC, Harrison WB *et al*. Renal biopsy findings and follow-up of renal function in rheumatoid arthritis patients treated with Cyclosporin A. An update from the International Kidney Biopsy Registry. *Arthritis Rheum* 1996; **39**: 1491–8.

Romano G, Claudio PP, Kaiser HE, Giordano A. Recent advances, prospects and problems in designing new strate-gies for oligonucleotide and gene delivery in therapy. *In Vivo* 1998; **12**: 59–67.

Sasaki T, Muroyi T, Takai O *et al*. Selective elimination of anti-DNA antibody producing cells by antiidiotypic anti-body conjugated with neocarcinostatin. *J Clin Invest* 1986; **77**: 1382–6.

Schreider M, Bering T, Waldendorf H *et al*. Immunoadsorbent plasma perfusion in patients systemic lupus erythematosus. *J Rheumatol* 1990; **17**: 900–7.

Schroeder JO, Euler HH, Loffler H. Synchronization of plasmapheresis and pulse cyclophosphamide in severe systemic lupus erythematosus. *Ann Intern Med* 1987; **107**: 344–6.

Schulze-Koops H, Lipsky PE, Kavanaugh AF *et al*. Elevated levels of Th1 and Th0-like cytokine mRNA in peripheral circulation of patients with rheumatoid arthritis: modula-tion by treatment with anti-ICAM-1 correlates with clinical benefit. *J Immunol* 1995; **155**: 5029–37.

Sieper J, Kary S, Sörensen H *et al*. Oral type II collagen treat-ment in early rheumatoid arthritis: double-blind placebo-controlled trial randomised trial. *Arthritis Rheum* 1996; **39**: 41–52.

Sigal NH, Dumont FJ. Cyclosporin A, FK506, and rapamycin: pharmacologic probes of lymphocyte transduction. *Ann Rev Immunol* 1992; **10**: 519–60.

Spina CA. Azathioprine as an immune modulating drug: clinical applications. *Clinics Immunol Allergy* 1984; **4**: 415–46.

Staines NA, Harper N, Ward FJ *et al*. Mucosal tolerance and suppression of collagen-induced arthritis induced by nasal inhalation of synthetic peptide 184-198 of bovine type II collagen expressing a dominant T cell epitope. *Clin Exp Immunol* 1996; **103**: 368–75.

Suzuki N, Kaneko S, Ichino M *et al*. In vivo mechanisms for the inhibition of T lymphocyte activation by long term therapy with Tacrolimus (FK-506). *Arthritis Rheum* 1997; **40**: 1157–67.

Tak PP, van der Lubbe PA, Cauli A *et al*. Reduction of synovial inflammation after anti-CD4 monoclonal antibody treatment in rheumatoid arthritis. *Arthritis Rheum* 1995; **38**: 1457–65.

Trentham DE, Dynesius-Trentham RA, Orav EJ *et al*. Effects of oral administration of type II collagen on rheumatoid arthritis. *Science* 1993; **261**: 1669–70.

Tugwell P, Bombardier C, Gent M *et al*. Low-dose cyclo-sporin versus placebo in patients with rheumatoid arthritis. *Lancet* 1990; **335**: 1051–5.

Tugwell P, Pincus T, Yocum D *et al*. Combination therapy with cyclosporin and methotrexate in severe rheumatoid arthritis. *New Eng J Med* 1995; **333**: 137–41.

Turk JL, Parker D. The effect of cyclophosphamide on the immune system. *J Immunopharmacol* 1979; **1**: 127–37.

Tyndall A, Black C, Finke J *et al.* Treatment of systemic sclerosis with autologous haemopoetic stem cell transplantation. *Lancet* 1997; **349**: 254.

van Laar JM, Miltenburg AMM, Verdonk MJA *et al.* Effects of innoculation with attenuated autologous T cells in patients with rheumatoid arthritis. *J Autoimmun* 1993; **6**: 159–67.

Vane JR. Mechanism of action of NSAIDs. *Br J Rheumatol* 1996; **35**(Suppl. 1): 1–3.

Verdengh M, Holmdahl R, Tarkawski A. Administration of antibodies to hyaluron receptor (CD44) delays the start and ameliorates the severity of collagen II arthritis. *Scand J Immunol* 1995; **42**: 353–8.

Waldmann H. Manipulation of T cell responses with monoclonal antibodies. *Ann Rev Immunol* 1989; **7**: 407–44.

Watts RA, Isaacs JD, Hale G *et al.* Peripheral blood lymphocytes subsets after CAMPATH-1H therapy for RA — a 3 year follow up. *Arthritis Rheum* 1994; **37**(Suppl.): S338.

Weiner HL, Friedman A, Miller A *et al.* Oral tolerance: immunologic mechanisms and treatment of animal and human organ specific autoimmune diseases by oral administration of autoantigens. *Ann Rev Immunol* 1994; **12**: 809–37.

Wicks I, Cooley H, Szer J. Autologous haemopoetic stem cell transplantation. A possible cure for rheumatoid arthritis. *Arthritis Rheum* 1997; **40**: 1005–11.

Williams RO, Ghrayeb J, Feldmann M *et al.* Successful therapy of collagen induced arthritis with TNF receptor-IgG fusion protein and combination with anti-CD4. *Immunology* 1995; **84**: 433–9.

Wofsy D, Seaman WE. Reversal of advanced lupus in NZB/NZW F1 mice by treatment with monoclonal antibody to L3T4. *J Immunol* 1987; **138**: 3247–53.

Wojtulewski JA, Schattenkirchner M, Barcelo P *et al.* A six month double blind trial to compare the efficacy and safety of meloxicam 7.5 mg daily and naproxen 750 mg daily in patients with rheumatoid arthritis. *Br J Rheumatol* 1996; **35**(Suppl. 1): 22–8.

Wraith DC. Antigen specific immunotherapy of autoimmune disease. *Clin Exp Immunol* 1996; **103**: 349–52.

Yanez RJ, Porter AC. Therapeutic gene targeting. *Gene Ther* 1998; **5**: 149–59.

Yoshino S, Cleland LG, Mayrhofer G. Treatment of collagen-induced arthritis in rats with a monoclonal antibody against the alpha/beta T cell antigen receptor. *Arthritis Rheum* 1991; **34**: 1039–47.

Yu DT, Clements PJ, Peter JB *et al. Arthritis Rheum* 1974; **17**: 37–45.

Zagon G, Tumang JR, Li Y *et al.* Increased frequency of Vβ17-positive T cells in rheumatoid arthritis. *Arthritis Rheum* 1994; **37**: 1431–40.

Zhang ZJ, Lee CSY, Lider O. Suppression of adjuvant arthritis in Lewis rats by oral administration of type II collagen. *J Immunol* 1990; **145**: 2489–93.

Zouali M, Isenberg DA, Morrow WJW. Idiotype manipulation for autoimmune diseases: where are we going? *Autoimmunity* 1996; **24**: 55–63.

4 | *Systemic lupus erythematosus*

Introduction

Systemic lupus erythematosus (SLE) is a syndrome of multifactorial aetiology, characterized by widespread inflammation, most commonly affecting women during the child-bearing years. Virtually every organ and/or system of the body may be involved, although the skin and joints are the most frequently affected. The course of the disease is typically one of remissions and exacerbations. With good management this disease, which was once widely regarded as fatal, has a 10 year survival figure of approximately 90%.

SLE is characterized serologically by autoantibodies to DNA, RNA, other nuclear antigens, cytoplasmic, and cell surface antigens. The diversity of its clinical features is thus matched by an apparent diversity among the autoantibodies detectable in the serum. There are, in addition, a large number of other immunological abnormalities that have been described in patients with SLE.

The term lupus (from the Latin meaning wolf) has been used since medieval times to describe the erythemic ulcerations which can 'eat away' the face. The potential for systemic involvement of lupus has been realized for approximately 130 years. In the past 30 years there has been an enormous effort by both clinical and basic scientists to dissect and understand the complex array of immunological disturbances that culminate in the diverse clinical features that characterize the disease.

As will be discussed later, a variety of murine and other animal models of lupus exist, and these have been used extensively to pursue the immunogenetic and cellular abnormalities that are characteristic of human SLE.

Milestones in the history of SLE

460–370 BC Herpes esthiomenos of Hippocrates. Probably a synonym for SLE — according to Lusitanus (1510–1568 AD).

1230–1611 Rogerius (*c.* 1230), Paracelsus (1493–1541), Manardi (*c.* 1500), Sennert (1611) all credited with mentioning lupus in their writings.

1845 Hebra first likened the facial rash to a butterfly shape.

1852 Cazenave and Clausit used the term 'lupus érythémateux'.

1875 Hebra and Kaposi differentiated discoid lupus from the systemic or 'aggregated' form.

1895–1903 Sir William Osler, in a series of articles, comprehensively described many of the clinical features now recognized as complicating SLE. These included arthralgia, CNS involvement, nephritis, gastrointestinal crisis, endo- and pericarditis.

1898 Boeck discussed the possibility that tuberculosis was the cause of many cases of discoid lupus. This was the first of many attempts to link lupus to infectious diseases.

1924 Libman and Sacks described an endocarditis now recognized as a form of SLE.

1935 Baehr, Klemperer, and Schifrin reported structural changes in the glomeruli of lupus patients.

1941 Klemperer, Pollack, and Baehr coined the term 'diffuse connective tissue disorder'.

1948   Discovery of the LE cell test by Hargreaves, Richmond, and Marks.

1949   Thorn and colleagues used cortisone therapy.

1951   Page employed quinacrine (mepacrine), an antimalarial drug, to control lupus with dermal lesions.

1954   Dustan, Taylor, Corcoran, and Page observed that hydralazine could induce LE cells: probably the first report of drug-induced lupus.

1957–1958   Friou and colleagues described anti-nuclear antibodies in SLE sera.

1959   Bielschowsky, Helyer, and Howie derived the NZB mouse, the first murine model of lupus.

1969   Koffler and colleagues correlated immunofluorescent staining patterns of the glomeruli with degree of proteinuria.

1971   American Rheumatism Association published criteria for the classification of SLE (revised in 1982).

1980–1983   Schwartz, Stollar, and colleagues dissected the spectrum of autoantibody-producing cells in both autoimmune mice and humans with SLE: many of the cloned antibodies were found to have cross-reacting idiotypes.

1980–1990   Physicians at the National Institutes of Health, including Klippel, Plotz, and Steinberg, demonstrated the use of combinations of prednisolone and intravenous cyclophosphamide given as boluses for the treatment of severe, especially renal, disease.
Hughes, Harris, and colleagues identified the important clinical associations of anti-phospholipid antibodies.

1987–1993   Combined international efforts undertaken to compare and validate disease activity indices, e.g. BILAG, SLAM, SLEDAI.

1996   Systemic lupus international collaborating clinics (SLICC) agree a validated damage index for SLE.

Definition and classification

The American Rheumatism Association (now the American College of Rheumatology, ACR) initially published a classification criteria set in 1971 which was revised in 1982 (Tan *et al.* 1982). Strictly speaking the criteria are for classification of the disease rather than for use as a diagnostic tool, although in practice there is a blurring of this distinction. The 1982 revised criteria are set out in Table 4.1. The chameleon-like nature of lupus means that patients with the disease may present to a wide variety of specialists, including rheumatologists, dermatologists, neurologists, cardiologists, and respiratory physicians. Since a minority of lupus patients present with the classic butterfly rash, it is important for all physicians to consider lupus within the differential diagnosis of a wide variety of complaints. A broad overview of the cumulative percentage incidence of the features of systemic lupus in five large published studies is shown in Table 4.2.

Epidemiology and natural history

Lupus is found world-wide. It is, however much more common among black females in the UK, the West Indies, and the United States, although, curiously, it remains rare in Africa (Nived and Sturfelt 1997). Thus, in a recent study from Birmingham, UK (Johnson *et al.* 1995) prevalence rates of 36.2, 90.6, and 206 per 100 000 among women of Caucasian, Asian, and Afro-Caribbean origin, respectively, were recorded. This study did not record prevalence rates among Chinese women, but the figure is likely to be approximately 100 in a 100 000.

It is widely agreed that lupus is between 10 and 20 times more common in women than in men. The overwhelming majority of patients will develop their disease between the ages of 15 and 40 years. In recent years, however, it has been recognized that in 10–15% of patients, the disease will begin after the age of 50. In

Table 4.1   Criteria of the American Rheumatism Association for the classification of SLE (Tan *et al.* 1982)*

1. Malar rash
2. Discoid rash
3. Photosensitivity
4. Oral ulcers
5. Arthritis
6. Serositis
    (a) Pleuritis
    (b) Pericarditis
7. Renal disorder
    (a) Proteinuria > 0.5 g/24 h or 3+, persistently
    (b) Cellular casts
8. Neurological disorder
    (a) Seizures
    (b) Psychosis (having excluded other causes, e.g. drugs)
9. Haemolytic disorder
    (a) Haemolytic anaemia
    (b) Leucopaenia or < 4.0×10^9/l on two or more occasions
    (c) Lymphopaenia or < 1.5×10^9/l on two or more occasions
    (d) Thrombocytopaenia < 100×10^9/l
10. Immunological disorders
    (a) Positive LE cell
    (b) Raised anti-native DNA antibody binding
    (c) Anti-Sm antibody
    (d) False-positive serological test for syphilis, present for at least six months
11. Anti-nuclear antibody in raised titre

* '... a person shall be said to have SLE if four or more of the 11 criteria are present, serially or simultaneously, during any interval of observation.'

this subgroup the female to male ratio falls to around 4:1.

Although 40 years ago lupus was widely regarded as a serious and frequently fatal disease (the five year survival was thought to be around 50% only), there has been a marked improvement in the last 20 years. This is probably the consequence of greater awareness of the condition, greater ease of performing relevant autoantibody tests to make the diagnosis earlier, the more judicious use of steroids and other immunosuppressive drugs, and, undoubtedly, the widespread availability of dialysis and renal transplantation. It does, however, remain a disease with the potential to cause considerable morbidity and increased mortality.

Clinical features

Non-specific features

Severe fatigue, fever, anorexia, weight loss, and lymphadenopathy are well recognized features of lupus. In our own experience fatigue is frequently the symptom that troubles the patients most, not least because they find it so difficult to persuade friends, relatives, and

their general practitioner to believe them! Active lupus is often associated with high fevers. These may cause diagnostic confusion, not least because the disease itself as well as its treatment makes patients more susceptible to infection. A careful infection screen is therefore mandatory, but more often than not no cause other than the disease is to be found. For reasons that remain uncertain, the C reactive protein (CRP) level is usually normal in patients with active lupus, but is raised in the presence of concomitant infection. Anorexia and weight loss are commonly found in the presence of active disease and indeed, in some patients, may be very useful markers of disease activity. Lymphadenopathy is frequently evident and many lupus patients who present with this feature end up having lymph node biopsy to exclude the possibility of an underlying malignancy.

Musculoskeletal involvement

Arthralgia is present in about 90% of patients with lupus. It is usually polyarticular, symmetrical, episodic and may be flitting in nature. Patients' symptoms usually exceed the objective clinical findings, and synovial effusions are rather uncommon in lupus patients

Table 4.2 Cumulative prevalence of clinical features in patients with SLE

Feature	ACP*	Feature	ACP*
Musculoskeletal		Cerebral	
Arthralgia/arthritis	90	Depression	15
Tenosynovitis	20	Psychosis	15
Myalgia	50	Seizures	20
Myositis	5	Hemiplegia	10
Cardiopulmonary		Cranial nerve lesions	10
Shortness of breath	40	Cerebellar signs	5
Pleurisy	35	Meningitis	1
Pleural effusion	25	Migraine	40
Lupus pneumonitis	5	Haematological	
Interstitial fibrosis	5	Anaemia (iron deficiency)	30
Pulmonary function abnormalities	85	Anaemia (of chronic disease)	75
Cardiomegaly	20	Autoimmune haemolytic anaemia	15
Pericarditis	15	Leucopaenia	60
Cardiomyopathy	10	Lymphopaenia	60
Myocardial infarction	5	Thrombocytopaenia	25
Gastrointestinal		Circulating anticoagulants	15
Anorexia	40	Dermatological	
Nausea	15	Butterfly rash	40
Vomiting	< 10	Erythematous maculopapular eruption	35
Diarrhoea	< 10	Discoid lupus	20
Ascites	< 10	Relapsing nodular non-suppurative panniculitis	< 5
Abdominal pain	30		
Hepatomegaly	25	Vasculitic skin lesions	40
Splenomegaly	10	Livedo reticularis	20
Renal		Purpuric lesions	40
Haematuria	10	Alopecia	70
Proteinuria	60		
Casts	30		
Serum albumin < 35 g/l	30		
Serum creatinine > 125 μmol/l	30		
Reduced 24-hour creatinine clearance	35		

* ACP: approximate cumulative prevalence.

and of small volume when they do occur. Clinically overt arthritis, with deformities and/or bone erosions, is found in no more than 5% of the patients. However cystic bone lesions have been reported in approximately 40% of patients with lupus (Laasonen *et al.* 1990). In fact, tenosynovitis is more intense than intra-articular synovial membrane reaction, though ironically this may cause 'Swan-neck' deformities and ulnar deviation which superficially resemble the changes of rheumatoid arthritis. Marked deformities in the hands are generally known as Jaccoud's arthropathy (Fig. 4.1) which is generally, but not always, a reversible subluxation (Spronk *et al.* 1992).

When synovial fluid can be removed from a lupus patient's joint, a white cell count of less than 3000 per ml is present, in which mononuclear cells predominate. The fluid is occasionally positive for rheumatoid factor or anti-nuclear antibodies. Histologically the 'lupus

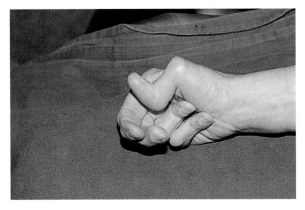

Fig. 4.1. Jaccoud arthropathy — a non-erosive condition, mimicking rheumatoid arthritis.

synovium' usually has minimal cellular inflammation, occasional haematoxylin bodies, and non-specific vasculitis and perivasculitis (Labowitz and Schumacher

1971). Electron microscopy may reveal cytoplasmic inclusions in vascular endothelial cells. Other less common musculoskeletal features include spontaneous tendon rupture (generally confined to the patella or Achilles tendons), subcutaneous nodules, calcinosis, chondritis, and avascular necrosis (Furie and Chartash 1988). The last of these features occurs in 5–10% of lupus patients, invariably associated with prior corticosteroid therapy and in many instances occurring at multiple sites.

Myalgia, muscle weakness, and tenderness have been reported in up to 60% of patients with lupus though true myositis is confined to about 5% of these patients (Isenberg *et al.* 1981). Treatment with corticosteroids and chloroquine may cause a myopathy, but in the main the myalgia experienced by patients seems to be a result of referred pain from adjacent joint involvement. Histologically, a vacuolar myopathy has been described in lupus. This is identified by the presence of plump, swollen sarcolemmal nuclei with other prominent vacuolated nuclei, centrally located within the muscle fibre. Immunoglobulin deposition is often seen in the muscles of patients with lupus (Isenberg 1983) but this is irrespective of whether they have clinically overt muscle disease and seems to relate more to minor fibre damage as a secondary event rather than to primary inflammatory myopathy.

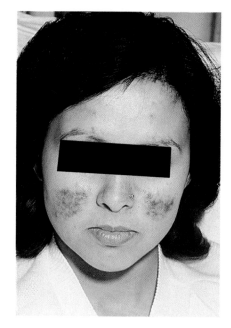

Fig. 4.2.   Malar rash — the 'classical' distribution in a patient with SLE.

Dermatological involvement

The classic butterfly rash found over the bridge of the nose and malar bones is actually present in only approximately one-third of patients with the disease (Fig. 4.2). However, dermatological abnormalities as a whole are present in up to 85% of lupus patients (Pistiner *et al.* 1991). In addition to maculopapular and discoid lesions, splinter haemorrhages, dilated capillaries at the nail base, bullous lesions, angioneurotic oedema and buckle, and nasal ulceration are all widely recognized. Vasculitic skin lesions are usually found at the finger tips or toes, or the extensor surface of the forearm. When they occur around the malleoli, they may lead to tender, deep leg ulcers which may take months to heal.

Many lupus rashes are exacerbated by ultraviolet light (and on occasion this exposure may lead to generalized flare of the disease) and thus sunbathing should be discouraged in patients with lupus, especially if no sunblocking agent has been applied. Not surprisingly, however, photosensitivity is more common among white females and even while driving with an arm exposed through an open window an adequate sunscreen should be used.

Alopecia is a common feature of lupus. It is often diffuse and non-scarring but psychologically may be upsetting to many patients. In contrast, severe scarring alopecia is quite uncommon but can be quite devastating when it does occur. Other dermatological features of lupus include hyperpigmentation and lupus panniculitis. The latter is a form of lipoatrophy which usually develops as a relapsing, nodular, non-suppurative lesion. A particular variant of systemic lupus known as subacute cutaneous lupus erythematosus is well recognized. The condition is associated with anti-Ro antibodies.

Immunoglobulin deposition at the dermal/epidermal junction has been recognized for over 30 years (Burnham *et al.* 1963). Immunoglobulins are usually of the IgG or IgM isotype (Fig. 4.3). Intriguingly, such deposition may be identified in lupus patients in the areas of skin that are not light exposed (e.g. the upper thighs and buttocks). This forms the basis of the so-called lupus band test. Complement components may also be found at this junction.

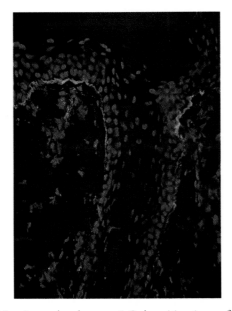

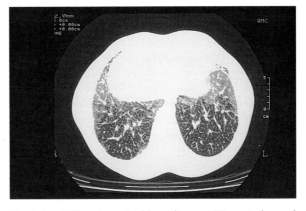

Fig. 4.4. Diffuse interstitial lung disease (CT scan) observed in a 24-year-old lupus patient with a one-year history of shortness of breath.

Fig. 4.3. Lupus band test — IgG deposition (green fluorescence) at the junction of the dermis and the epidermis, from a non-lesional skin biopsy.

Cardiovascular and pulmonary involvement

The most common feature of pulmonary disease is pain due to pleurisy, which affects approximately 40% of lupus patients at some time. This may be uni- or bilateral, and is often present at the costophrenic angles anteriorly or posteriorly. It may be associated with pleural effusions, which tend to be relatively small. The protein content of these effusions is generally greater than 3 gm/dl and they have a high mononuclear cell count with occasional anti-nuclear antibodies being present.

Parenchymal involvement owing to lupus has been reported in up to 18% of patients (Haupt *et al.* 1981). These patients had interstitial fibrosis, pulmonary vasculitis, and interstitial pneumonitis. However, these authors argued cogently that many pulmonary lesions such as alveolar haemorrhage, alveolar wall necrosis, and oedema are probably secondary to factors such as concomitant infection, congestive heart failure, and even oxygen toxicity. True lupus pneumonitis is rare (probably less than 2% of patients). Clinically symptomatic diffuse interstitial lung disease is also very uncommon (Fig. 4.4). Its manifestations resemble those found in patients with scleroderma and rheumatoid arthritis and tend to be of slow onset, with a chronic non-productive cough and shortness of breath.

In the past 10 years there has been a great interest in the links between thrombotic events and phospholipid antibodies. Perhaps as many as 10% of patients with lupus develop a thrombophlebitis and/or pulmonary embolus. Anti-phospholipid antibodies should certainly be sought in these patients and also in the small number who present with pulmonary hypertension. Also well recognized, though rare, among pulmonary lesions is the so-called 'shrinking lung syndrome' (Hoffbrand and Beck 1965). In these patients it is evident that diaphragmatic dysfunction is making a significant contribution.

Abnormal pulmonary function tests are present more frequently than clinical features suggest. In particular, diminished total lung volumes and flow rates have been reported, although these changes often appear to stabilize over time (Martens *et al.* 1983). Haemoptysis is, however, most unusual. Involvement of the heart in patients with lupus may take a variety of forms with disease affecting the pericardium, myocardium, and valves. A detailed review of the pleuropulmonary manifestations of SLE has been published recently (Orens *et al.* 1994).

Pericardium

Pericardial disease is the most common component of heart involvement. The frequency with which pathology is implied by various tests far outweighs the number of patients with clinically evident involvement. Pericardial rub is also more common than significant accumulations of pericardial fluid. Thus, Mandell (1987), in reviewing over 20 studies of pericardial involvement, concluded that whereas 29% of the patients have clinical evidence of cardiac disease, echocardiography revealed abnormalities in 37% and necropsy studies showed that 66% of patients have some pericardial involvement. Abnormalities of the electrocardiogram, notably the T waves, may be detectable in up to 75% of the patients. Studies of pericardial fluid have shown the presence of anti-nuclear antibodies, LE cells, and even hypocomplementaemia.

Large pericardial perfusions are uncommon in lupus and their presence suggests that there may be a complicating factor such as uraemia or concurrent infection. Histological abnormalities vary from occasional foci of fibrinoid degradation and inflammatory infiltrates to far more extensive lesions. Immune complex components have been found throughout the pericardial tissue even in areas that look normal histologically.

Myocardial disease

True myocardial involvement is less frequent than pericardial disease. Dubois and Tuffarelli (1964) reported such involvement in just 8% of 520 patients. However, as with pericardial disease, the results of investigations and necropsy studies suggest that involvement is more common than is suspected on clinical examination (Fig. 4.5). Clinical myocarditis, as defined by combinations of unexplained tachycardia, congestive heart failure, arrhythmias, prolongation of the PR interval on electrocardiography, or cardiomegaly without pericardial effusion, occurs in about 15% of patients with lupus.

Electrocardiographic studies have suggested that myocardial function can deteriorate reversibly in parallel with flares of generalized lupus activity. A link between corticosteroid therapy and an increase in atherosclerosis in these patients has been suggested. In their literature review, Doherty and Siegel (1985) studied the features of 33 patients with SLE reported to have had coronary artery disease under the age of 35. One-third of the patients had atherosclerosis.

Histological studies of the myocardium have indicated that mild, non-specific perivascular infiltration with lymphocytes and neutrophils is relativelycommon. Intimal proliferation of the smaller intramyocardial arteries is also reported fairly commonly, together with hyalinized vessels that may reflect either previous arthritis or primary thrombosis. The latter is of interest in view of its link to anti-phospholipid antibodies.

Valves

Conduction defects and rhythm disturbances are an occasional feature of lupus, and systolic murmurs have been recorded in up to 30% of the patients. In most cases this probably simply represents a hypodynamic circulation secondary to the chronic anaemia commonly found in patients with lupus. Diastolic murmurs are rather rare.

The classic endocarditis described by Libman and Sacks (1924), although identified in up to 50% of cases at autopsy, rarely causes significant lesions. Histologically small (1–4 cm) vegetations comprising proliferating degenerative valve tissue with fibrin and thrombi are seen. A recent prospective echocardiographic study of 132 consecutive patients with lupus reported a prevalence of 22.7% (Khamashta *et al.* 1990). These lesions were most commonly found at the edges of the mitral and aortic valves and were shown to contain immunoglobulin and complement components.

Bacterial endocarditis has been reported on a number of occasions in patients with lupus. It is probably a consequence of both the underlying immunopathology of the disease and the predisposition to infection induced by its therapy.

Gastrointestinal involvement

Abdominal pain occurs sporadically in up to 20% of patients. Because of its tendency to settle sponta-

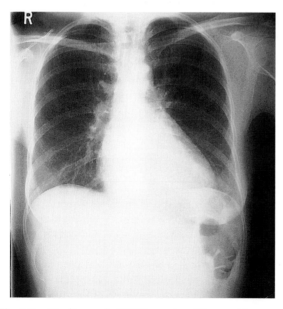

Fig. 4.5. Cardiomegaly (CXR) seen in a 36-year-old woman with lupus and significant mitral incompetence.

neously, its precise cause is rarely determined. Rare cases of ileal and colonic perforation and regional enteritis have been described. Pathologically necrotizing vasculitis may be found when perforation occurs. Ascites, dysphagia, pharyngitis, and oesophagitis are occasional accompaniments (Dubois and Tuffarelli 1964).

Hepatomegaly and/or persistent liver function test abnormalities are found in up to 10% of patients. The latter in many cases are due to concomitant drug therapy. A form of lupoid hepatitis was first distinguished by Mackay *et al.* (1959). Similarly, splenomegaly is present in approximately 10% of patients (Fishman and Isenberg 1997) but pancreatitis is even less common (Watts and Isenberg 1989).

Haematological abnormalities

A normochromic, normocytic anaemia is present in up to 70% of patients with lupus. The levels of ferritin in these patients are usually normal, however. There are a number of other factors that may contribute to the anaemia, including end stage renal disease and gastrointestinal blood loss owing to the prescription of non-steroidal anti-inflammatory drugs (NSAIDs). In addition, a Coombs positive haemolytic anaemia occurs in up to 10% of all patients. A rare association between pure red cell aplasia and systemic lupus has also been reported.

Leucopaenia (less than 4×10^9 white blood cells per litre) and lymphopaenia (less than 1.5×10^9 per litre) are the most frequent abnormalities of the white blood cell count in patients with lupus. Estimates have ranged from approximately 45–65% for the former and up to 80% for the latter. Both T and B cells are reduced. Lymphocytotoxic antibodies have been found in over one-third of patients with lupus. Leucocytosis is rare in lupus.

There are at least three types of thrombocytopaenia associated with lupus. Chronic thrombocytopaenia (platelet count less than 100×10^9/litre) has been reported in approximately 20% of several studies. This is hardly ever associated with bleeding disorders. Rarely, an acute thrombocytopaenia can occur in a matter of days during which the fall in platelet count may be both dramatic and life threatening. Finally, some patients present with what is initially diagnosed as idiopathic thrombocytopaenia, usually treated successfully with corticosteroids or splenectomy, who some years later go on to develop further manifestations of the disease. [A detailed overview of the haematological manifestations of lupus is reported elsewhere (Keeling and Isenberg 1993)].

Nervous system involvement

In perhaps no other system is the ability of lupus to mimic other diseases more evident. Virtually every feature of central nervous system disease, from migraine to madness, has been associated with lupus (reviewed in West 1994). Approximately 30% of lupus patients suffer from migraine (Isenberg *et al.* 1982), but of much greater concern are the *grand mal* seizures (fits) which may be an initial manifestation of lupus in perhaps 5% of patients, though as many of 20% may develop them in due course. Convulsions may be a manifestation of more general problems (Sibley *et al.* 1992). For example, they could be secondary to uraemia or other biochemical disturbances. Similarly, hemiplegia (stroke) may be consequent upon primary neurological involvement or secondary to hypertension associated with renal disease. Movement disorders in lupus, including chorea, hemiballismus, Parkinsonism, and blepharospasm are recognized but rare (Tam *et al.* 1995; Liang and Karlson 1996). A variety of syndromes with impaired temporal-spatial orientation, poor memory, and intellectual deficit are well recognized and are difficult to manage.

Anxiety and depression are common features of patients with lupus, though again these may be secondary, rather than primary effects (Shortall *et al.* 1995). On occasion, lupus may mimic mania or schizophrenia, though in the latter case a degree of insight is invariably retained that distinguishes the patients from schizophrenics. Far more common is the presence of cognitive deficit although estimates of its prevalence vary considerably, dependent in part upon the complexity and range of tests used to identify it (Hanley *et al.* 1993, Hay *et al.* 1994).

A recent report of suicides in patients with lupus serves to emphasize that depression must be taken very seriously in patients with systemic lupus (Matsukawa *et al.* 1994). Although investigations of CNS (central nervous system) disease, including CT (Kaell *et al.* 1986), MRI (Chinn *et al.* 1997), and SPECT (Griffey *et al.* 1990) scanning, all provide far greater non-invasive insight into the central nervous system, correlation with neuropsychological testing remains poor. Examination of the cerebrospinal fluid in lupus patients with neuropsychiatric disease may help to exclude infection but often adds little to management. Many patients show moderately raised cell counts and moderately increased protein and IgG levels.

Although corticosteroids were once believed to be a major cause of diagnostic confusion, the report of

Table 4.3   Potential antigenic targets in CNS lupus

Phospholipids ± β_2-glycoprotein-1
Glycolipids
Neurofilaments
Ribosomal P
50/52 kDa (lymphatic, synaptic)
97 kDa (neuronal)
GMP-140 (endothelial)
Limbic system/specific antigen

Feinglass *et al.* (1976) concluded that only two of 140 patients actually had a true steroid-induced psychosis.

Approximately 10% of patients with lupus develop a peripheral neuropathy in the course of their disease, which is usually sensory or, occasionally, sensorimotor. Cranial nerve involvement is less common and is usually associated with active systemic disease, manifested by visual defects, tinnitus, vertigo, nystagmus, ptosis, and facial palsies. Optical neuritis is also recognized though very uncommon. Transverse myelitis is similarly recognized but rare and is usually linked to the presence of anti-phospholipid antibodies (Hardie and Isenberg 1985).

Apart from the CSF (cerebrospinal fluid) examination there has been a great deal of interest in trying to associate autoantibodies with CNS disease. The list of potential target antigens is shown in Table 4.3. Of these antibodies, those binding the ribosomal P protein have been the focus of considerable interest. However, approximately 15% of Caucasians appear to have these antibodies (the figure is twice as high in Chinese/Malaysian populations studied) and, on balance, measuring these antibodies provides very little help to the clinician (Fox and Isenberg 1997).

Electroencephalographic studies may help to demonstrate focal change. Computerized tomography (CT) has been used to analyse patients with lupus for some 10 years. This form of scanning together with nuclear magnetic resonance imaging (MRI), is often used to investigate patients with central nervous system involvement. Too often, unfortunately, there is a disparity in the results obtained compared with the clinical features (Fig. 4.6).

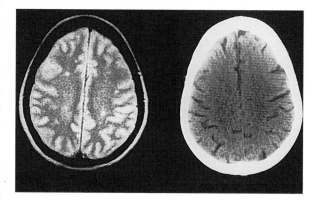

Fig. 4.6.   CNS involvement (CT/MRI). On the right a CT scan from a 40-year-old woman with severe organic depressive disease. The scan is normal, unlike the MRI scan on left which shows several areas of high signal, compatible with vasculitis.

Table 4.4   Major forms of renal lupus

World Health Organization classification	Deposits			Proliferation			
	Mesangial	Subendothelial	Subepithelial	Mesangial	Endocapillary	Extracapillary	Necrosis
Class I	–	–	–	–	–	–	–
Class IIA	+	–	–	–	–	–	–
Class IIB	+	–	–	+	–	–	–
Class III	++	+	±	+	+ Focal	+ Focal	+ Focal
Class IV Diffuse proliferative Membranoproliferative	++	++	+	++	++	+	+
Class V Pure membranous	–	–	+++	–	–	–	–
With II, III, IV	+	±	+++	+	±	±	±

Renal involvement

Until very recently, renal disease has been the most common cause of death in patients with lupus. Ironically, clinical symptoms directly owing to renal involvement, notably swelling of the ankles, shortness of breath, and 'frothy' urine, are not evident until substantial damage has been done to the kidneys. It is thus mandatory that careful monitoring of the urine for protein and red cells and casts, checking the blood pressure for hypertension, and the plasma for raised creatinine and urea levels is performed regularly. The World Health Organization (WHO) has subdivided renal lupus into five major categories based on renal biopsy results (see Table 4.4 and Fig. 4.7). In addition, end-stage renal disease with completely sclerosed glomeruli may occur but kidneys with this appearance are essentially non-functional. It is our practice to use disease activity and damage scores when reporting renal biopsy results. Although some authorities (e.g. Schwartz *et al.* 1992) doubt the value of pathology

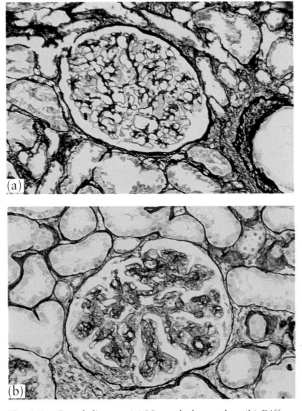

Fig. 4.7. Renal disease. (a) Normal glomerulus. (b) Diffuse proliferative glomerulonephritis.

indices, most reports indicate that they are of use (McLaughlin *et al.* 1991) and supplement the ability of clinicians to predict outcome in lupus nephritis (Esdaile *et al.* 1992). Thus, patients with a high activity index but low damage score should be treated aggressively with immunosuppressive therapy, but a patient with a low activity index and a high damage score does not require immunosuppressive therapy — there is nothing left to treat.

Although these kinds of assessments are useful and do have therapeutic implications, it must be remembered that renal biopsy appearances may not be uniform and may well change with time. In addition, the WHO score does not consider tubular interstitial disease, nor does it recognize the recently described overlap of lupus nephritis and the multiple small thrombi associated with anti-phospholipid antibodies.

The role of renal biopsy in the management of lupus nephritis

About 30% of lupus patients overall will develop significant renal disease. It is thus not justified to biopsy every patient with lupus — the biopsy procedure is not without side effects, including major blood loss. It is most important to assess the clotting capability of the patient before performing the biopsy. We recommend that patients with lupus who have anything more than trivial and transient proteinuria or haematuria and those with diminished glomerular filtration rates should seriously be considered for renal biopsy. The opinion of a pathologist with experience in assessing kidney biopsies from lupus patients is strongly advised.

Overall clinical assessment

In order to reflect the totality of the effects of any disease upon a patient, it is necessary to distinguish disease activity (clinical features that are essentially reversible) from damage (irreversible features). In addition, an understanding of the disease from the patient's perspective is also important. This final point was emphasized in a study of 100 patients with lupus who were asked to list the clinical features of the disease that troubled them the most. Instead of the anticipated fear of death or facial disfigurement, severe fatigue was by far the most common complaint (D.A. Isenberg, personal observations). In the past 10 years there have been major developments in the establishment of disease activity indices. Several reliable and validated

Table 4.5   Demonstration of the use of the BILAG disease activity index a study of patient AC

Date	Organ/System							
	General	Mucocutaneous	CNS	Musculoskeletal	CVS/Resp.	Vasculitis	Renal	Haematological
10 January 1997	C	D	E	C	D	D	D	C
30 January 1997	A	D	E	A	D	D	B	B
20 February 1997	B	D	E	B	D	D	B	B
20 March 1997	C	D	E	B	D	D	C	C
17 April 1997	C	D	E	B	D	D	C	C

A = 'active', the most active disease state requiring major immunosuppressive drugs; B = 'beware', patient is known to have active disease but is already on immunosuppressive therapy; C = 'contentment', patient has relatively mild disease controlled by little specific therapy if any; D = 'discount', there is no activity in this system now; E = no 'evidence' of activity in this system now or previously.

global activity scores have been developed, including the SLAM (systemic lupus activity measures) (Liang *et al.* 1988) and SLEDAI (systemic lupus erythematosus disease activity index) (Bombardier *et al.* 1992). While robust and easy to use, these instruments remain relatively blunt tools and to provide a more detailed analysis distinguishing activity in eight organs or systems, the BILAG (British Isles Lupus Assessment Group) (Hay *et al.* 1993) index provides a more comprehensive approach based on the principle of the physician's intention to treat. It provides an accurate means of grading disease activity from the most active (grade A, requiring major immunosuppression) to grade E (no evidence of disease activity currently or previously in an organ or system). Thus at a glance (see Table 4.5) it can be discerned not only that a lupus patient is flaring but also in which particular system and over what period of time. The utility of this approach was perhaps best shown by Ehrenstein and colleagues (1994), who showed that the levels of a DNA antibody idiotype (B3Id) did not correlate with disease activity overall but was very closely associated with disease activity in the musculoskeletal system. For the purposes of comparison, the BILAG system can be converted into a global score (A grade = 9 points, B = 3, C = 1, D and E = 0) and the value of international clinical collaboration has perhaps never been better demonstrated than in a long series of studies over the past decade that has shown strong correlations between a BILAG global score and SLAM and SLEDAI scores. Furthermore, the Systemic Lupus International Collaborating Clinics group (SLICC) has also collectively devised a damage score for lupus that has been recognised by the American College of Rheumatology (Gladman *et al.* 1997). The details of this index are shown in Table 4.6. This has now been used in a

variety of studies and appears to have gained international recognition.

Several health assessment questionnaires have been utilized in the study of patients with lupus. John Ware and colleagues from the Rand Corporation developed a series of questionnaires designed to measure health attributes, using multi-item scales that are scored using a method of summated ratings (Ware *et al.* 1980). This method is based on certain scaling assumptions that can be tested. A considerable amount of research has been undertaken in this area to try to determine the reliability and validity. Starting from a questionnaire that incorporated over 200 different questions, the so-called 'short form' (SF-20) was developed and used in a number of studies. However it was felt that the SF-20 was failing to capture certain important problems (e.g. by not asking explicitly about limitations owing to emotional problems, the SF-20 may not distinguish role limitation owing to physical health or mental problems) and the slightly longer SF-36 is generally regarded as preferable. The SF-36 includes multi-item scales, measuring eight different health concepts. In addition, the SF-36 includes a further general health rating item that asks respondents to indicate a change in their health over a one-year period. This item is not used to score any of the eight multi-item scales, however. In a cross-sectional study of 150 lupus patients (Stoll *et al.* 1997a), it has been shown that the SF-36 domains were internally consistent and significant associations of the SF-36 domains with the corresponding SF-20+ sections (this is the SF-20 questionnaire together with a particular question relating to fatigue) were found. Although the SF-20+ is a little shorter, the SF-36 is to be preferred because of its broader scale of questions and its widespread acceptance. In a separate study Stoll *et al.* (1997b) demon-

Table 4.6 The Systemic Lupus International Collaborating Clinics/American College of Rheumatology damage index

Systemic Lupus International Collaborating Clinics

Patient name: Study no:

Assessment date: /   /

Damage occurring since diagnosis of lupus ascertained by clinical assessment and present for at least 6 months unless otherwise stated. Repeat episodes mean at least 6 months apart to score 2. The same lesion cannot be scored twice.

Item	Score (circle)		
OCULAR (Either eye by clinical assessment)			
Any cataract ever	0	1	
Retinal change or optic atrophy	0	1	
NEUROPSYCHIATRIC			
Cognitive impairment (e.g. memory deficit, difficulty with calculation, poor concentration, difficulty in spoken or written language, impaired performance level)			
OR major psychosis	0	1	
Seizures requiring therapy for 6 months	0	1	
Cerebral vascular accident ever (score 2 if > 1) resection not for malignancy	0	1	2
Cranial or peripheral neuropathy (excluding optic)	0	1	
Transverse myelitis	0	1	
RENAL			
Estimated or measured GFR < 50%	0	1	
Proteinuria 24 h > 3.5 g	0	1	
OR			
End-stage renal disease (regardless of dialysis or transplantation)	3		
PULMONARY			
Pulmonary hypertension (right ventricular prominence or loud P2)	0	1	
Pulmonary fibrosis (physical and X-ray)	0	1	
Shrinking lung (X-ray)	0	1	
Pleural fibrosis (X-ray)	0	1	
Pulmonary infarction (X-ray) or resection not for malignancy	0	1	
CARDIOVASCULAR			
Angina OR coronary artery bypass	0	1	
Myocardial infarction ever (score 2 if < 1)	0	1	2
Cardiomyopathy (ventricular dysfunction)	0	1	
Valvular disease (diastolic murmur or a systemic murmur > 3/6)	0	1	
Pericarditis × 6 months or pericardectomy	0	1	
PERIPHERAL VASCULAR			
Claudication × 6 months	0	1	
Minor tissue loss (pulp space)	0	1	
Significant tissue loss ever [e.g. loss of digit or limb, resection (Score 2 if > 1)]	0	1	2
Venous thrombosis with swelling ulceration or venous stasis	0	1	
GASTROINTESTINAL			
Infarction or resection of bowel [below duodenum, spleen, liver or gall bladder ever (Score 2 if > 1)]	0	1	2
Mesenteric insufficiency	0	1	
Chronic peritonitis	0	1	
Stricture or upper gastrointestical tract surgery ever	0	1	
Pancreatic insufficiency requiring enzyme replacement or with pseudocyst	0	1	

Table 4.6   *Continued*

MUSCULOSKELETAL			
Atrophy or weakness	0	1	
Deforming or erosive arthritis (including reducible deformities, excluding avascular necrosis)	0	1	
Osteoporosis with fracture or vertebral collapse (excluding avascular necrosis)	0	1	
Avascular necrosis (score 2 if > 1)	0	1	2
Osteomyelitis	0	1	
Ruptured tendons	0	1	
SKIN			
Alopecia	0	1	
Extensive scarring or panniculum other than scalp and pulp space	0	1	
Skin ulceration (excluding thrombosis) for more than 6 months	0	1	
PREMATURE GONADAL FAILURE	0	1	
DIABETES (regardless of treatment)	0	1	
MALIGNANCY (exclude dysplasia)	0	1	2

strated that there is little overlap between the BILAG disease activity measure, the SLICC/ACR damage index, and the SF20+, confirming the requirement for all three types of index to assess the full range of effects of lupus on a patient.

SLE in children

It is generally reported that about 20% of all cases of lupus have an onset before the age of 18. Silverman and Eddy (1998) in reviewing the literature estimated that the true incidence of lupus in this age group is between 8 and 18.9 cases per 100 000 in white females and 20–30 per 100 000 in black females.

The sex ratio of male to female differs between childhood onset and adult onset cases, with a relatively high number of boys with SLE presenting in childhood. Thus the boy:girl ratio in childhood lupus is probably about 1:5 (i.e. about half that seen in adults). Tucker *et al.* (1995) reviewed the major clinical and haematological features of childhood- and adult-onset lupus. There is a lower frequency of arthritis and cardiopulmonary disease in the childhood onset patients, with a higher frequency of renal disease in this group. There is also a trend towards a higher incidence of fever in childhood onset disease. Other clinical features such as rash, oral ulcers, and central nervous system involvement appear with equal frequency. Major haematological disease was found in about 20% of adult patients and about 40% of childhood onset patients, although no differences have really emerged with

respect to the incidence of leucopaenia or lymphopaenia. Among immunological studies, anti-dsDNA antibodies appear to be more prevalent in childhood-onset cases and a trend towards an increased prevalence of anti-RNP but reduced anti-La antibodies has been noted. There is a much higher frequency of Coombs' positivity among the childhood onset cases, i.e. 55–73%, compared with 17–27% in adults.

A neonatal lupus syndrome has been well described. This disease of the newborn is defined by the demonstration of maternal autoantibodies to Ro and/or La, being detectable in the neonate (following transplacental passage), together with complete congenital heart block (Buyon *et al.* 1989), which may be permanent, and subacute cutaneous lupus rashes, which are transient (Fig. 4.8). Much more rarely, haemolytic

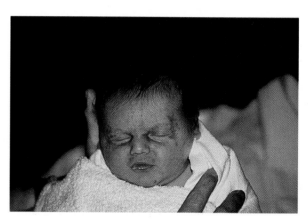

Fig. 4.8.   Facial rash of neonatal lupus.

anaemia, thrombocytopaenia, urinary abnormalities, and liver dysfunction have been described. Only 1:20 of mothers who have antibodies to Ro and/or La have children with the syndrome and it still remains obscure as to why these 5% of children remain are affected but not the others.

SLE and pregnancy

Most recent studies have concluded that fertility is little changed by lupus, although patients in renal failure are less likely to become pregnant. There is a diversity of opinion in the literature as to whether lupus patients who become pregnant are more likely to flare during the pregnancy. In a case–control study of 46 patients with 79 pregnancies, lupus flares occurred no more frequently than in non pregnant lupus controls (Urowitz *et al.* 1993]. In contrast Petri *et al.* (1991) found a higher rate of flare during pregnancy compared with the rate in the same patients post partum or in the Johns Hopkins University lupus cohort overall. Our own experience resembles the report from Urowitz and colleagues. In practice, most pregnant lupus patients need close observation throughout the duration of their pregnancy. The final trimester of pregnancy can be a particularly difficult period for patients with renal lupus, though an increase in proteinuria may be a result of pre-eclampsia rather than a major exacerbation of lupus nephritis. Distinguishing the two may be difficult.

A combination of spontaneous abortion and still birth causes a fetal mortality of around 20%. Furthermore, perhaps as many as one-quarter of babies born to mothers with lupus are delivered prematurely. Despite the panoply of antibodies associated with lupus, only those binding phospholipids and the Ro antigen have an important effect during or just after pregnancy. Patients with the phospholipid variant of lupus are, like patients with primary anti-phospholipid syndrome, more prone to developing recurrent miscarriages and anti-Ro/La antibodies are associated with the neonatal lupus syndrome (see above).

Lupus in other situations

Gender and age

Although lupus in males, especially Caucasian males, is relatively uncommon, as discussed by Isenberg and Malick (1994), no clearly defined criteria distinguishing male from female lupus have been identified. Individuals with Klinefelter's syndrome, who have an XXY karyotype, are thought to be more susceptible to systemic lupus. Abnormalities in oestradiol metabolism in these patients may be linked to persistent oestrogenic stimulation, which might explain the predisposition.

In most large studies, lupus with an onset after age 50 represents approximately 10% of the study population. On the whole it appears that the onset of lupus in this group is likely to be more insidious, with a lower incidence of severe renal and neurological complications and a lower frequency of antibodies to double stranded DNA and hypocomplementaemia, but probably an increased frequency of serositis, interstitial lung disease, and antibodies to Ro and La. The last of these features suggests that an overlap between lupus and Sjögren's syndrome may be more frequent in the elderly population.

The anti-phospholipid antibody variant of lupus

As discussed in Chapter 9, the clinical features that are linked to the presence of anti-phospholipid antibodies include venous and arterial thromboses, thrombocytopaenia, cerebral disease (including cerebrovascular accident, transient ischaemic attacks, chorea, amaurosis fugax), recurrent fetal loss, pulmonary hypertension, and livedo reticularis. A meta-analysis undertaken by Love and Santoro (1990) of 29 published series estimated an average frequency of 34% of lupus patients having lupus anticoagulant and 44% having anticardiolipin antibodies. However, the anti-cardiolipin antibodies that appear to be linked to the presence of the above clinical features are probably binding a complex, or a neo-epitope, formed by phospholipid and a plasma co-factor β_2-glycoprotein 1 (Galli *et al.* 1990). These observations are discussed in more detail on p. 224.

More recent studies reviewed by Alarcon-Segovia and Cabral (1996) have proposed that there are other co-factors and indeed that antibodies to the co-factor may even be a better marker for the thrombotic tendency than antibodies to the phospholipid alone or the complex.

Lupus and malignancy

A rather low frequency of malignancy has been noted in most studies of patients with SLE. However, two recent large studies have focused on this issue. From a cohort of 1585 patients Mellemkjaer *et al.* (1997) reported that there was a significant excess of non-Hodgkin's lymphoma among SLE patients (although it was not clarified in this paper how hard the authors had looked for the presence of Sjögren's syndrome which is well known to be linked to this tumour) and also an increased risk of cancers of the lung, liver, and vagina/vulva. In the study by Urowitz and colleagues the link with non-Hodgkin's lymphoma was also emphasized (Abu-Shakra *et al.* 1996).

Drug-induced lupus

Since 1945 when Hoffman (reported by Gold 1951) described a young man with clinical features of skin rash, haematological and renal disease that resembled systemic lupus erythematosus after he had been treated with sulphadiazine, over 70 drugs have been identified as inducing lupus-like features and/or anti-nuclear antibodies. In addition, other drugs, including antibiotics, hormones, non-steroidal anti-inflammatory drugs, and gold salts, may exacerbate the true systemic disease.

It has been suggested that there may be up to 20 000 new cases of drug-induced lupus in the United States per annum, the majority accounted for by procainamide, isoniazid, chlorpromazine, hydralazine, methyl dopa, and D-penicillamine. Drug-induced lupus commonly causes arthralgia and arthritis, pleuritis, fever, and weight loss, but glomerulonephritis and central nervous system disease are extremely rare.

Over 95% of these patients have an anti-nuclear antibody whose principal specificity is to histones and single stranded DNA but not, unlike SLE, to double stranded DNA. Rheumatoid factor may be present in 20–30% of these patients but anti-cardiolipin antibodies and antibodies to the extractable nuclear antibodies are uncommon. Once the diagnosis has been made the offending drug must be stopped. However, this may not be sufficient on occasion to cause a rapid cessation of the clinical features, which may require a short course of corticosteroid therapy.

Reviews of drug-induced lupus have been published elsewhere (e.g. Fritzler 1994) and have emphasized that genetic factors are likely to be important in the expression of drug-induced disease. Thus symptomatic drug-induced lupus is rare in the black population. It is also somewhat more common in women (approximately 2–4 times greater than in men) and does seem to be associated with HLA-DR4 (reviewed in Adams and Mongey 1984). There is a significant increase in C4

null alleles among these patients compared with normal controls.

Perry *et al.* (1970) were the first to show that levels of hepatic acetyltransferase activity in the acetylator phenotype of individuals are linked to the development of drug-induced lupus. These observations depend upon the fact that the acetyl group of procainamide and the hydralazine group of hydralazine and isoniazid appear to be central to the pathogenesis of drug-induced lupus. Individuals may be distinguished on the basis of their slow or fast ability to activate acetyl transferase. Slow acetylators are homozygous for a recessive gene that controls hepatic acetyl transferase and in these individuals autoantibodies and clinical symptoms develop more rapidly once they have been started on the above named drugs.

Although several hypotheses have been put forward to explain the pathogenesis of drug-induced lupus, including immune complex deposition (invoking anti-histone antibodies in the complex) and molecular mimicry, no universally accepted theory has emerged.

Immunogenetics

An increased frequency of HLA-DR2 and DR3 was first reported in Caucasian SLE patients in 1978 (Reinertsen *et al.* 1978). Many subsequent studies confirmed this observation. In some Caucasian populations, both DR2 and DR3 are increased while in others only DR3 (Reveille *et al.* 1991; Skarsvag *et al.* 1992) or only DR2 is increased (Ahearn *et al.* 1982). Studies from the US and Canada found differing HLA associations when Caucasian patients were categorized according to their ancestry (e.g. French Canadian, English etc), (Goldstein and Sengar 1993; Schur *et al.* 1990). There is variability in the frequency of HLA antigens in differing Caucasian populations, for example between Northern and Southern Europeans (Tsuji *et al.* 1992) and this variability may contribute to differences in HLA antigens that are found in association with a disease. Among black patients with SLE an increase of DR3 and DR2 has also been described (Kachru *et al.* 1984) although not in all studies (Howard *et al.* 1986). In Asian populations (where DR3 is uncommon) an increase of DR2 has been found among Chinese (Hawkins *et al.* 1987), Malay (Kong *et al.* 1994) and Japanese (Hashimoto *et al.* 1994) patients with SLE. Despite the consistency with which DR2 and DR3 have been described in association with SLE the following observations merit emphasis. In most studies less than 50% of all SLE patients have DR2 or DR3 and in most studies the relative risk associated with these antigens is modest, in the range of 2.0 to 3.0.

Some studies have suggested stronger HLA associations when SLE patients are categorized by clinical subsets. In patients with subacute cutaneous lupus a relative risk of 11 has been reported for DR3 (Sontheimer *et al.* 1981). DR2 and some alleles of DQ1 have been reported in association with lupus nephritis in some studies (Fronek *et al.* 1990; Freedman *et al.* 1993), but not in others (Lu *et al.* 1997). Patients with overlap syndromes often have DR4, in contrast to patients with SLE without overlap (Dong *et al.* 1993). Many studies have found no significant correlation of HLA antigens with clinical subsets of SLE.

Recent studies have applied DNA typing techniques to investigate HLA associations in patients with SLE. If a study utilized DNA-typing the gene that encodes, for example the DR3 molecule, is designated as DRB1*03. There is strong linkage disequilibrium in the HLA class II region particularly among DRB genes (DRB1, DRB3, DRB4, DRB5) and DQ genes (DQA1 and DQB1) so that particular combinations of alleles are often inherited as extended haplotypes i.e. 'en bloc' (see Chapter 1). The DRB1*03 haplotype that has been identified is DRB1*03, DRB3*0101, DQA1*0501, DQB1*0201, described in Caucasians from Scandinavia and in a large European multicenter study (Skarsvag *et al.* 1992; Yao *et al.* 1993). The DRB1*02 haplotype DRB1*02, DQA1*0102, DQB1*0602 was also increased in the European multicenter study. This haplotype is similar to that identified in Japanese SLE patients where typing included further definition of the allelic variant of DRB1*02 as DRB1*1501, and the allelic variant of DRB5 (DRB5*0101) that is also present on haplotypes with DRB1*02 (Hashimoto *et al.* 1994). While some reports have indicated the strongest association is with a particular DQB1 allele (Lu *et al.* 1997), and others with a DQA1 allele (Skarsvag *et al.* 1992), there is strong linkage disequilibrium among class II genes and it has generally been difficult to determine whether a particular locus is of primary importance.

There is no specific amino acid sequence that is common between any DRB1*02 and DRB1*03 allele, nor to the DQA1 or DQB1 alleles in linkage disequilibrium with DRB1*02 and DRB1*03. Thus in contrast to studies of patients with rheumatoid arthritis where a theme emerges of a shared amino acid stretch expressed by a number of differing alleles, the theme that emerges with SLE is that of the extended haplo-type and of genes in linkage disequilibrium in the MHC complex. In addition to extended HLA class II haplotypes, other MHC genes that are in linkage disequilibrium with class II genes have been investigated including HLA class I genes, genes of the complement families, and genes encoding tumor necrosis factor.

Some class I antigen associations have been described in SLE patients. However, no specific class I gene has consistently been identified in SLE patients. Also, studies across differing ethnic groups have generally demonstrated that associations with class I antigens are secondary to those with class II antigens. For example, DRB1*03 occurs on an extended haplotype with A1 and B8 that is very common in Caucasian populations; however, in a study of blacks with SLE, whereas DR3 was significantly increased, no increase of A1 or B8 was found (Kachru *et al.* 1984).

In contrast to HLA class I antigens, genes encoding components of the complement system have consistently been shown to be important in SLE. The genes that encode for complement proteins C4A, C4B, Factor B and C2 are located between the class I and class II genes in the MHC complex. Many patients with SLE with complete deficiencies of complement components, including C2, have been described, however the most common inherited abnormality of complement that has been identified in SLE patients is a C4A null allele. Because a null allele at the C4A locus is in strong linkage disequilibrium with DRB1*03, to address whether the C4A null allele is independently associated with risk of SLE Batchelor *et al.* (1987) examined DR3-negative patients and controls. They found that significantly more patients than controls had a C4A null allele (60% vs. 37%) and concluded that null alleles of complement genes are independently associated with SLE. The C4A null allele has been observed in association with SLE in numerous racial/ethnic groups, including blacks (Petri *et al.* 1993; Howard *et al.* 1986), Chinese and Japanese (Hawkins *et al.* 1987; Dunckley *et al.* 1987). Homozygosity for C4A null, although present in only a small number of patients, has been described with a relative risk of almost 17 (Howard *et al.* 1986). Although the mechanism is not known, a potential explanation for the role of complement deficiency in SLE is impaired solubilization and clearance of immune complexes.

In addition to complement, the HLA class III region also contains genes for tumor necrosis factor (TNF). Immunomodulatory properties of TNF are well recognized so that TNF genes are of interest in the investigation of susceptibility to SLE. Most studies have not identified a contribution of TNF genes that is independent of the previously identified HLA class II and complement haplotypes (Bettinotti *et al.*, 1993; D'Alfonso *et al.*, 1996; Hajeer *et al.* 1997). However, in a study that examined levels of TNF-α inducibility, low levels of TNA-α were found in SLE patients with DR2 and DQ1, and normal or high levels in patients with DR3 and DR4 (Jacob *et al.* 1990*b*). These results are potentially of interest in light of the prior report that DR2, DQ1 haplotype correlated, whereas DR3 and DR4 did not correlate, with lupus nephritis.

HLA associations have also been investigated with autoantibodies in SLE patients. Antibodies to Ro and La are found with increased frequency in SLE patients who have both DQ1 and DQ2 (Harley *et al.* 1989), similar to patients with Sjögren's syndrome who have these antibodies (see Chapter 6). Because the strongest association is found with this heterozygous combination it has been proposed that 'hybrid' DQ molecules might be responsible. Both the DQα and DQβ chains have variability so that a hybrid molecule can be created by pairing of a chain encoded by a gene inherited from one parent with the chain encoded by a gene inherited from the other parent. Additional work has investigated the specificity of antibodies to Ro and La for correlation with HLA antigens. Antibodies to a 52kD Ro and La antigen correlated with DR3 in one study (Ehrfeld *et al.* 1992), and in another antibodies to an N-terminal epitope of the 52kD Ro antigen correlated with the DR3 haplotype DRB1*0301, DQA1*0501, DQB1*0201 (Buyon *et al.* 1994). In other studies, among patients with antibodies to Ro, DQA1*0501 and DQB1*0201 were most frequent (encoding DQ2), followed by DQA1 and DQB1 alleles that encode a molecule in the DQ1 family; the strongest association was found in patients with DQA1 and DQB1 alleles that encode both DQ2 and DQ1, confirming prior reports (Reveille *et al.* 1991). Antibodies to Ro and La have also been studied in mothers with or without SLE who have infants with neonatal and lupus (see below) and in patients with Sjögrens syndrome (see Chapter 8). An association with particular DQB1 alleles has been reported with antiphospholipid antibodies (see Chapter 9).

As summarized above, significant associations have been described in the MHC complex in patients with SLE (Table 4.7). Nevertheless in most studies less than half of patients have any given gene. Most investigators believe that genetic contributions to SLE are likely to be complex and multiple. Summaries in this book are limited to the MHC complex, but numerous invest-

igations are currently underway to identify genes outside of the MHC complex and on other chromosomes in susceptibility to SLE. Another interesting hypothesis that is currently being investigated is whether persistence of maternal cells that have trafficked into the fetal circulation during pregnancy might contribute to risk of subsequent SLE in her progeny (Nelson 1998).

Neonatal lupus syndrome and immunogenetics

Neonatal lupus (NLE) and complete heart block (CHB) are most frequently observed in neonates of women who have antibodies to both Ro and La. Because DR2, DQ1 was associated with a subgroup of patients who made antibodies to Ro, but not to La (Hamilton *et al.* 1988), it would be expected that NLE and CHB might occur more frequently for mothers with DR3, DQ2. This expectation has been confirmed in a number of studies (Julkunen *et al.* 1995). In an Italian population, in addition to DR3, an increased frequency of DR5 was found (Brucato *et al.* 1995a). DR3 was not found in mothers of infants with NLE in a Japanese study (Kaneko *et al.* 1992) where instead, an increase of DR12 was observed in mothers (although HLA results were available for only eight women). DR3, DR5, and DR12 are in linkage disequilibrium with DQA1*0501, thus raising the question as to whether DQA1*0501 is the maternal risk factor for a child with NLE and/or CHB.

Some investigators have asked whether fetal HLA antigens contribute to NLE or CHB. (Arnaiz-Villena *et al.* 1989; Watson *et al.* 1984; Lee *et al.* 1983; Brucato *et al.* 1995b). With the exception of a small study in Japanese in which DR12 was increased in neonates (Kaneko *et al.* 1992), no increase of any specific HLA antigen has been observed. It has therefore generally been concluded that neonatal HLA antigens do not affect risk of NLE or CHB. However, until recently, no study addressed the question as to whether the maternal-fetal HLA relationship might affect risk. In a small study from Japan significantly more children with CHB were HLA class II identical with their mothers for DRB1, DQA1 and DQB1 than children without CHB (Miyagawa *et al.* 1997). Reports from other investigators have also suggested a possible role for complement genes in NLE and CHB (Arnaiz-Villena *et al.* 1989; Watson *et al.* 1992).

Experimental models of SLE

Although canine models of lupus have been described, it is mainly the spontaneous mouse models of lupus that have been used to study the immunopathology of the disease. In Table 4.8 the major biological and immunological features of these lupus-prone strains are shown.

New Zealand black mice

The New Zealand black (NZB) mouse is one of the best known models of human lupus. It was derived and partially characterized by Dr Marianne Bielschowsky and her colleagues at the University of Dunedin, New Zealand, and selected for inbreeding on the basis of a solid coat colour (black) (Bielchowsky *et al.* 1959; Helyer and Howie 1963). These animals are primarily a model for autoimmune haemolytic anaemia, although they are often considered together with the NZB/W hybrid (see below) which develops a more complete form of lupus.

Disease in the NZB mice is not sex linked and 50% survival is approximately 18 months. Anaemia starts to develop at the age of nine months and by 12 months virtually 100% of the animals have an erythrocyte-bound antibody as detected by the direct Coombs test. Anaemia is most severe in virgin females. Splenomegaly is seen commonly in these animals. As well as anti-erythrocyte antibodies, antibodies binding to double- and single-stranded DNA and other nuclear components may be found, as may circulating immune complexes. Kidney disease, though less frequent than in the NZB/W mouse, often develops, particularly in the virgin females. The kidneys, which are enlarged and pale, show a membranous form of glomerulonephritis and immunofluorescent studies reveal deposits of IgG, indicating that the inflammation is due to localization of immune complexes on the glomerular basement membrane.

Lymphoid hyperplasia develops in the medulla of the thymus, as well as in the germinal centres of the spleen and cortices of the lymph nodes. In later life, when autoimmune disease is severe, plasma cells can be seen throughout the medullary region of the spleen and in most lymph nodes. Lymphoid neoplasia occurs in 10–20% of these animals, although it has been suggested that these are often pseudo-lymphomas. Treatment with azathioprine causes a considerable increase in the appearance of thymic lymphomas.

NZB/W mice

The NZB/W mouse is the progeny of an NZB and New Zealand white (NZW) mouse (Fig. 4.9a). Although the NZW does not develop overt autoimmunity, the hybrid has proved an excellent model of human lupus. The lupus-like disease develops principally in the female with clinical symptoms becoming apparent from six months of age, and most animals dying of an immune complex nephritis by nine months. In males the disease becomes apparent after approximately 10 months, with the majority of animals dying around 15 months.

The renal dysfunction is accompanied by an increase in autoantibody positivity (notably ANA and anti-dsDNA). The kidneys may become enlarged and develop subcapsular haemorrhages. Concomitant with the appearance of the anti-nuclear antibodies, foci of glomerulonephritis can be seen, especially in the peripheral loops that are associated with regions of endothelial and mesangial hypercellularity. Small

Table 4.7   MHC immunogenetics in SLE

- Risk of SLE is associated with particular extended MHC haplotypes in most studies.
- The haplotypes that are increased in SLE patients are those with DRB1*02 and DRB1*03. These haplotypes are: DRB1*02, DRB5*0101, DQA1*0102, DQB1*0602 and DRB1*03, DRB3*0101, DQA1*0501, DQB1*0201, the latter frequently with a null allele at C4A.
- HLA class II associations nevertheless account for 50% or less of SLE patients in most studies.
- The relative risk associated with HLA class II genes in most reports is modest (often 2.0–3.0).
- Stronger HLA associations have generally not been evident when patients are categorized by clinical subsets, although lupus nephritis may be increased among patients with DR2 and particular alleles of the DQ1 family.
- Specific HLA-associations have been found with some autoantibodies. Antibodies to Ro and/or La are found in individuals who have DQA1 and DQB1 alleles that encode for DQ1 and DQ2.
- Genetic abnormalities of complement are associated with SLE and a null C4A allele is probably an independent risk factor for SLE.
- Currently available data does not indicate a major independent role for alleles at TNF loci.
- There is a general consensus that multiple genes contribute to susceptibility to SLE.

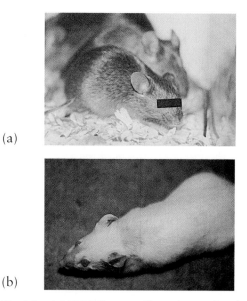

(a)

(b)

Fig. 4.9.   (a) NZB/W mouse. The patient preferred to remain anonymous! (b) MRL/*lpr* mouse.

quantities of immunoglobulin and complement are deposited along the mesangium and capillary basement membranes. These deposits increase as the mice age, and distortion and damage of the capillary basement membrane becomes evident. As the disease advances the membrane becomes fibrous and necrotic and epithelial cells fill the capsular space and tubular casts appear.

Haematological disease may occur, with marked reticulocytosis and a positive Coombs test. Lymphocytic infiltration of the lachrymal and parotid glands occurs in both this mouse and the NZB, indicating that they also develop a disease analogous to Sjögren's syndrome.

As well as antibodies to DNA (single- and double-stranded), these mice develop antibodies to RNA, synthetic polynucleotides, and heat shock protein 90. In addition, antibodies to gp70, the glycoprotein envelope of the endogenous retrovirus, are also identified. During the first few months of life, anti-DNA antibodies of the IgM isotype predominate. However, a class switch occurs and IgG becomes the dominant isotype (Steward and Hay 1976); this change is associated with the development of clinical features.

MRL/lpr/lpr mice

The MRL/*lpr/lpr* (usually abbreviated to MRL/*lpr* or simply *lpr*) mouse was derived 20 years ago (Murphy

and Roths 1978). Females of this strain develop a fatal immune complex glomerulonephritis with the disease becoming evident at two to three months of age (Fig. 4.9b). Most of the animals are dead within six months. These mice develop a broad range of immunological abnormalities. Perhaps the most remarkable physical feature is the development of massive lymphoproliferation. This characteristic (*lpr* refers to lymphoproliferation) is manifest in the development of enormous peripheral lymph nodes, particularly in the axillary and cervical regions, and gross splenomegaly. There is considerable laboratory to laboratory variation but some of these mice also develop articular lesions resembling rheumatoid arthritis. Hind limb swelling can be seen together with a deforming arthritis, synovitis, pannus formation, and joint effusions. Although obvious clinical symptoms only occur in a small percentage of animals it has been claimed that up to 75% of joint lesions resembling rheumatoid arthritis are detected under electron microscopy (Hang *et al.* 1982). Other clinical features include vasculitic skin lesions (particularly of the ear), hair loss, and necrotizing arteritis.

MRL+/+ mice

The MRL+/+ mice develop a similar but milder and later onset form of lupus, with a 50% survival time of 18 months. They differ from the MRL/*lpr* mice by one gene (the *lpr* gene). The MRL/*lpr* mice have an endogenous retroviral DNA sequence integrated into the *fas* gene, which results in incorrect membrane expression of Fas protein and loss of apoptosis. This abnormality results in the failure of self-reactive T cells to undergo apoptosis in the thymus, and may well be the cause of the accumulation of double negative T cells (CD4⁻, CD8⁻) which infiltrate in many tissues in these mice. Wu *et al.* (1994) ameliorated disease in CD2–Fas transgenic MRL/*lpr* mice. CD2 promoter and enhancer were used to restore Fas expression in these animals and this resulted in greatly reduced features of autoimmune disease, antibody production, and a complete elimination of lymphoproliferation.

NZB/SWR F₁ mice

F₁ hybrids between the autoimmune strain (NZB) and a non-autoimmune strain (SWR) have an accelerated autoimmune disease with a high incidence of nephritis. All females are dead by one year of age. These mice have IgG2b anti-dsDNA antibodies that are cationic and deposit in their glomerular basement membrane. The pathogenic antibodies derive from the normal SWR parent and carry a nephritogenic idiotypic marker that is not found in the circulation of either parent. Normal parents have deleted 50% of their T cell receptor β chains and are I–E-negative (equivalent to HLA-DR in humans), thus they have peripheral T cells with I–E-reactive T cell receptors. The autoimmune parent and the F_1 offspring are I–E-positive. Autoimmunity arises from the expression of forbidden T cell receptors by double negative T helper cells and this suggests an abnormality in thymic selection or deletion (Gavalchin and Datta 1987).

BXSB mice

The BXSB mouse is a recombinant inbred strain resulting from crossing C57 BL/6J females with SB/le males (the latter being a model for Chediak–Higashi immunodeficiency syndrome). The BXSB is unique in that males develop the most severe form of the disease. The disease is characterized by haemolytic anaemia, splenomegaly, lymphadenopathy, a severe exudative proliferative nephritis, and serological abnormalities (beginning at age two months), including the presence of antibodies to DNA and anti-erythrocyte antibodies. In addition, immune complexes and hypocomplementaemia are noted and thymic atrophy is evident at an early age.

Moth-eaten mice

The moth-eaten mouse was developed from a mutation in C57 BL/6J strain mice (Schultz and Zurier 1978). The moth-eaten trait is recessive. Heterozygous animals develop lesions on their limbs and skin and exhibit patchy loss of hair. Although the mice show a wide variety of autoimmune lupus-like phenomena, including anti-DNA antibodies, anti-erythrocyte antibodies, circulating immune complexes, and glomerulonephritis, they are seriously immunocompromised with a life span of little over one month. This characteristic limits their experimental usefulness.

Palmerston North mice

Of all the lupus-like murine models, the Palmerston North (PN) strain is probably the least well known. Like the NZB and related hybrids it was derived in New Zealand (at the Palmerston North Hospital), though it remains genetically distinct. Originally,

outbred PN mice were described as developing polyarteritis nodosa (Widgley and Couchman 1966). Since these early studies the strain has been inbred and studied further, revealing an autoimmune pathology resembling lupus. As with NZB/W and MRL/*lpr* mice, the most severe form of disease is seen in females — 50% survival being 11 months. The animals die of an immune complex nephritis. Glomerular lesions can be found in very young animals. Thickened basement membranes and segmental hypercellularity have been found in 45% of renal glomeruli from one-month-old mice. Over the next few months glomerular hypercellularity, fibrinoid degeneration, and crescent formation are found. Immunofluorescent staining reveals deposits of IgG, IgM, and C3 and arteritis also occurs in the renal tissue characterized by fibrinoid necrosis of the arterial walls of small and medium vessels. As well as in the kidney, arteritis is also seen in the thymus, lymph nodes, spleen, and ovaries. Extensive vasculitis is also evident, notably in the blood vessels of the thymus, spleen, ovaries, skeletal tissue, and kidneys. The thymus becomes enlarged and hyperplastic up to the age of five months. After nine months involution occurs with the loss of Hassall's corpuscles. Hyperplastic lymph nodes occur in animals of all ages. Neoplastic malignancies, notably lymphomas, are found in up to 14% of the mice.

Anti-DNA antibodies can be detected in the sera of some newborn animals and by two months of age almost 60% have such antibodies. In addition, antithymocyte antibodies, anti-erythrocyte antibodies and hypergammaglobulinaemia are all recognized features.

Swan mice

Swan mice (Swiss anti-nuclear) were originally developed in Switzerland and selected for breeding because of ANA positivity. This strain develops a relatively mild form of glomerulonephritis which becomes apparent around 10 months of age. The glomerular basement membrane thickens owing to subendothelial deposits of immunoglobulin and complement and there is associated hypertrophy and hyperplasia of the mesangium. The thymus atrophies early, Hassall's corpuscles are rarely found, thymic hormone secretion is terminated, and thymic epithelium cells exhibit ultrastructural abnormalities. Anti-DNA antibodies can be detected in most animals. Relatively little is known about the T cell compartment. Swan mice are similar to the PN strain in that they express very small quantities of xenotropic type C retrovirus. This strain is not a widely used model, mainly because the onset is slow and the disease rather mild.

Other models of lupus-like disease

Although really a veterinary oddity rather than a practical model for SLE it is now acknowledged that dogs regularly develop lupus-like disorders. The clinical spectrum appears to be wide and thus analogous to the human condition. The incidence of lupus in domestic dogs has been estimated at approximately 1 in 5000 (see Quimby et al. 1978). It is sex linked, occurring in females four times as often as in males. The onset varies from six months to 14 years. No breed seems to be particularly at risk. The clinical manifestations include polyarthritis, butterfly rash, photosensitivity, CNS involvement, cardiac complications, haemolytic anaemia, thrombocytopaenia, and, in half of the cases, glomerulonephritis. As with human lupus the cause of disease is variable, with remissions and exacerbations. The 50% survival time is around three years. The glomerulonephritis has been noted to be either membranous or membranoproliferative, with deposition of immunoglobulin and complement on the glomerular basement membrane.

Several other animal strains can be used as models for syndromes resembling lupus. However, they are virus induced and cannot be regarded as true models of lupus and offer no real advantages over the auto-immune mouse strains described above. Rather, they are models of immune complex disease induced by chronic infection. Notable examples are lymphocytic choriomeningitis (LCM) virus in mice, Aleutian virus disease in mink, and equine infectious anaemia virus in horses.

A contentious animal model of lupus said to be induced in healthy strains of mice by injections of human monoclonal antibodies bearing a particular idiotype designated 16/6 has been reported. The principal advocates of this model, have published a series of papers describing both the clinical features and therapy of the disease thus induced (e.g. Mendelovic et al. 1988; Shoenfeld 1994). In essence the authors reported that 1 μg of 16/6 idiotype-positive DNA-binding antibodies given on two occasions (the first in the presence of complete Freund's adjuvant) intradermally and three weeks apart, will, after approximately three to four months, induce a disease whose features include skin rashes, glomerulonephritis, leucopaenia, thrombocytopaenia, and a full panoply of lupus-related autoantibodies, including antibodies to DNA, Ro, La,

Sm, RNP, and cardiolipin. It is now 10 years since the original claims were made for this model, and given the apparent ease with which the researchers claim to induce the model it is very striking that no other group has been able to reproduce it (Isenberg et al. 1991). It was, however, suggested that there must be a critical environmental factor that determines the development of the disease.

The importance of environmental factors, even if unknown in the development of murine models, is emphasized by the recent description of Governman et al. (1993) of a transgenic model of experimental allergic encephalomyelitis which developed only in mice kept in a non-sterile environment. This example provides a useful analogy. The topic is reviewed in detail elsewhere (Williams and Isenberg 1994). On balance it is evident that the 'idiotype' model of lupus is not easily exportable and thus is of limited utility.

The severe combined immunodeficient (SCID) mouse has been used to study the effects of human monoclonal anti-DNA antibodies (Ehrenstein et al, 1995). Some, but not all of the antibodies tested induced proteinuria and early changes of glomerulonephritis seen under electron microscopy (Ravirajan et al. 1998).

Immunopathology of SLE

The remarkable diversity among the clinical features found in lupus patients (Fig. 4.10) is matched by the diversity among the immunological abnormalities reported. These will be considered initially in the context of the experimental models.

Serology

A multitude of abnormalities can be found in the sera of patients with lupus (Table 4.9) and they are characterized as follows.

Autoantibodies

The lupus erythematosus (LE) cell
This classic phenomenon of lupus erythematosus was first described by Hargreaves et al. (1948) and became the basis of the laboratory test which for many years was the standard criterion for diagnosing SLE. Although the LE cell test has been superseded by the anti-nuclear antibody and antibodies to dsDNA,

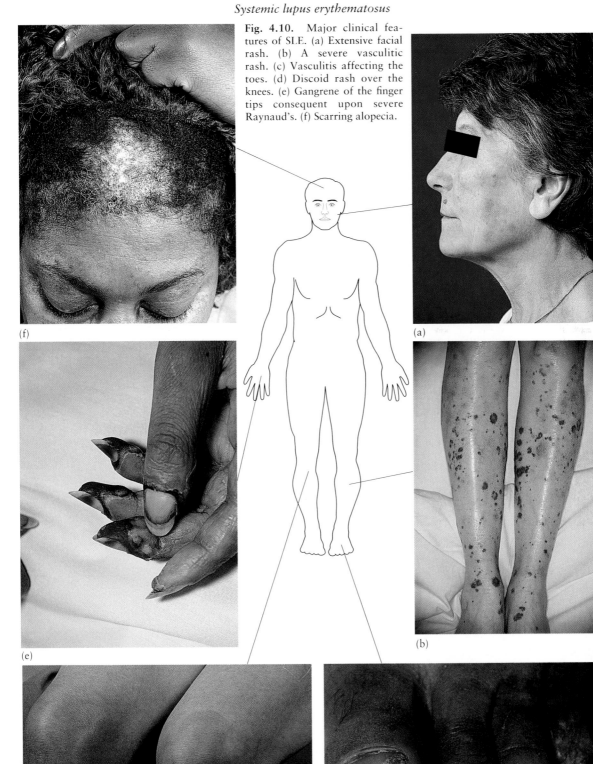

Fig. 4.10. Major clinical features of SLE. (a) Extensive facial rash. (b) A severe vasculitic rash. (c) Vasculitis affecting the toes. (d) Discoid rash over the knees. (e) Gangrene of the finger tips consequent upon severe Raynaud's. (f) Scarring alopecia.

(f)

(a)

(e)

(b)

(d)

(c)

it is worthy of note for historical reasons. Poly-morphonuclear leucocytes from the blood or bone marrow are seen to ingest large quantities of homogeneous nuclear material from other leucocytes, presumably damaged by the action of anti-nuclear antibodies.

Anti-nuclear antibodies

It is now over 40 years since the discovery of anti-nuclear and anti-DNA antibodies in the serum of patients with lupus. Since these seminal observations, numerous diverse autoantibodies have been described, including those of various forms of DNA, RNA, histones, and synthetic polynucleotides. These are summarized in Table 4.8. The biological significance of these antibodies is discussed later in this section, and

the details of the detection of many of them have been discussed in Chapter 2.

Friou and colleagues, in a series of articles, described and partially characterized a phenomenon by which serum from patients with SLE would bind to nuclear antigens. Using fluorochrome-labelled antisera, it was shown that the component binding to the nucleus was in fact antibody from the patient (Friou 1957; Friou *et al.* 1958). This finding clearly demonstrated that an autoimmune pathology was underlying the disease and heralded a new era of research in SLE.

Screening for anti-nuclear antibodies (ANA) is an important primary step in the diagnosis of lupus, though to some extent this test has been superseded by the easy availability of DNA-binding assays. Ninety-five per cent or more of patients with lupus have a

Table 4.8 Features of lupus-prone mouse strains

Strain	Haplotype	Sex in which disease is most severe	50% survival time	Major clinical features	Major immunological features
NZB	H-2^d	M and F	18 months	Haemolytic anaemia, glomerulonephritis, lymphomas	Anti-erythrocyte antibodies IgM hyperproduction Generalized lymphocyte dysfunction
(NZB × NZW)F$_1$	H-2$^{d/z}$	F	7–8 months	Severe immune complex nephritis	Anti-nuclear and anti-DNA autoantibodies Generalized lymphocyte dysfunction
MRL/*lpr/lpr*	H-2^k	F	2–4 months	Lymphoproliferation, immune complex nephritis, rheumatoid arthritis, vasculitis	Anti-nuclear antibodies and rheumatoid factors Proliferation of Ly1 cells, generalized lymphocyte dysfunction
MRL+/+	H-2$^\kappa$	F	18 months	As for MRL/*lpr* but less severe	As for MRL/*lpr*
BXSB	H-2^b	M	2–4 months	Haemolytic anaemia, lymphadenopathy, glomerulonephritis	Anti-DNA, NTA, and erythrocyte antibodies, Thymic atrophy occurs early
Moth-eaten	H-2^b	M and F	1 month	Hair loss, glomerulonephritis, infections	Anti-DNA, NTA, and erythrocyte antibodies Immunosupression
Palmerston–North	H-2^q	F	11 months	Polyarteritis nodosa, immune complex nephritis	Anti-DNA autoantibodies, B cell hyperactivity
Swan	H-2^k	M and F	18 months	Mild glomerulonephritis	Anti-DNA autoantibodies, early thymic atrophy
(SWR × NZB)F$_1$	H-2$^{d/q}$	F	4–8 months	Severe glomerulonephritis	Anti-DNA, anti-nucleosome antibodies

NTA = natural thymocytotoxic antibody.

positive anti-nuclear antibody. Immunofluorescent assays screened for anti-nuclear antibodies appear in various patterns (see Chapter 2). The homogeneous pattern corresponds with antibodies binding to double-stranded DNA and/or histones. The speckled pattern, which is also commonly found, does not distinguish antibodies binding to a variety of determinants, including Sm, Ro, La, or RNP. Nucleolar fluorescence is seen occasionally in SLE, but occurs more frequently in scleroderma.

Of the few patients who remain persistently ANA-negative, most have antibodies to Ro (SS-A) or La (SS-B). These patients are less likely to have renal disease (Maddison *et al.* 1981). The approximate prevalence of anti-nuclear and other autoantibodies detectable in the serum of patients with lupus is shown in Table 4.10.

DNA autoantibodies

Coincident with Friou's notable observations on anti-nuclear antibodies, were reports from other laboratories in Europe and America describing antibodies in the sera of lupus patients that would bind to DNA (Cepellini *et al.* 1957; Miescher and Straessle 1957; Robbins *et al.* 1957; Seligman 1957). Since then the dsDNA-binding test [carried out by various techniques (see Chapter 2)] has remained the single most import-

ant laboratory test for the diagnosis of SLE. Its discriminating ability for patients with lupus is illustrated in Fig. 4.11a.

Assessment of the clinical associations with anti-dsDNA antibodies was hampered until recently by the lack of validated and reliable disease activity indices. With this caveat in mind, most large cohort studies have tended to confirm that in the majority of cases, anti-dsDNA antibodies are linked most closely to the occurrence and severity of renal involvement. Thus, Swaak *et al.* (1979) contrasted 51 patients with SLE and 660 patients who had autoimmune conditions. Fifty of the sera from lupus patients contained anti-dsDNA antibodies, in contrast to just one of the control sera. Furthermore, in many patients with renal exacerbations of their lupus a sharp fall in the anti-dsDNA level was usually preceded by a rise — an observation suggesting that the antibodies were being deposited in an organ such as the kidney. Lloyd and Schur (1981) found that complement depletion and raised anti-dsDNA antibodies were associated more closely with renal than non-renal exacerbations in lupus. Ter Borg *et al.* (1990), in a prospective study of 72 patients, showed that active lupus nephritis was usually associated with high anti-dsDNA antibody titres. More recently, Okamura *et al.* (1993) demonstrated a close relationship between renal disease activ-

Table 4.9 Autoantibodies in SLE

Antibodies to cell nucleus components	Anti-nuclear antibodies
	Anti-dsDNA antibodies
	Anti-ssDNA antibodies
	Anti-ssRNA antibodies (including anti-poly A, -poly C, -poly I, -poly U)
	Anti-ssRNA antibodies (including anti-poly-rU, -poly-rA)
	Anti-poly (ADP-ribose) antibodies
	Antibodies to extracellular nuclear antigens, anti-ribonucleoprotein antibodies, anti-Sm antibodies
	Anti-SS-A(Ro) antibodies
	Anti-SS-B(La) antibodies
Antibodies to cytoplasmic antigens	Heat shock proteins
Antibodies to cell membranes	Lymphocytotoxic antibodies
	Anti-neurone antibodies
	Anti-erythrocyte antibodies
	Anti-platelet antibodies
	Anti-phospholipid antibodies
Antibodies to serum components	Anticoagulants
	Antiglobulins (rheumatoid factor)
	Clq

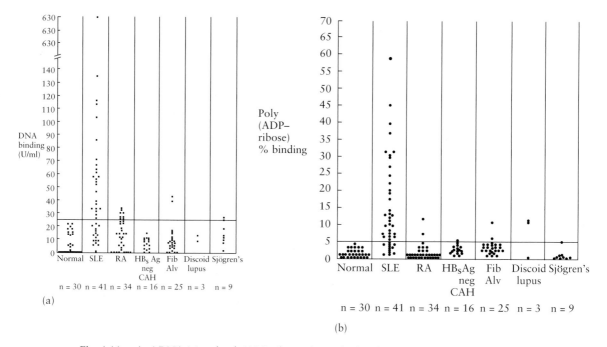

Fig. 4.11.   Anti-DNA (a) and poly(ADP-ribose) (b) antibodies distinguish SLE from other diseases.

ity assessed on biopsy, with IgG anti-dsDNA levels but not with IgM anti-dsDNA or antibodies to single-stranded DNA of either isotype.

Recently, Bootsma *et al.* (1995), utilizing the concept of a rise in anti-dsDNA antibody levels as a means of predicting a clinical relapse, showed that treating these patients with high levels of prednisolone (30 mg/day) reduced the relapse rate compared with a control group treated with more conventional therapy ($p > 0.001$). In an attempt to overcome the problems of defining disease activity referred to above, a serial longitudinal study of 14 Afro-Caribbean lupus patients has utilized the British Isles Lupus Assessment Group's (BILAG) detailed activity score (Isenberg *et al.* 1997). Anti-bodies to dsDNA were shown to be correlated with renal disease ($p = 0.0006$), cardiopulmonary disease ($p = 0.0004$), and global score ($p = 0.02$), but not with musculoskeletal, central nervous system, or haematological involvement. This study assessed blood samples taken over periods of follow-up ranging from three to 15 years.

While the mere detection of anti-DNA antibodies in the kidneys of lupus patients does not prove that they were responsible for the development of this complication, it does place them at 'the scene of the crime'. Koffler *et al.* (1967) were able to elute IgG, complement, and IgM antibodies from the kidneys of

patients who had died from lupus nephritis. These eluates were found to have anti-nuclear binding activity and, although a specific test for anti-DNA binding was not performed, the anti-nuclear binding of the eluates could be partially inhibited by adding dsDNA.

Among a number of studies that have reported the deposition of anti-DNA antibodies in the kidneys of murine lupus models, the study of Pankewycz *et al.* (1987) was of particular interest, showing that eluted immunoglobulin from the kidney cortices of female MLR/*lpr/lpr* mice with early nephritis was predominantly IgG with antibody activity against DNA. Intriguingly, these eluted antibodies also reacted with multiple nucleic antigens, including cardiolipin, suggesting that polyreactivity might be a distinguishing feature of nephritogenic autoantibodies.

In a study of over 40 lupus families, whereas 21% of 147 relatives had antibodies detectable to ssDNA, only two had antibodies to dsDNA, strongly suggesting that these latter antibodies were implicated in the disease process and not simply bystanders (Isenberg and Collins 1985).

Antibodies to the extractable nuclear antigens
These are conventionally divided into Ro (SS-A), La (SS-B), Sm, and RNP. Antibodies to La are particularly

associated with the coincidence of Sjögren's syndrome and lupus. Patients with anti-La antibodies are less likely to have renal disease (Maddison *et al.* 1988). Anti-Ro antibodies are associated with photosensitive rashes, the so-called subacute cutaneous form of lupus, and vasculitis. As indicated earlier in this chapter, antibodies to Ro and La are both associated with neonatal lupus syndrome. Immune complexes containing Ro may participate occasionally in renal inflammation, as increased Ro activity has been found in glomerular eluates in the kidneys of two patients who died with severe lupus nephritis (Maddison and Reichlin 1979). Antibodies to RNP are not associated with any particular disease features in patients with lupus, and their role in the so-called mixed connective tissue disease is controversial (see Chapter 10). Antibodies to Sm have periodically been linked to particular clinical features, e.g. central nervous system involvement, but, on balance, while their presence is virtually diagnostic of patients with lupus, they do not have a strong association with any particular disease feature. For reasons that remain to be elucidated, anti-Sm antibodies are found in approximately 30% of black lupus patients, but in only approximately 5% of Caucasians. Similarly obscure is the reason why only 30% of MRL/*lpr* mice have anti-Sm antibodies.

Antibodies to RNA

Autoantibodies to RNA can be found in SLE in a higher incidence than in patients with other autoimmune diseases. They appear to have relatively little clinical significance in lupus, though it has been suggested that they may represent, in part, an immune response to a virus (Schur and Monro 1969).

Antibodies to poly(ADP-ribose)

Some years ago Morrow *et al.* (1982) confirmed and extended the findings of other groups (Kanai *et al.* 1977; Okolie and Shall 1979) in demonstrating the presence of antibodies to this nuclear polymer in the sera of lupus patients. Poly(ADP-ribose) is formed from nicotinamide adenine dinucleotide (NAD) by the action of a chromatin-bound enzyme, poly(ADP) polymerase, for the loss of the nicotinamide moiety. Our data showed that sera from lupus patients binds to poly(ADP-ribose) as often as to DNA, with slightly fewer false-positives (Fig. 4.11b). Furthermore, in serial studies, binding to poly(ADP-ribose) appeared to reflect the clinical activity of patients somewhat more accurately than antibodies to ds or ssDNA — though relatively crude methods of assessing clinical activity

were used in that study. The origin of these antibodies is uncertain. However, the function of poly(ADP-ribose) is probably concerned with chromatin regulation and DNA repair. It may thus be irrelevant that studies with mouse monoclonal antibodies binding to poly(ADP-ribose) have shown a significant cross-reaction with DNA (Sibley *et al.* 1986). Alternatively, anti-DNA and anti-poly(ADP-ribose) antibodies could share idiotypes.

Lymphocytotoxic antibodies

These are mostly of the IgM class and affect B and T cell populations equally. These antibodies react most effectively at 4°C, unlike the IgG isotype which has a tropism for B cells and is not cold reactive. The immunopathological role of lymphocytotoxic antibodies is still obscure although they have been correlated with lymphopaenia. They have also been known to react with brain cells, probably because of a shared antigenic determinant analogous to the cross-reaction between antigens on brain- and thymus-derived cells seen in mice.

Antibodies to ribosomal P protein

The ribosomal P proteins consist of three acidic phosphoproteins, P0, P1, and P2, with molecular weights of 38, 19, and 17kDa, respectively. They are required for protein synthesis and ribosome-associated GTPase activity. Anti-ribosomal P antibodies react to at least one common immunodominant epitope common to all three proteins corresponding to a single linear antigenic determinant, present in the carboxyl terminal 22 amino acid sequence. In 1987, Bonfa *et al.* suggested that there was a strong association between neuropsychiatric lupus and the presence of these antibodies. This claim has generated much controversy (reviewed in Teh and Isenberg 1994). The prevalence of these antibodies appears to be higher in Japanese (30–42%) and Malaysian Chinese (38%) than in Caucasians and African-Americans. These data may reflect genetic and/or environmental risk factors. On balance, it is evident that although these antibodies appear relatively specific for lupus they are not specific for neuropsychiatric disease and do not reliably predict neuropsychiatric flares. We believe that there is no value in routinely measuring anti-ribosomal P antibodies in the management of patients with neuropsychiatric lupus.

In an extension of the work on antibodies to ribosomal P, Arnett and Reichlin (1995) performed a retrospective study of liver dysfunction in 131 patients with lupus and identified unexplained liver dysfunction in four patients, all four of whom had ribosomal P antibodies. The significance of this observation remains to be determined. However, neither Petri (1996), in an analysis of 393 patients, nor Fox *et al.* (1997), in a retrospective study of 200 patients, were able to confirm a link between unexplained abnormal liver function tests and anti-ribosomal P antibodies. To complete the controversial picture of anti-ribosomal P antibodies, there are also conflicting studies about the possible role of these antibodies in renal lupus! (discussed in Fox and Isenberg 1997).

Anti-erythrocyte antibodies

Autoantibody activity directed against red blood cells can be seen in some patients. Using the direct Coombs test, Estes and Christian (1971) detected erythrocyte-binding antibodies in 38 out of 1250 patients. However, overt haemolytic anaemia appears to be a rare complication of lupus. In their study, Estes and Christian identified haemolytic anaemia in only 13 of the 38 patients who were Coombs-positive. The pathogenic antibodies are usually of the IgG class.

Anti-platelet antibodies

Between 25 and 50% of lupus patients have a degree of thrombocytopenia at some stage of their disease. This is usually a result of anti-platelet antibodies (reviewed in Keeling and Isenberg 1993). The opsonized platelets appear to be destroyed primarily by splenic macrophages rather than by complement-mediated lysis.

Anti-cardiolipin antibodies and lupus anticoagulants

Anti-cardiolipin antibodies are present in 20–50% of lupus patients, and lupus anticoagulants in 15–35%. In the past 15 years they have been associated with a group of clinical features, including recurrent spontaneous abortion, recurrent thrombosis, and thrombocytopaenia. These antibodies also occur independently of lupus and in the presence of the above clinical features constitute the primary anti-phospholipid syndrome (see Chapter 9). Recently, an important co-factor known as β_2-glycoprotein-1 has been identified. Binding of β_2-glycoprotein-1 to cardiolipin induces change in the phospholipid conformation from the bilayer to the hexagonal form. Antibodies that recognize this conformation, especially of an IgG isotype, seem to be those most commonly associated with the clinical features described above.

The lupus anticoagulant blocks the activation of the prothrombin-activated complex that comprises factor Xa, V calcium, and a phospholipid. Other antibodies have been reported to inhibit factors VII, VIII, XI, and XIII. Lupus anticoagulant may be of the IgG or IgM class, and it is identified by a marked prolongation of the partial thromboplastin time, which is currently corrected by adding an equal volume of normal plasma to the patient's plasma. Paradoxically, this anticoagulant is not usually associated with an increased bleeding tendency and biopsies may be performed safely in these patients.

False-positive tests for syphilis are frequently found in patients with lupus anticoagulant. It has now been shown that certain monoclonal anti-DNA antibodies can react with cardiolipin (which is the test antigen in the Wassermann reaction) and also have anticoagulant properties.

Other autoantibodies

Smolen and colleagues identified an antibody known as RA 33 which was subsequently shown to be identical to the A2 protein of the heterogeneous nuclear RNP complex in patients with rheumatoid arthritis (Steiner *et al.* 1992). However, it has now been associated with a subset of lupus patients who have an erosive arthropathy (Isenberg *et al.* 1994; Richter-Cohen *et al.* 1998).

Approximately 25% of patients with lupus also have rheumatoid factor. These antibodies are usually, though not always, present in low titre and do not appear to have an obvious role in the pathology of the disease and have no apparent relevance to prognosis.

Several of the lupus autoantibodies appear to be linked. The most obvious 'subsets' (see Fig. 4.12) are those linking anti-DNA and anti-phospholipid antibodies. Indeed, Diamond and Scharff (1984) showed that a mutant of antibody S107, known as U4, differs from the parent clone by a single amino acid (alanine is substituted for glutamic acid at position 35 on the heavy chain) and, in consequence, did not bind phosphocholine but did bind dsDNA, cardiolipin, and protamine. There is also an apparent link between subgroups of antibodies to the extractable nuclear antigens. Thus, anti-La antibodies are invariably accompanied by anti-Ro, and anti-RNP by anti-Sm.

Idiotypic considerations

Antibodies are usually defined by the antigens to which they bind. Another way of distinguishing antibodies

a

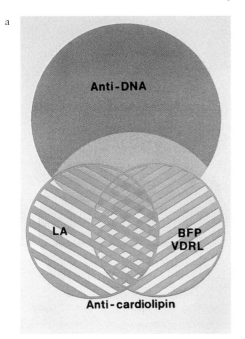

b

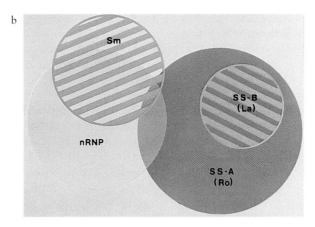

Fig. 4.12. Overlapping relationships between lupus autoantibodies. (a) Shows links between anti-DNA and anti-phospholipid antibodies. LA = lupus anticoagulant; BFPVDRL = biologically false positive venereal disease research laboratory. (b) Links between antibodies to the extractable nuclear antigens.

serologically involves an analysis of their idiotypes, which are essentially phenotypic markers of the variable (V) region genes used to encode the antigen-binding Fab region of immunoglobulin molecules (see also Chapter 1). These regions encode tertiary structures termed idiotopes. A collection of these idiotopes together may be called an idiotype. Idiotypes may represent amino acid sequences located on light or heavy chains alone or in combination. Idiotypes may be categorized into two main groups, depending on how they are recognized by anti-idiotypic antibodies. Restricted, or private, idiotypes are defined by anti-idiotypic antibodies that react only with the immunizing immunoglobulin. Public, or cross-reactive, idiotypes may reflect common amino acid sequences within the framework regions, of the complementarity determining regions and may be present on antibodies with similar or different antigenic specificity. However, in some cases, public idiotypes may actually be more properly thought of as isotypes or possibly autotypes. A cautionary review on the definition of antibody idiotypes has been published recently (Jefferies 1993).

Several groups have investigated the idiotypes associated with anti-DNA antibodies. Thus Rauch *et al.* (1982) prepared an anti-idiotype by immunizing rabbits with an MRL/*lpr* monoclonal DNA-binding antibody designated H130. This reagent detected cross-reactions with eight out of 12 other MRL/*lpr* mono-clonal antibodies, as well as the presence of the H130 idiotype in 40/40 MRL/*lpr* sera.

Other groups have reported the presence of public idiotypes on human monoclonal DNA antibodies, and

Table 4.10 Approximate prevalence of antibodies detectable in the serum of patients with SLE

Antibody specificity	Literature	BRU (%)
ANA	> 90	96
dsDNA	40–90	52
ssDNA	up to 70	–
Histone	30–80	–
Sm	5–30	10
RNP	20–35	20
Ro	30–40	35
La	10–15	15
Cardiolipin	20–50	24 (G) 10 (M)
LAC	10–20	16
Fc IgG (RF)	25	23
hsp 90	5–50	25 (G) 35 (M)
hsp 70	5–40	5
Thyroid Ags	up to 35	21
Clq	20–45	–

The 'literature' column refers to an approximate range from several published studies.

The BRU column is based on the first 200 patients with SLE under long-term follow-up in the Bloomsbury Rheumatology Unit, Middlesex hospital.

LAC = lupus anticoagulant.

G = IgG; M = IgM; Ags = antigens

a comprehensive review of their frequency in the sera of patients with lupus and other groups is shown in Table 4.10. In an international collaborative study of human sera from 180 individuals (Isenberg *et al.* 1990), 18 DNA antibody idiotypes were analysed. In this study the strongest correlations of the idiotype levels were with anti-single-stranded DNA antibodies (in 13 cases) and a total serum IgM (11 cases). Only three human idiotypes tested correlated with anti-dsDNA antibody levels (AM, BEG 2, and 3I). The level of the 124, 3I, PR4, and AM idiotypes correlated with disease activity in some of the patients bled sequentially. However, none of these idiotype studies was disease specific and it is evident that idiotypes, even if initially identified on DNA antibodies, may not be confined to antibodies of that specificity. However, in several cases DNA antibody idiotypes have been identified on immunoglobulins deposited in the renal lesions of lupus patients, suggesting that they may have pathological significance. Thus, in a study of 26 lupus renal biopsies, 12 were shown to contain either or both the 16/6 and 32/15 idiotypes (Isenberg and Collins 1985) (see Fig. 4.13). The idiotypes were identified in the glomerular basement membrane, mesangial cell cytoplasm, and in focal tuft proliferations. In contrast, neither idiotype could be identified in immunoglobulin-positive non-SLE renal biopsies. The 9G4 idiotype has similarly been identified in three of 11 kidney biopsies, and in none of the controls (Isenberg *et al.* 1993). Fascinatingly, an idiotype GN2, first identified on a murine monoclonal DNA antibody has been found in 15 of 20 lupus kidney biopsies but in only 1 of 17 controls (Kalunian *et al.* 1989). Further assessments of the structural basis of idiotypy and other typical and therapeutic considerations are reviewed elsewhere (Staines

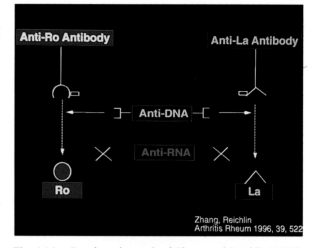

Fig. 4.14. Based on the work of Zhang and Reichlin (1996) it is evident that anti-DNA antibodies (but not anti-RNA) may act as anti-idiotypes to anti-Ro and anti-La antibodies.

1992; Williams and Isenberg 1994). A potential idiotypic linkage between DNA and other lupus autoantibodies has been identified by Zhang and Reichlin (1996) who have shown that anti-DNA antibodies may act as anti-idiotypes for anti-Ro and anti-La antibodies (Fig. 4.14).

Immune complexes

The presence of circulating immune complexes in the sera of lupus patients is one of the most important immunopathological characteristics of the disorder. Immune complexes appear to be damaging by depositing in the kidney, skin, choroid plexus of the brain, and other tissues. From these sites they are thought to initiate a number of inflammatory mechanisms including 'bystander lysis', whereby tissues surrounding the deposited complexes are damaged by complement after it has been fixed to the complexes, and also the recruitment of inflammatory cells.

During the late 1970s and early 1980s there was a tremendous interest in immune complexes and their role in autoimmune rheumatic diseases. Lupus was a particular focus of attention as it was (and still is) considered to be a model for an immune complex-mediated disorder. Numerous studies, including several by ourselves, attempted to correlate levels of circulating complexes with clinical status or use them as disease predictors. These investigations met with only limited success. While it was clear that patients with lupus

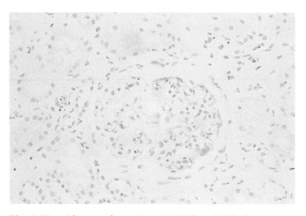

Fig. 4.13. Idiotype deposition (16/6 Id) in SLE kidney.

generally had elevated levels of circulating immune complexes there was no clear picture regarding clinical correlates. This finding most probably reflects the diverse nature of immune complexes and their pathogenic potential is likely to be regulated by their physicochemical properties, including size, antibody class subclass, and affinity, as well as the bound antigen. Although anti-dsDNA antibodies are the serological hallmark of lupus it should be noted that this antigen could not consistently be demonstrated within circulating immune complexes: a finding that suggested that these entities might be aggregates of idiotype–anti-idiotype antibodies. We no longer use immune complex measurements in routine patient assessments.

As discussed in detail elsewhere (Vaishnaw and Walport 1995) patients with lupus may have a failure of the physiological clearance mechanisms of immune complexes. Under normal circumstances the generation of immune complexes leads to activation of complement and opsonization of these complexes, which then bind via C3b to the complement receptor CR1 on red blood cells. This combination is then transported to the fixed mononuclear phagocyte system in the liver and spleen for further processing. Complement deficiencies, which are known to exist in at least some patients with lupus, will result in the defective binding of certain complement components (notably C3 and C4) to immune complexes. Persistently circulating immune complexes may stimulate autoimmunity through antigen associated with the immune complex or as a consequence of antigens released after immune complex-mediated tissue injury. However, relatively few patients with lupus have a total inherited deficiency of individual complement components, but, as indicated earlier in this chapter, many lupus patients do have a C4 null allele which may be sufficient to inhibit immune precipitation of immune complexes and their normal adherence to erythrocytes. It is conceivable that the reduction of CR1 on erythrocytes, which is observed in patients with active lupus, may contribute to disease persistence in a similar manner to reduced C4 levels.

Complement

The complement system is involved in the sequence of inflammatory events seen in SLE and historically has been well studied. Numerous reports have demonstrated that complement is fixed or consumed by immune complexes and localized in the tissues, particularly the kidney. Also, the cleavage fragments C3a and C5a cause the release of vasoactive amines from mast cells. Furthermore, vascular permeability can be increased from fragments of C2 with kinin-like activity. This allows localization of immune complexes as well as causing acute inflammation *per se*. It has been known for over 40 years that reduced complement levels are associated with SLE (Elliott and Mathieson 1953). Not only is the overall haemolytic ability (as usually measured by the CH_{50} test) of the complement system decreased, but levels of most of the major components are also reduced.

Early reacting components of the classical pathway, C1 (and its subcomponents, C1q and C1s), C4, C2, and C3 are frequently reduced in active disease, notably nephritis (Morse *et al.* 1962; Gotoff *et al.* 1969). The final component, C9, has been observed to be elevated in non-renal forms of the disease, although levels become subnormal with glomerulonephritis (Ruddy *et al.* 1971). Following earlier observations that patients with homozygous C1q deficiency develop a form of lupus (albeit with reduced prevalence of ANA and anti-dsDNA antibodies) Walport and collegues have developed a C1q 'knockout' mouse. About 25% of these mice develop glomerulonephritis and anti-Sm antibodies have been identified in their serum but not anti-dsDNA (Walport personal communication).

Kohler and Ten Bensel (1969) and Schur and Sandson (1968) observed that, in some cases, levels of total haemolytic complement fell prior to worsening of the clinical condition. C4 levels are apparently reduced first, followed sequentially by C3, CH_{50}, C1q, and C9 (Ruddy *et al.* 1971). However, the complement profile may be highly variable from patient to patient, and the activation and subsequent utilization is clearly different according to the nature of the disease.

Although activation of the complement cascade usually occurs by way of immune complexes and the classical pathway, there is evidence to suggest that the alternative pathway is also involved. Factor B, one of the components of this pathway, has been shown to be present at the dermal–epidermal junction (Rothfield *et al.* 1972).

Homozygous C2 deficiency is occasionally seen in lupus patients. This defect has been described in patients prior to developing the disease (Agnello *et al.* 1973; Day *et al.* 1973). A range of other complement component deficiencies has also been reported for SLE (for review, see Glass and Schur 1977). All these observations are consistent with the views of Schifferli and Peters (1983) that deficiency in the complement pathway can predispose an individual to immune complex disease.

Acute phase proteins

Unlike patients with rheumatoid arthritis, C-reactive protein (C-RP) is not generally present in high concentrations (usually less than 100 mg/ml) in the sera of lupus patients unless there is superimposed infection (Honig *et al.* 1977; Becker *et al.* 1980). However, exceptions occur on occasions (Lauter *et al.* 1979), and we have noted that modest increases of C-RP accompany disease exacerbations in some patients (Morrow *et al.* 1981). Similarly, the serum amyloid P component is often seen to be elevated in autoimmune diseases, but levels are not raised in lupus.

Cellular dysregulation

The diversity of clinical features observed in patients with lupus is matched by the many functional defects identified in cells of the immune system. In Table 4.12 the major cellular and cytokine abnormalities that have been reported in patients with lupus are shown. There is a notable increase in activated B lymphocytes, which contributes to the frequently observed hypergammaglobulinaemia. On circulating B cells, receptors for the cytokine IL-2 are increased while the CR-1 (receptor for C3b) expression is decreased. There is increased cytoplasmic and surface expression of heat shock protein 90 on B cells (and CD4+ T cells) compared with normal cells (reviewed in Twomey *et al.* 1996). The mechanism for the surface expression

is uncertain but may be analogous to the surface expression of nuclear antigens that is a feature of apoptosis. CD4+ cells bearing the CD45R+ phenotype show a marked reduction in patients with lupus. This population of cells is important as it helps to induce suppression by providing a signal to the CD8+ T cell population. This may explain why hyperactive B cells are not suppressed. Alternatively, anti-T cell antibodies may be playing a critical role. Indeed, the titres of such antibodies have been reported to show a correlation with disease activity (Yamada *et al.* 1993).

Rajagopalan *et al.* (1990), in a study of activated T cells cloned *in vitro* from patients with lupus, reported that only 15% provided help for B cells to make pathogenic DNA antibodies. Most of these cells were CD4+ T lymphocytes expressing the classical α,β T cell receptor, but 17% were CD4-, CD8- (double negative), many of which expressed the alternative γ,δ T cell receptor, which proliferated in response to endogenous heat shock or stress proteins of the hsp60 family expressed by lupus B cells. Sequencing of the T cell receptors showed Vδ and Vγ gene usage, not found in normal healthy adults and resembling that of fetal lymphocytes in early ontogeny.

T cells from patients with lupus have been shown to have increased DNA mutations, which might result in T cell death and an increased release of non-degraded DNA by necrosis rather than apoptosis, which could in turn contribute to the production of anti-DNA antibodies.

Table 4.11   Common DNA antibody idiotypes in patients with SLE and control groups

Idiotype	SLE	SLE relatives	SLE spouses	RA	Normals
16/6	40	24	10	25	4
32/15	23	7	NK	11	1
134	45	30	0	NK	1
37	90	85	NK	NK	NK
AM	85	NK	NK	90	0
PR4	70	4	0	40	3
BEG-2	8	5	0	23	7
F4	59	NK	NK	NK	2
8.12	48	NK	NK	NK	0
TOF	91	NK	NK	NK	4
4.6.3	90	NK	NK	NK	24
B3	20	NK	NK	1	0
9G4	45	NK	NK	4	2

Values shown are percentages.
NK = not known.
Original references to all of these idiotypic frequencies are reported in Watts and Isenberg (1990), except for B3 (see Ehrenstein *et al.* 1994) and 9G4 (Isenberg *et al.* 1993).

Several authors have suggested that a biochemical defect of T cells underlies the impairment of T cell responses in patients with systemic lupus. There are two possible defects in the T cell cAMP pathway. The first occurs at the level of adenylate cyclase and the other at the level of cAMP-dependent protein kinase. Cross-linking of surface receptors and lymphocyte movement to sites of inflammation (homing) have effects on the cAMP pathway. These events enhance the intracellular turnover of cAMP, promote occupancy of cAMP receptors, activate cAMP-dependent phosphorylation, and induce directed mobility of surface molecules to a pole of the cell (capping). The cAMP pathway thus mediates the mobility of certain transmembrane and glycolipid-anchored cell surface molecules, resulting in ligands bound to T cell membrane molecules being selectively internalized or cleared from the cell surface by capping and endocytosis, or by shedding.

T cells from lupus patients (unlike those from normal individuals) show markedly abnormal capping of cell surface proteins (CD4 and CD8) during active and inactive disease and show decreased cAMP production in response to adenosine, associated with an inability to switch phenotype and express suppressor activity. Cell-permeable cAMP does not bypass potential adenylate cyclose defects or restore suppressor activity (reviewed by Kammer and Stein 1990).

The appearance of class II molecules, usually HLA-DR, on T cells is taken as a mark of activation. Peripheral T cells with increased expression of HLA-DP at the cell surface and as mRNA transcripts have been found in patients with lupus. The frequency of HLA-DP expression has been reported to exceed that of HLA-DR and to correlate with disease activity. The ratio of HLA-DP+ T cells is inversely proportional to the extent of IL-2 production during *in vitro* response to mitogens (Kanai *et al.* 1993).

Antigen-specific T cells have been cloned from patients with lupus. Patients who have circulating antibodies to ribosomal P2 proteins have T cells that can proliferate *in vitro* to recombinant P2 and are inhibited in the presence of antibodies to MHC class II antigens. These T cells were CD4-positive and thus may help B cells to produce adjuvant-specific antibodies (Crow *et al.* 1994). HLA-DR-restricted T cells have also been cloned from a patient with lupus and shown to induce IgG antibodies *in vitro* from high density, activated B cells from DR-matched patients with lupus, and IgM anti-DNA antibodies from B cells from DR-matched normal individuals (Murakami *et al.* 1992).

For the last few years there has been an increasing focus on the role of cytokines in patients with lupus. The major cytokine effects are shown in Table 4.12. Of the interleukins, there has been particular emphasis on IL-2, IL-6, and IL-10. Studies *in vitro* on the response to IL-2 of the CD4+ T cell subset indicate that there is altered expression of IL-2 receptors. The CD8+ T cell subset has IL-2 receptors but fails to respond if there is no IL-2 signal from CD4+ T cells. This is a secondary defect. The primary disorder relates to the CD4+ subset which expresses IL-2 receptors of low affinity. Functional IL-2 receptors are of high affinity. Variable synthesis of both types of receptors may be governed by altered intracellular synthesis and transport.

IL-10 is a potent *in vitro* inducer of B lymphocyte differentiation as well as an inhibitor of T cells and antigen-presenting cells. It has been shown that the peripheral blood mononuclear cells in treated lupus patients express the IL-10 gene at higher levels than normal controls and that these cells in lupus patients spontaneously release large amounts of IL-10 (Llorente *et al.* 1995). Furthermore, spontaneous immunoglobulin production from peripheral blood mononuclear cells on lupus patients is increased in response to IL-10 and inhibited in response to an anti-IL-10 monoclonal antibody. There is also evidence that disease severity in patients with lupus correlates with an increased ratio of IL-10-secreting PBMCs. It has been shown that treatment of NZ/BW F_1 mice with an anti-IL-10 monoclonal delayed the onset of autoimmune manifestations including peripheral blood mononuclear cells autoantibodies. Interestingly, IL-10 has also been shown to enhance the expression of Hsp90 in PBMCs from normal individuals and may thus be linked to the overexpression of Hsp90 in lupus patients (A Stefanou, DA Isenberg, DS Latchman, unpublished observations).

Tumour necrosis factor-α (TNF-α) is produced by T and B lymphocytes, natural killer cells, and mononuclear phagocytic cells. TNF-β, originally called lymphotoxin, is produced by activated lymphocytes. The genes for both TNF-α and -β are closely linked and located within the MHC. Elevated production is found in DR3- and DR4-positive subjects, whereas low production was found in DR2- and DQW1-positive donors. The DR2, DQ1 genotype in patients with lupus is associated with lupus nephritis in some populations. It is intriguing that monoclonal antibodies to TNF-α have been used as a form of treatment for rheumatoid arthritis (discussed in detail in Chapter 5) and that a side-effect seen in 5–10% of these patients is

Table 4.12   Cellular abnormalities and cytokine dysregulation

Cell type/cytokine	Dysregulation
Monocyte/macrophages	↓ TNF-α production — genetic defect
Lymphocytes	
B cells	↑ Numbers, activated B cells → hypergammaglobulinaemia → IgG autoantibodies reactive with self-antigens (cell membrane, cytoplasmic proteins, nuclear antigens, extracellular proteins) and non-self (polyclonal)
	↑ IL-2R, ↓ CR1 expression, ↑ surface expression of hsp90 but not hsp70 compared with normal cells
T cells	↓ CD4⁺CD45R⁺ (subset Th, suppressor/inducer)
	↑↑ CD4–8-TCR-αβ⁺Th (escape thymic deletion since double negative?)
In vivo	IFN-γ-activated T cells are class II + (DP, DR)
	Defective suppression
	Impaired cytotoxicity
	Activated peripheral T cells (only 15% → anti-DNA help),
	cloned → Tγ∂ cells reactive with hsp60
In vitro	and → help to anti-DNA+ B cells (not class II restricted) (blocked by Ab to hsp65 but not hsp70)
Cytokines	
IL-1	↓ Does not activate T cells? insufficient production by accessory cells or defective T cell IL-1 receptor. Not corrected by addition of IL-1 *in vitro*.
IL-2	Normal or ↓ IL-2 production by CD4⁺ and CD8⁺ T cells. Impairment not reversed by addition of IL-2. IFN-γ +IL-2 restores T cell proliferation *in vitro*? functional activity v/s level of IL-2. Low affinity IL-2 R [receptors] expressed on CD4⁺ T cells.
IL-4	↑ IL-4 (Ag primed T cells → IL-4 → all B cells)
IL-6	↑ in many patients.
IL-10	↑ in patients. Administration accelerates disease in NZB/W mice.
	Antibodies against IL-10 delay disease onset and ↑ TNF-α.
TNF-α	MHC-linked production, probably protective, therefore levels may be critical.
IFN-γ	Normal levels produced. NK cells refractory.
	Administration of rIL-2 exacerbates disease.

TNF-α, tumour necrosis factor; IL-2R: interleukin-2 receptor; hsp, heat shock protein; Th, T helper cell; TCR, T-cell receptor; IFN-γ, interferon-8; MHC, major histocompatibility complex; NK, natural killer cells; rIL-2, recombinant interleukin 2.
[Adapted from Table 14, Chapter 5.7.1 in *Oxford Textbook of Rheumatology*, 2nd edn. Oxford University Press, with permission.]

the production of anti-DNA antibodies. The reasons for this remain tantalizing but may be due to increased production of IL-10.

Both macrophage- and natural killer cell-mediated cytotoxicity are frequently impaired in patients with lupus. Gamma-interferon-induced enhancement of both types of cytotoxicity is also impaired despite normal levels of IFN-γ production by lupus Th1 cells. Lupus natural killer cells fail to release soluble factors necessary for killing. Recombinant FN-γ has been shown to exacerbate disease in patients with lupus (Machold and Smolen 1990) and in lupus-prone mouse strains (Jacob *et al.* 1990).

Cell adhesion molecules

As leucocytes in the peripheral blood roll in the direction of blood flow, random contact is made with the blood vessel endothelium. Transient adhesion of leucocytes to the endothelium occurs by low-affinity binding to E-selectins. The cells become activated and then bind with higher affinity to vascular integrins. When cells are firmly attached, transendothelial migration occurs and, under the influence of extravascular chemoattractants, some endothelial migration into the extracellular matrix follows.

Ng *et al.* (1998) have described a intracellular signalling defect associated with a β1 integrin and autoantibody production in 20% of SLE patients studied.

Upregulation of the surface expression of E-selectin, VCAM-1, and ICAM-1 has been shown in biopsies of clinically uninvolved skin from 16 patients with lupus. Levels of adhesion molecules were directly correlated with disease activity and in serial biopsy specimens they decrease with clinical improvement (Belmont *et al.* 1994). These findings suggest that excessive complement activation in association with primed endothelial cells, can induce leucocyte endothelial cell adhesion and leuco-occlusive vasculopathy. Furthermore, ultraviolet radiation of keratinocytes *in vitro* induces the release of epidermal and dermal cytokines and increases ICAM-1 expression, which, *in vivo*, may lead to vascular activation, culminating in a photosensitivity typical of some patients with lupus.

Soluble forms of adhesion molecules are elevated in the circulation of patients with lupus, compared with healthy controls. Elevated levels of soluble ICAM-1 have been reported to show significant association with skin involvement in disease activity (see Sfikakis *et al.* 1994). Lupus patients also have elevated levels of a soluble form of VCAM-1 (Wellicome *et al.* 1993). The importance of these observations may become apparent from studies in murine lupus which have demonstrated upregulation of ICAM in nephritic MRL/*lpr*/*lpr* and NZB/W kidneys, particularly in the brush borders of proximal tubules, the glomerular mesangium, and the endothelium of large vessels (Wuthrich *et al.* 1990). Similarly, VCAM-1 is also upregulated in MRL/*lpr*/*lpr* kidneys, not only in the endothelium, but also in cortical tubules and glomeruli. Kidney tissue sections from nephritic MRL/*lpr*/*lpr* mice also display increased adhesiveness for T cell and macrophage cell lines, which can be blocked by monoclonal antibodies to ICAM-1 and VCAM-1 (Wuthrich 1992).

Apoptosis

In the last few years it has become clear that the process of programmed cell death, or apoptosis, is likely to be dysfunctional in a variety of autoimmune diseases. It is thought to be the mechanism of T cell depletion in the thymus and is the cytotoxic mechanism induced by cytotoxic T cells, natural killer cells, and cytokines such as lymphotoxin and tumour necrosis factor. Thus, inappropriate deletion or lack of depletion of certain lymphocyte subpopulations is likely to lead to immune dysregulation.

The intracellular signalling pathways that lead to apoptosis are not fully elucidated but are thought to follow the pathways indicated in Figure 4.15. The cell surface receptors associated with apoptosis, Fas (APO-1 or CD95), and tumour necrosis factor receptor-1 (TNFR-1), upon activation by their cognate ligands, become attached to cytosolic adaptor proteins which then recruit FLICE (caspase-8) to activate the interleukin-1β-converting enzyme (ICE) family protease (caspase) cascade. Activation of these caspases

during apoptosis results in the cleavage of crucial cellular substrates including poly-ADP-ribose polymerase and lamins, leading to the dramatic morphological changes seen in apoptosis. The receptor-interacting protein (RIP), associated with both receptors, may also play a part in apoptosis through the activation of sphingomyelinase and the subsequent release of ceramide from membrane-associated sphingolipids, as shown in the figure. The part played by Bcl-2 in these pathways, either as a suppressor or promoter of cell death, is not yet clear; this molecule is discussed further below.

Rose *et al.* (1997) have recently reviewed defects in the regulation of lymphocyte survival in patients with SLE. It is now recognized that mice with mutations of the *Fas* gene product (*lpr* and *lpr*[cg]) or the Fas ligand (C3H*gld*) and mice transgenic for overexpression of *bcl*-2 develop prolonged B cell survival and other features in common with SLE patients, suggesting that these molecules, which both play critical roles in apoptosis, may play a role in the pathogenesis of SLE. To date however, there is no good evidence that patients with SLE have any mutations of the genes for *Fas* or the Fas ligand. However two recent reports describe a total of eight children (two siblings, and six unrelated children) with mutations in *Fas* (Fisher *et al.* 1995; Rieux-Laucat *et al.* 1995). All patients had clinical and immunological features similar to those seen in *lpr* mice, i.e. lymphoproliferative syndrome and a large proportion of peripheral and splenic T cells expressing neither CD4 nor CD8. Fas-mediated apoptosis was detected in T cells from all eight children. Some of the children had clinically significant autoimmune disorders, including haemolytic anaemia, neutropaenia, and thrombocytopaenia.

Bcl-2

Bcl-2 was identified originally because of its involvement in the majority of non-Hodgkin's B cell lymphomas, where a (14:18) interchromosomal translocation juxtaposes the *bcl*-2 gene with the immunoglobulin heavy chain locus, leading to transcription of high levels of *bcl*-2, which enhance cell survival. Strasser *et al.* (1991) maintained *bcl*-2 transgenic mice for long enough periods to show that those mice expressing the transgene in their B cells were prone to developing an autoimmune disease resembling lupus. After one year 60% were terminally ill, with death primarily resulting from an immune complex glomerulonephritis.

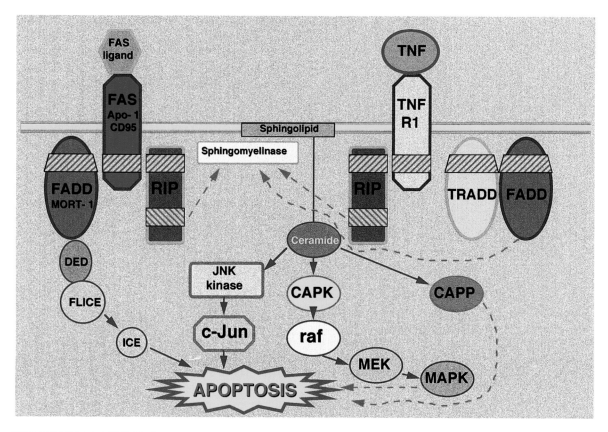

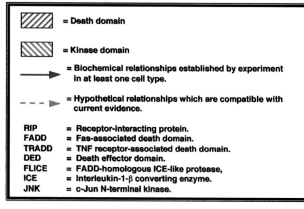

Fig. 4.15. Signal transduction pathways leading to cellular dysregulation and apoptosis.

There have been a number of studies with rather different results about whether bcl-2 expression is altered in lymphocytes from patients with lupus and healthy controls. On balance, the evidence favours the notion that bcl-2 expression is enhanced in a proportion of T cells, but not in B cells in the peripheral blood of patients with SLE. Enhanced bcl-2 expression by T cells in patients with lupus correlates somewhat with overall disease activity, regardless of the activity index employed. However, bcl-2 is simply one of a family of closely related molecules some of which, e.g. bcl-X$_L$, also suppress cell death while others, e.g. Bax, promote cell death. These bcl-2 family members are known to dimerize (hence the alliterative title 'the duelling dimers of death'!) and the mechanisms by which they regulate apoptosis are the subject of considerable scrutiny. Bcl-2, for example, can function both as an ion channel and as an adaptor or docking protein (Reed 1997).

Heat shock proteins

As mentioned in Chapter 1, heat shock proteins (hsps) are a group of proteins with major physiological roles, particularly concerning the folding and unfolding of proteins. Extensive studies reviewed elsewhere (Twomey *et al.* 1996) have shown that there is a notable association between hsp90 and SLE. In brief, approximately 30% of lupus patients, especially those with active cardiovascular, respiratory, and central nervous system involvement, are liable to overexpress hsp90 in their peripheral blood mononuclear cells. Furthermore, some 20% of lupus patients have been shown to surface express this protein, which is usually found in the cytoplasm, and between 25% and 35% of lupus patients have antibodies to the protein. These phenomena are particularly associated with lupus patients who lack the HLA A1 B8 DR3 haplotype commonly found among Caucasian lupus patients. As hsps have been shown to be immunodominant antigens during bacterial and mycobacterial infections, it may be hypothesized that, provided the other predisposing factors are present, following an initial exposure to exogenous hsps, a second event, such as a viral infection, could lead to the up-regulation of human hsp90 and/or surface localization, which could in turn induce antibodies and T cells primed against the bacterial or even protozoan protein to react against the human protein and thus be an important triggering event in autoimmunity.

The potential importance of hsp90 in at least a subset of patients is emphasized by observations in the MRL/*lpr* mouse, which confirm that hsp90 was elevated in the splenocytes of these animals (when compared with the MRL[+/+] and BALB/c controls) and that this increased expression preceded the onset of the disease. In addition, antibodies to hsp90 were detected in these mice shortly before the development of antibodies to double stranded DNA. There are also some theoretical reasons for believing that hsp90 expression may be linked to that of the Fas antigen.

Management of SLE

The treatment of patients with lupus not only includes drug therapy but certain general advice. These include avoidance of undue stress, infection, diet, and photoprotection (Table 4.13). A significant problem facing physicians caring for patients with lupus is trying to be sure which of their symptoms are actually a result of the disease. On occasion this can be difficult.

Modern pharmacological treatment of SLE began in the 1950s with the introduction of corticosteroids, nitrogen mustards, antibiotics, and anti-inflammatory drugs. Four main groups of drugs are used in the treatment of lupus patients — non-steroidal anti-inflammatory drugs (NSAIDs), antimalarials, corticosteroids, and immunosuppressives. The general indications for the use of each class of drug is given in Table 4.14, together with more specific considerations regarding initial doses and duration of treatment in Table 4.15.

The treatment of lupus patients must be tailored to suit each individual with appropriate combination of drugs to control the disease manifestations present. The patient with mild disease can usually be managed with NSAIDs together with antimalarials. Cutaneous disease

Table 4.13   General measures in treatment of SLE

Avoid stress	Rest as appropriate
Photoprotection	Avoid bright sunlight Use high factor (25–30) sun blocks
Infection control	High index of suspicion in febrile patients Vaccination for foreign travel Influenza and pneumococcal vaccine Consider prophylaxis for dental and GU procedures

Pregnancy	Contraception when active disease
	Contraception when using cytotoxic drugs
	Avoid medium or high oestrogen contraceptive pills — progesterone
	   only or the lowest possible oestrogen pill
	   (or other methods) are advised

Hormone replacement	Controversial, many patients tolerate without exacerbating disease activity
Diet	Use a low fat diet and consider adding fish oil derivatives

Table 4.14   Drug therapy in systemic lupus erythematosus

Feature	NSAID	Antimalarial	Corticosteroid	Immunosuppressive drugs
Malaise	−	+	+	−
Fever	+	−	+	−
Serositis	+	−	+	−
Arthralgia	+	+	+	−
Arthritis	+	+	+	+
Myalgia	+	+	+	−
Myositis	−	−	+	+
Malar/discoid rash	−	+	+[a]	−
Pneumonitis	−	−	+	+
Carditis	−	−	+	+
Vasculitis	−	−	+	+
CNS disease	−	−	?[b]	?
Renal	−	−	+	+
Haemolytic anaemia	−	−	+	+
Thrombocytopaenia	−	−	+	+
Raynaud's	−	−	?	?
Alopecia	−	−	?	?

+ = usually beneficial; − = not beneficial; ? = dubious/controversial.
NSAID = non steroidal anti-inflammatory drug.
[a] Widely prescribed but doubts remain that corticosteroids are beneficial in many cases.
[b] May use topical corticosteroids.

Table 4.15   Recommendations for drug usage in systemic lupus erythematosus

Symptom	Drugs to try	Comment
Arthralgia	NSAIDs	No special recommendations.
Myalgia Lethargy Arthralgia	Hydroxychloroquine	Start at 400 mg/day for 3–4 months, reducing to 200 mg/day for 3–4 months, then to 200 mg 5 × per week for 3–4 months. Repeat courses may be necessary. Pretreatment ophthalmological checks are generally recommended. For cutaneous skin disease summertime treatment only may be neccesary.
Arthritis Pleuritis Pericarditis	Prednisolone	20–40 mg/day initially for 2–4 weeks, reducing in 5–10 mg steps each week, if patient responds; treatment likely to be needed for several months.
Autoimmune haemolytic anemia/thrombocytopaenia	Prednisolone +/− azathioprine	60–80 mg/day prednisolone for 1–2 weeks, reducing in 10 decrements in response to blood tests; aim to use 2.5–3.0 mg/kg azathioprine; treatment will last several months.
Renal	Prednisolone + azathioprine or cyclophosphamide	Depending on severity of renal lesion, anything from 30 to 80 mg/day prednisolone is required; cyclophosphamide can be given by intravenous bolus (750–1000 mg) monthly for 6 months, then every 3 months for up to 2 years; alternative to cyclophosphamide is azathioprine 2.5–3.0 mg/kg; treatment is likely to last several years.
Central nervous system	Prednisolone + appropriate other drugs, e.g. antidepressants, anticonvulsants	Controversial — but prednisolone (20–100 mg/day) has been used together with azathioprine or cyclophosphamide.

can be treated with topical corticosteroids combined with antimalarials. Hydroxychloroquine or mepacrine are the favoured antimalarials. Hydroxychloroquine can cause a retinopathy but this is very rare at the doses used in SLE. Patients should have a pre-treatment ophthalmological assessment.

Oral corticosteroids are required when NSAIDs and antimalarials have failed to control the disease or there is major organ involvement. Low dose prednisolone (<0.5 mg/kg/day) is often sufficient to gain control. Severe organ involvement (nephritis, vasculitis) requires treatment with a combination of corticosteroids and either azathioprine or cyclophosphamide.

The treatment of lupus nephritis is surrounded by controversy, particularly regarding the place of cyclophosphamide and azathioprine. The introduction of aggressive therapy with prednisolone, azathioprine, and cyclophosphamide has helped to improve the prognosis of SLE, with significant improvement in survival rates (Austin *et al.* 1986; Boumpas *et al.* 1992) although these claims are not universally accepted. Renal biopsy is often performed to confirm the diagnosis of lupus nephritis and to stage the renal disease. The risk of renal progression depends on the degree of sclerosis, atrophy, and fibrosis (i.e. signs of chronicity) rather than the extent of active disease (Austin *et al.* 1994). Cyclophosphamide slows progressive renal scarring (Balow *et al.* 1984) and reduces the risk of end-stage renal failure requiring dialysis or renal transplantation (Austin *et al.* 1986).

Cyclophosphamide given as intravenous boluses at monthly intervals (for 6 months, then 3 monthly for 2 years) can be added to daily oral prednisolone (Boumpas *et al.* 1992). This regimen is associated with certain toxicity particularly infertility (Boumpas *et al.* 1993), and infection (Bradley *et al.* 1989). The major risk factors for infection are nadir white count and dose of corticosteroids (Pryor *et al.* 1996). In younger female patients many groups prefer to use azathioprine as a first cytotoxic agent for lupus nephritis. Azathioprine can also reduce proteinuria and stabilize renal function (Felson and Anderson 1984).

The management of neuropsychiatric lupus is also controversial. High dose corticosteroids and immuno-suppressive agents may be helpful in treatment of encephalopathies but it must be remembered that corticosteroids, particularly in high doses, are associated with mood disturbances. Convulsions should be treated with anticonvulsants while depression responds to antidepressants.

Arterial and venous thrombosis should be treated in the conventional manner using heparin followed by warfarin. Patients with anti-phospholipid antibodies are at risk of recurrent episodes and prolonged prophylaxis is required. The risks of long-term anticoagulation must be balanced against the risks, particularly of haemorrhage. Aspirin is often used in these patients.

Treatment of pregnant lupus patients

Management of flares of lupus during pregnancy follows a similar pattern to that of the non-pregnant patient. Corticosteroids have been used extensively in pregnant SLE patients. There is now considerable experience with the use of azathioprine in pregnancy (if the maternal SLE requires it) and there has been no increased risk of congenital malformations in the exposed fetus. Other immune suppressives are contraindicated in pregnancy. Only corticosteroids should be used during lactation (reviewed in Ramsey-Goldman and Schilling 1997).

Management of neonatal lupus

Mothers known to be positive for anti-Ro and/or anti-La should have regular fetal echocardiography to detect complete heart block. Dexamethasone and plasmapheresis have both been tried in attempts to prevent development of complete heart block (Tseng and Buyon 1997). The rationale is that heart block is consequent to an inflammatory process. Permanent cardiac pace-makers may be required.

Infants with the rash of neonatal lupus need little specific therapy except avoidance of sunlight until nine months of age. The rash will fade once maternal autoantibodies have disappeared from the neonatal circulation.

Management of childhood SLE

The basic principles of treatment for SLE in childhood are the same as for adult-onset disease, although children seem to have more severe disease (Tucker *et al.* 1995), and may therefore be treated with steroids more frequently and in higher doses. There are no controlled trials of therapeutic regimes in childhood SLE, and the results from adult experience are extrapolated to child patients. Outcome data are difficult to interpret because of the small number of children at each centre (reviewed in Silverman and Lang 1997).

Experimental treatment

There is increasing interest in using other immuno-suppressive agents, such as methotrexate and the immunophilin ligands cyclosporin and tacrolimus. Methotrexate appears to be effective in controlling dermatitis and arthritis with modest steroid sparing potential (Wise *et al.* 1996). Initial studies with cyclosporin at high doses (10 mg/kg/day) were associated with significant renal impairment (Isenberg *et al.* 1981). The renal side effects have been overcome using lower doses (<5 mg/kg/day). Low dose cyclosporin can normalize complement levels, improve disease activity, lower DNA binding titres, and improve platelet and lymphocyte counts. Careful monitoring of renal function and blood pressure is necessary even with low dose treatment (Manger *et al.* 1996; Caccavo *et al.* 1997). Tacrolimus has recently been used in three cases as an alternative to cyclosporin with encouraging results (Duddridge and Powell 1998). Rapamycin has not been used in human SLE but prolongs survival in the MRL/*lpr* mouse (Warner *et al.* 1994).

Plasma exchange was popular in the 1970s, the concept being that removal of circulating, presumably pathogenic, immune complexes would be therapeutically helpful. While some patients respond well within a few days or weeks there is often a rebound with worsening of disease. Although some initial trials claimed modest benefit, six controlled studies revealed no advantage to this approach (reviewed in McClure and Isenberg 1997). For example, a controlled trial involving sham exchange in mild lupus showed that plasma exchange was of no value (Wei *et al.* 1991). Plasma exchange is now reserved for patients who are refractory to conventional immunosuppressive therapy. Synchronization of plasmapheresis with pulse cyclophosphamide (three daily plasma exchanges followed by pulse cyclophosphamide therapy) has showed promising initial results but subsequent studies have been controversial. Schroeder *et al.* (1987) demonstrated some benefit but with significant toxicity. Euler and Guilleuin (1994) produced impressive improvement in 12 of 14 patients with plasmapheresis followed by high dose (12 mg/kg) cyclophosphamide during the period of presumed clonal viability. However, in a prospective, randomized study of 151 patients from 37 centres, Schroeder and colleagues found that repeated plasma exchanges combined with subsequent pulse cyclophosphamide did not confer any additional benefit compared with cyclophosphamide alone (Schroeder *et al.* 1997). Thus the rationale for using this form of treatment seems to be even further diminished. It is possible that selective apheretic techniques in which cryoproteins, single stranded and double stranded DNA antibodies, cardiolipin antibodies, and lupus anticoagulant are removed on immunoadsorbent columns may be of benefit (Schreider *et al.* 1990). To date some promising results have been obtained using this strategy and this highly selective removal does not seem to be followed by a rebound in titres of the removed autoantibody.

Intravenous gammaglobulins are a successful treatment for autoimmune disease, including thrombocytopaenia (Dwyer 1992) and have also been used for other manifestations including neutropenia and neurological disease. Use of IVIg in severe, active SLE has produced conflicting results, including both resolution of lupus nephritis (Akashi *et al.* 1990) and exacerbation of proteinuria and renal damage (Jordan 1989) owing to glomerular deposition of immune complexes of polyreactive, non-idiotype specific IgG. There is little controlled data to support its use in conditions other than autoimmune thrombocytopaenia. More recently, IVIg has been combined with specific anti-idiotype therapy. Commercial IVIg was absorbed to produce anti-idiotype IgG to specific DNA idiotypes (F4 and 8.12). In two patients with lupus nephritis this approach resulted in a decrease in both DNA binding titres and proteinuria (Silvestris *et al.* 1996).

Diet plays a role in the therapy of lupus. All patients should be encouraged to consume a low fat diet to lessen the risk of atherosclerosis as a consequence of the disease and long term corticosteroid therapy. Diet can also affect disease activity. In a double blind, crossover study, patients taking 10 g of fish oil in addition to a low fat diet were significantly better over a three month period (Walton *et al.* 1991).

Monoclonal antibody therapy directed against T cells (anti-CD4) or B cells (anti-CD5) has been used experimentally in lupus with encouraging results (Stafford *et al.* 1994).

Recombinant IFN-γ exacerbates disease both in lupus patients (Machold and Smolen 1990) and in lupus prone mice (Jacob *et al.* 1990*b*).

Lupus has a pronounced female bias and therefore attempts have been made to treat the condition by manipulation of sex hormones. A recent double-blind, placebo controlled trial of dehydroepiandrosterone showed benefit to patients with mild to moderate SLE (van Vollenhoven *et al.* 1995).

Extracorporeal photochemotherapy (photophoresis) has been used to avoid the potentially harmful effects of light (reviewed in Cohen and Isenberg 1996). Photophoresis of MRL/l mice delays disease progression. Phototherapy improves cutaneous lesions, constitutional symptoms, and arthritis, without activating systemic disease.

Experimental therapeutics in animal models of SLE

The existence of spontaneous lupus in mice of various strains provides the opportunity to test experimental therapies *in vivo*, and a number of techniques have been explored. Initial studies were directed at the T cell, CD4 Mab ameliorated disease in both NZB/W and MRL *lpr/lpr* mice (Wofsy and Seaman 1985), with reduced autoantibody production, retardation of renal disease, and prolongation of survival (Wofsy and Seaman 1987).

Selective inhibition of the B7–CD28 or B7–CTLA4 interaction using the B7-binding protein, CTLA4–Ig, resulted in marked improvement with prolongation of life and decreased autoantibody production in NZB/W F$_1$ mice (Finck *et al.* 1994).

In NZB/W mice, administration of anti-idiotypic antibody suppress both production of anti-DNA antibodies and nephritis, however, the effect was transient and anti-DNA antibodies appeared that did not bear the idiotype (Hahn and Ebling 1984). Conjugation of anti-idiotypic antibody to neocarcinostatin (a cytotoxic agent) eliminated anti-DNA producing cells *in vitro* (Sasaki *et al.* 1986). However, Teitlebaum *et al.* 1984 reported that anti-idiotypic therapy resulted in elevation of idiotype and DNA antibody levels. Modulation of the DNA idiotype–anti-idiotype network will perturb other idiotype–anti-idiotype systems. It must be remembered that such manipulation may induce disease rather than suppress it.

The idiotypic model of autoimmune disease has been used to explore many novel treatments for autoimmune disease; however, as the model is not readily reproducible these findings have not been replicated. These approaches are reviewed in Shoenfeld *et al.* (1997).

Antibodies to dsDNA are deposited in the renal lesions, causing glomerulonephritis. Anti-DNA antibodies may cross react with renal antigens and be deposited in the kidney. Inhibition of this cross reaction could ameliorate renal lupus. Soluble peptides that inhibit renal binding of the mouse anti-DNA antibody R4A also protect mice from renal lupus (Gaynor *et al.* 1997).

An alternative approach has been to block the generation of pro-inflammatory complement components. In NZB/W female mice a Mab specific for the C5 component of complement (which blocks cleavage of C5 and prevents generation of potent pro-inflammatory factors C5a and C5b-9) was used for six months with significant amelioration in glomerulonephritis and markedly increased survival (Wang *et al.* 1996).

Somatic gene therapy is an approach to increasing circulating levels of peptide hormone cytokines. cDNA expression vectors for TGF-β and IL-2 were administered monthly to MRL/*lpr/lpr* mice. TGF-β had beneficial effects, with decrease in renal inflammation and prolongation of survival, while IL-2 resulted in an exacerbation of renal disease (Raz *et al.* 1995).

Infection of BALB/c mice with the parasite *Plasmodium chabaudi* induces high production of autoantibodies. In NZB/WF$_1$ mice, infection with the parasite retards development of autoimmune disease (Hentati *et al.* 1994). Both survival and development of proteinuria and DNA antibodies were delayed for six months when parasite inoculation was given either before (three months) or after (seven months) the onset of clinical symptoms. Similar beneficial effects, albeit less marked, were observed when mice were treated with IgG or IgM, or cryoglobulin preparations isolated from *Plasmodium chabaudi*-infected BALB/c mice. Levels of anti-DNA antibodies, particularly of the IgG1 isotype, were reduced. Preparations from uninfected mice were not effective. The mode of action is thought to arise from malarial induction of high levels of natural antibodies bearing the D23 idiotype, characteristic of polyreactive natural autoantibodies with enhanced activity against the Fab and Fc fragments of IgG. These antibodies have immunoregulatory properties and attempt to rescue a natural autoantibody network that is deficient in B/W mice (Hentati *et al.* 1994).

Cytokine manipulation has been explored as a means of therapeutic intervention. In female NZB/W mice, soluble IFN-γ R or anti-IFN-γ Mab inhibited the onset of glomerulonephritis while IFN-γ accelerated the process (Ozmen *et al.* 1995). Replacement therapy with recombinant IFN-γ delayed disease development (Jacob and McDevitt 1988). TNF-α levels in serum increased in anti-IL-10-treated NZB/W mice, while disease onset was delayed. Recombinant IL-10-accelerated disease onset (Ishida *et al.* 1994). Similarly, IL-6 promoted disease onset, but anti IL-6 Mab prevented anti-dsDNA antibody production, decreased proteinuria, and prolonged life, provided that mice attained tolerance to rat immunoglobulin by a single injection of anti-CD4 Mab at the start of therapy (Finck *et al.* 1994*b*). Treatment of MRL *lpr/lpr* mice with neutralizing antibodies to IL-6 for five weeks at 15 weeks of age improved glomerular function and histological appearance and initially decreased DNA antibodies, but these increased again by week 4 (Kiberd 1993). Disease in the MRL *lpr/lpr* mouse can be reversed by the introduction of the *fas* gene under the control of the CD2 promoter and enhancer (Wu *et al.* 1994).

Summary

SLE has been recognized for centuries, although, owing to the great diversity of symptoms and previously problematical therapy, it has been studied in depth only in relatively recent years. It may appear in a number of organ systems, although joint and skin involvement are most common. In advanced disease, almost any system in the body may be involved, with renal, cerebral and pulmonary manifestations being most dangerous to the patient. SLE has the ability to masquerade as other diseases and great care must be taken with differential diagnosis.

Typically, the disease affects women, particularly of child-bearing age, and progresses in a series of exacerbations and remissions. The 10-year survival may be as high as 95% for mild cases. The aetiology is unclear but hormonal, genetic, viral, and environmental factors seem to influence the disease. The incidence of the disorder is greatest in non-Caucasian women, although no striking association with other HLA class I or II antigens or haplotype has been demonstrated.

The disease is characterized by disorders throughout all arms of the immune response. Serologically, autoantibodies directed towards components of the cell nucleus can be detected including anti-ds and ssDNA, RNA, nucleoproteins, and histones. Anti-lymphocyte, NK cell, and neuronal antibodies may also be present. Other serological abnormalities include circulating immune complexes, hypocomplementaemia, hypergammaglobulinaemia, and occasionally, levels of acute phase protein. At the cellular level, several independent defects are evident including B cell hyperactivity, a loss of T cell suppression, and resistance to undero programmed cell death.

Animal models of spontaneously occurring lupus have helped greatly in the understanding of the disease. The NZB/W F_1 hybrid mouse has served as an excellent system for therapeutic manipulation and investigations on the immunopathology of the disease for almsot four decades. More recently, the MRL/*lpr* strain has become the favoured model as it offers a number of advantages over NZB/W, including a shorter life span (with more aggressive disease) and a congenic strain, the MRL/n, which does not develop disease and serves as a useful control. Other strains that have also proved useful are BXSB, moth-eaten, Palmerston North, and Swan.

SLE can now be diagnosed quite easily, but the assessment of disease flare has proved to be difficult. However considerable progress has been made with clinical grading schemes; the relative ease with which computerized databases can be established has greatly aided this task.

Clinical therapy is still based on a strategy of generalized immunosuppression of the unbalanced immune system. Usual treatment of the patient who does not have severe disease consists of non-steroidal anti-inflammatory drugs, salicylates, and antimalarial preparations used alone or in combination. Acute exacerbation of disease is usually controlled by increasing doses of corticosteroids or cytotoxic agents such as azathioprine or cyclophosphamide. In addition, bolus doses of intravenous steroids have also proved to be effective. The use of apheretic techniques, notably plasma exchange, which were fashionable in the 1970s and 1980s has now greatly diminished.

References

Abu-Shakra, Gladmer DD, Urowitz M. Malignancy systemic lupus erythematosus. 1996; **39**: 1250–6.

Adams LE, Mongey AB. Role of genetic factors in drug related autoimmunity. *Lupus* 1994; 3: 443–7.

Agnello V, Koffler D, Kunkel HG. Immune complex systems in the nephritis of systemic lupus erythematosus. *Kidney Int* 1973; 3: 90–9.

Ahearn JM, Provost TT, Dorsch CA *et al.* Interrelationships of HLA-DR, MB and MT phenotypes, autoantibody expression and clinical features in systemic lupus erythematosus. *Arthritis Rheum* 1982; **25**: 1031–40.

Akashi K, Nagasawa K, Mayimi T *et al.* Successful treatment of refractory systemic lupus erythematosus with intravenous immunoglobulins. *J Rheumatol* 1990; **17**: 375–9.

Alarcon-Segovia D, Cabral AR. The antiphospholipid/cofactor syndromes. *J. Rheum* 1996; **8**: 1319–20.

Andrews BS, Eisenberg RA, Theofilopoulos AN *et al.* Spontaneous murine lupus-like syndromes. Clinical and immunopathological manifestations in several strains. *J Exp Med* 1978; **148**: 1198–215.

Arnaiz-Villena A, Vazquez-Rodriguez JJ, Vicario JL *et al.* Congenital heart block immunogenetics: Evidence of an additional role of HLA class III antigens and independence of Ro autoantibodies. *Arthritis Rheum* 1989; **32**: 1421–6.

Arnett FC, Reichlin M. Lupus hepatitis: an under-recognised disease feature associated with autoantibodies to ribosomal P. *Am J Med* 1995; **99**: 465–72.

Austin HA, Boumpas DT, Vaughan EM, Balow JE. Predicting renal outcomes in severe lupus nephritis: contributions of clinical and histologic data. *Kidney Int* 1994; **45**: 544–50.

Austin HA III, Klippel JH, Balow ED *et al*. Therapy of lupus nephritis: controlled trial of prednisolone and cytotoxic drugs. *N Eng J Med* 1986; **314**: 614–9.

Balow JE, Austin HA, Muenz LR et al. Effect of treatment on the evolution of renal abnormalities in lupus nephritis. *N Engl J Med* 1984; **311**: 491–5.

Batchelor JR, Fielder AHL, Walport MJ *et al*. Family study of the major histocompatibility complex in HLA-DR3 negative patients with systemic lupus erythematosus. *Clin Exp Immunol* 1987; **70**: 364–71.

Becker GJ, Waldburger M, Hughes GRV, *et al*. Value of serum C-reactive protein measurement in the investigation of fever in systemic lupus erythematosus. *Ann Rheum Dis* 1980; **39**: 50–2.

Belmont HM, Buyon J, Giorno R *et al*. Upregulation of endothelial cell adhesion molecules characterizes disease activity in systemic lupus erythematosus. The Schwartzman phenomenon revisited. *Arthritis Rheum* 1994; **37**: 376–83.

Bettinotti MP, Hartung K, Deicher H *et al*. Polymorphism of the tumour necrosis factor beta gene in systemic lupus erythematosus: TNFB-HMC haplotypes. *Immunogenetics* 1993; **37**: 449–54.

Bielchowsky M, Helyer BJ, Howie JB. Spontaneous haemolytic anaemia in mice of the NZB/BL strain. *Proc Univ Otago Med School* 1959; **37**: 9–11.

Bombardier C, Gladman D, Urowitz MB *et al*. The development and validation of the SLE Disease Activity Index (SLEDAI). *Arthritis Rheum* 1992; **35**: 630–40.

Bonfa E, Golombek SJ, Kaufman LD *et al*. Association between lupus psychosis and anti-ribosomal P protein antibodies. *N Eng J Med* 1987; **317**: 265–71.

Bootsma H, Spronk P, Derksen R *et al*. Prevention of relapses in systemic lupus erythematosus. *Lancet* 1995; **345**: 1595–9

Boumpas DT, Austin HA III, Vaughan EM *et al*. Controlled trial of methyl prednisolone versus two regimens of pulse cyclophosphamide in severe lupus nephritis. *Lancet* 1992; **340**:741–5.

Boumpas DT, Austin HA, Vaughan EM *et al*. Risk of sustained amenorrhoea in patients with SLE receiving intermittent pulse cyclophosphamide. *Ann Intern Med* 1993; **119**: 366–9.

Bradley JD, Brandt KD, Katz BP. Infectious complications of cyclophosphamide therapy for vasculitis. *Arthritis Rheum* 1989; **32**: 45–53.

Brucato A, Franceschini F, Gasparini M *et al*. Isolated congenital complete heart block; long-term outcome of mothers, maternal antibody specificity and immunogenetic background. *J Rheumatol* 1995a; **22**: 533–40.

Brucato A, Gasparini M, Vignati G *et al*. Isolated congenital complete heart block: longterm outcome of children and immunogenetic study. *J Rheumatol* 1995b; **22**:541–3.

Burnham TK, Neblett TR, Fine G. The application of the fluorescent antibody technique to the investigation of lupus erythematosus and various dermatoses. *J Invest Dermatol* 1963; **41**: 451–6.

Buyon JP, Ben-Chetrit E, Karp S *et al*. Acquired congenital heart block. *J Clin Invest* 1989; **84**: 627–634.

Buyon JP, Slade SG, Reveille JD, Hamel JC, Chan EKL. Autoantibody responses to the 'native' 52-kDa SS-A/Ro protein in neonatal lupus syndromes, systemic lupus erythematosus, and Sjögren's syndrome. *J Immunol* 1994; **152**: 3675–84.

Caccavo D, Lagana B, Mitterhofer AP *et al*. Long-term treatment of systemic lupus erythematosus with cyclosporin A. *Arthritis Rheum* 1997; **40**: 27–35.

Cepellini R, Polli E, Celeda F. DNA-reacting factor in a serum of a patient with lupus erythematosus diffusus. *Proc Soc Exp Biol Med* 1957; **96**: 572–4.

Chinn RJS, Wilkinson ID, Hall-Craggs MA *et al*. Magnetic resonance imaging of the brain and cerebral proton spectroscopy in patients with SLE. *Arthritis Rheum* 1997; **40**: 36–46.

Cohen MR, Isenberg DA. Ultraviolet radiation in systemic lupus erythematosus: friend or foe. *Br J Rheumatol* 1996; **35**: 1002–7.

Crow MK, DelGiudice-Asch G, Zehetbauer JB *et al*. Autoantigen-specific T cell proliferation induced by the ribosomal P2 protein in patients with systemic lupus erythematosus. *J Clin Invest* 1994; **94**: 345–52.

D'Alfonso S, Colombo G, Della Bella S *et al*. Association between polymorphisms in the TNF region and systemic lupus erythematosu in the Italian population. *Tissue Antigens* 1996; **47**: 551–5.

Day NK, Geiger H, McLean R, Michael A, Good RA. C2 deficiency. Development of lupus erythematosus. *J Clin Invest* 1973; **52**: 1601–7.

Diamond B, Scharff M. Somatic mutation of the T15 heavy chain gives rise to an antibody with autoantibody specificity. *Proc Natl Acad Sci USA* 1984; **81**: 841–4.

Doherty NE, Siegel RJ. Cardiovascular manifestations of systemic lupus erythematosus. *Am Heart J* 1985; **110**: 1257–65.

Dong RP, Kimura A, Hashimoto H *et al*. Difference in HLA-linked genetic background between mixed connective tissue disease and systemic lupus erythematosus. *Tissue Antigens* 1993; **41**: 20–5.

Dubois EL, Tuffanelli DL. Clinical manifestations of systemic lupus erythematosus. Computer analysis of 520 cases. *JAMA* 1964; **190**: 104–11.

Duddridge M, Powell RJ. The treatment of severe and difficult cases of systemic lupus erythematosus with tacrolimus — a report of three cases. *Ann Rheum Dis* 1997; **58**: 125–7.

Dunckley H Gatenby PA, Hawkins B *et al*. Deficiency of C4A is a genetic determinant of SLE in three ethnic groups. *J Immunogen.* 1987; **14**: 209–18.

Dwyer JM. Manipulating the immune system with immune globulin. *N Eng J Med* 1992; **326**: 107–11.

Ehrenstein MR, Longhurst CM, Latchman DS *et al*. The serologic and genetic characterisation of a human monoclonal anti-DNA idiotype. *J Clin Invest* 1994; **93**: 1787–97.

Ehrenstein MR, Katz DR, Griffiths M *et al*. Human IgG anti-DNA antibodies deposit in kidneys and induce proteinuria in SCID mice. *Kid Intn* 1995; **48**: 705–11.

Ehrfeld H, Hartung K, Renz M *et al*. MHC associations of autoantibodies against recombinant Ro and La proteins in systemic lupus erythematosus. *Rheumatol Int* 1992; **12**: 169–73.

Elliot JA, Mathieson DR. Complement in disseminated (systemic) lupus erythematosus. *Arch Derm* (Chicago) 1953; **65**: 170–6.

Esdaile JM, Mackenzie T, Barré P *et al*. Can experienced clinicians predict the outcome of lupus nephritis. *Lupus* 1992; **1**: 205–14.

Estes D, Christian CL. The natural history of systemic lupus erythematosus by prospective analysis. *Medicine* 1971; **50**: 85–95.

Euler HH, Guillevin L. Plasmapheresis and subsequent pulse cyclophosphamide in severe systemic lupus erythematosus. An interim report of the Lupus Plasmapheresis Study Group. *Ann Intern Med* 1994; **145**: 296–302.

Feinglass EJ, Arnett FC, Sorsch CA *et al*. Neuropsychiatric manifestations of systemic lupus erythematosus: diagnosis, clinical spectrums, and relationship to other features of the disease. *Medicine* 1976; **66**: 323–32.

Felson DT, Anderson J. Evidence for the superiority of immunosuppressive drugs and prednisolone over prednisolone alone in lupus nephritis. Results of a pooled analysis. *N Eng J Med* 1984; **311**: 1528–33.

Finck BK, Chan B, Wofsy D. Interleukin-6 promotes murine lupus in in NZB/NZW F1 mice. *J Clin Invest* 1994a; **94**: 585–91.

Finck BK, Linsley PS, Wofsy D. Treatment of murine lupus with CTLA4Ig. *Science* 1994b; **265**: 1225–7.

Fisher GH, Rosenberg FJ, Straus SE *et al*. Dominant interfering Fas gene mutations impair apoptosis in a human autoimmune lymphoproliferative syndrome. *Cell* 1995; **81**: 935–46.

Fishman D, Isenberg DA. Splenic involvement in the autoimmune rheumatic diseases. *Sem Arthritis Rheum* 1997; **27**: 141–55.

Fox R, Isenberg DA. Antibodies to ribosomal P — where are we now. *Jap J Rheumatol* 1997; **7**: 235–46.

Fox R, Reichlin MW, Reichlin M *et al*. Liver function test abnormalities in systemic lupus erythematosus (SLE) (abst). *Brit J Rheumatol* 1997; **36**: S16.

Freedman BI, Spray BJ, Heise ER *et al*. A race-controlled human leukocyte antigen frequency analysis in lupus nephritis. *Am J Kid Dis* 1993; **21**: 378–82.

Fronek Z, Timmerman LA, Alper CA *et al*. Major histocompatibility complex genes and susceptibility to systemic lupus erythematosus. *Arthritis Rheum* 1990; **33**: 1542–53.

Friou GJ. Clinical applications of lupus serum–nucleoprotein reaction using fluorescent antibody technique. *J Clin Invest* 1957; **86**: 890.

Friou GJ, Finch SC, Detre KD. Interaction of nuclei and globulin from lupus erythematosus serum demonstrated with fluorescent antibody. *J Immunol* 1958; **80**: 224–9.

Fritzler MJ. Drugs recently associated with lupus syndromes. *Lupus* 1994; **3**: 445–9.

Furie RA, Chartash EK. Tendon rupture in systemic lupus erythematosus. *Sem Arthritis Rheum* 1988; **18**: 127–33.

Galli M, Compurius P, Maassen C *et al*. Anticardiolipin antibodies (ACA) directed not to cardiolipin but to a plasma protein co-factor. *Lancet* 1990; **335**: 1544–7.

Gavalchin J, Datta SK. The NZB x SWR model of lupus nephritis II. Autoantibodies deposited in renal lesions show a distinctive and restricted idiotypic diversity. *J Immunol* 1987; **138**: 138–46.

Gaynor B, Putterman C, Valadon P *et al*. Peptide inhibition of glomerular deposition of an anti-DNA antibody. *Proc Natl Acad Sci USA* 1997; **94**: 1955–60.

Gladman DD, Urowitz MB, Goldsmith CH. The reliability of the systemic lupus international collaborating clinics/ American College of Rheumatology damage index in patients with systemic lupus erythematosus. *Arthritis Rheum* 1997; **40**: 809–13.

Glass D, Schur P. Autoimmunity and systemic lupus erythematosus. In *Autoimmunity. Genetic, Immunologic, Virologic and Clinical Aspects*.

Gold S. Role of suphonamides and penicillin in the pathogenesis of systemic lupus erythematosus. *Lancet* 1951; **1**: 268–72.

Goldstein R, Sengar PS. Comparative studies of the major histocompatibility complex in French Canadian and Non-French Canadian Caucasians with systemic lupus erythematosus. *Arthritis Rheum* 1993; **36**: 1121–7.

Gotoff SP. Isaacs EW, Mvchrcke RC *et al*. Serum beta Ic globulin in glomeronephritis and systemic lupus erythematosus. *Am Intern Med* 1969; **71**: 327–33.

Governman J, Woods A, Larson L *et al*. Transgenic mice that express a myelin basic protein-specific T cell receptor develop spontaneous autoimmunity. *Cell* 1993; **72**: 551–60.

Griffey EH, Brown MS, Bankhurst AD *et al*. Depletion of high energy phosphates in the central nervous system of patients with systemic lupus erythematosus, as determined by phosphorus-31 nuclear magnetic spectroscopy. *Arthritis Rheum* 1990; **73**: 827–33.

Hahn BH, Ebling FM. Suppression of NZB/NZW murine nephritis by administration of a synergeic monoclonal antibody to DNA. *J Clin Invest* 1983; **71**: 728–36.

Hahn BH, Ebling FM. Suppression of murine lupus nephritis by administration of an anti-idiotype to anti-DNA. *J Immunol* 1984; **134**: 187–90.

Hajeer AH, Worthington J, Davies EJ *et al*. TNF microsatellite a2, b3 and d2 alleles are associated with systemic lupus erythematosus. *Tissue Antigens* 1997; **49**: 222–7.

Hamilton R, Harley J, Bias W *et al*. Two Ro (SS-A) autoantibody responses in systemic lupus erythematosus. Correlation of HLA-DR/DQ specificities with quantitative expression of Ro (SSA) autoantibody. *Arthritis Rheum* 1988; **31**: 496–505.

Hang LH, Theofilopoulos AN, Dixon FJ. A spontaneous rheumatoid arthritis-like disease in MRL/l mice. *J Exp Med* 1982; **155**: 1690–1701.

Hanley JG, Walsh NMG, Risk JD *et al*. Cognitive impairment and autoantibodies in systemic lupus erythematosus. *Br J Rheumatol* 1993; **31**: 1472–9.

Hardie R, Isenberg DA. Tetraplegia as a presenting feature of systemic lupus erythematosus complicated by pulmonary hypertension. *Ann Rheum Dis* 1985; **44**: 491–3.

Hargreaves MM, Richmond H, Morton R. Presentation of two bone marrow elements: the 'tart' and 'L.E.' cell. *Proc Staff Meet Mayo Clin* 1948; **23**: 25–8.

Harley BJ, Sestak AL, Willis LG *et al*. A model for disease heterogeneity in systemic lupus erythematosus. *Arthritis Rheum* 1989; **32**: 826–36.

Hashimoto H, Nishimura Y, Dong RP *et al*. HLA antigens in Japanese patients with systemic lupus erythematosus. *Scan J Rheumatol* 1994; **23**: 191–6.

Haupt HM, Moore WG, Hutchins GM. The lung in systemic erythematosus. Analysis of the pathologic changes in 120 patients. *Am J Med* 1981; **71**: 791–7.

Hawkins BR, Wong KI, Wong RWS *et al*. Strong association between the major histocompatibility complex and SLE in Southern Chinese. *J Rheumatol* 1987; **14**: 1128–31.

Hay EM, Bacon PA, Gordon C et al. The BILAG index: a reliable and valid instrument for measuring clinical disease activity in systemic lupus erythematosus. *Q J Med* 1993; **86**: 447–58.

Hay EM, Black D, Huddy A et al. A prospective study of psychiatric disorder and cognitive function in systemic lupus erythematosus. *Ann Rheum Dis* 1994; **53**: 298–303.

Helyer BJ, Howie JB. Renal disease associated with positive lupus erythematosus tests in cross-bred strains of mice. *Nature* 1963; **197**: 197.

Hentati B, Sato MN, Payelle-Brogard B et al. Beneficial effect of polyclonal immunoglobulins from malaria infected BALB/c mice on the lupus-like syndrome of (NZB × NZW)F1 mice. Eur J Immunol 1994; **24**: 8–15.

Hochberg MC. Updating the American College of Rheumatology revised criteria for the classification of systemic lupus erythematosus. *Arthritis Rheum* 1997; **9**: 1725.

Hoffbrand BI, Beck ER. 'Unexplored' dyspnoea and shrinking lungs in systemic lupus erythematosus. *Br. Med J* 1965; **1**: 1273–7.

Honig S, Gorevic P, Weissman G. C-reactive protein in systemic lupus erythematosus. *Arthritis Rheum* 1977; **20**: 1065–9.

Howard PF, Hochberg MC, Bias WB et al. Relationship between C4A null genes, HLA-D region antigens and genetic susceptibility to SLE in Caucasian and Black Americans. *Am J Med* 1986; **81**: 187–93.

Isenberg DA, Collins C. Detection of cross-reactive anti-DNA idiotypes on renal tissue bound immunoglobulins from lupus patients. *J Clin Invest* 1985; **76**: 287–94.

Isenberg DA. Immunoglobulin deposition in skeletal muscles in primary muscles disease. *Quart J Med* 1983; **52**: 297–310.

Isenberg DA, Malick J. Male lupus — the Loch Ness syndrome revisited. *Br J Rheumatol* 1994; **33**: 307–8.

Isenberg DA, Snaith ML, Morrow WJW et al. Cyclosporin A for the treatment of systemic lupus erythematosus. *Int J Immunopharmacol* 1981; **3**: 163–5.

Isenberg DA, Meyrick-Thomas D, Snaith ML et al. A study of migraine in SLE. *Ann Rheum Dis* 1982; **41**: 33–5.

Isenberg D, Williams W, Axford J et al. Comparison of DNA antibody idiotypes in human sera: an international collaborative study of 19 idiotypes from 11 different laboratories. J Autoimmun 1990; **3**: 393–414.

Isenberg DA, Katz D, Le Page S et al. Independent analysis of the 16/6 idiotype lupus model. *J Immunol* 1991; **147**: 4172–7.

Isenberg DA, Spellerberg M, Williams W et al. Identification of a role for the 9G4 idiotope in systemic lupus erythematosus. *Br J Rheumatol* 1993; **32**: 876–82.

Isenberg DA, Steiner G, Smolen J. Clinical utility and serological connections of RA-33 antibodies in SLE. *J Rheumatol* 1994; **32**: 1515–20.

Isenberg DA, Garton M, Reichlin MW et al. Long term follow up of autoantibody profiles in black female lupus patients and clinical comparison with Caucasian and Asian patients. *Br J Rheumatol* 1997; **36**: 229–33.

Isenberg DA, Shoenfeld Y, Walport M et al. Detection of cross-reactive anti-DNA antibody idiotypes is the serum of patients who have systemic lupus erythematosus and their relatives. *Arthritis Rheum* 1985; **28**: 999–1207.

Ishida H, Muchamuel T, Sakaguchi S et al. Continuous administration of anti-interleukin-10 antibodies delays onset of autoimmunity in NZB/W F1 mice. *J Exp Med* 1994; **179**: 301–10.

Jacob CO, McDevitt HO. Tumour necrosis factor α in murine autoimmune 'lupus' nephritis. *Nature* 1988; **331**: 356–8.

Jacob CO, Fronek Z, Lewis GD et al. Heritable major histocompatiblity complex class II-associated differences in production of tumor necrosis factor : Relevance to genetic predisposition to systemic lupus erythematosus. *Proc Natl Acad Sci, USA* 1990a; **87**:1233–7.

Jacob CO, van der Meide PH, McDevitt HO. In vivo treatment of (NZBxNZW)F1 lupus-like nephritis with monoclonal antibody to γ interferon. *J Exp Med* 1990b; **166**: 798–803.

Jefferies R. Idiotypes and idiotypic networks: a time to redefine concepts. *Clin Exp Immunol* 1993; **91**: 193–5.

Johnson AE, Gordon C, Palmer RG et al. The prevalence and incidence of systemic lupus erythematosus (SLE) in Birmingham UK, related to ethnicity and country of birth. *Arthritis Rheum* 1995; **38**: 551–8.

Jordan SC. Intravenous gamma globulin therapy in systemic lupus erythematosus and immune complex disease. *Clin Immunol Immunopathol* 1989; **53**: S164–9.

Julkunen H, Siren MK, Kaaja R et al. Maternal HLA antigens and antibodies to SS-A/Ro and SS-B/La. Comparison with systemic lupus erythematosus and primary Sjögren's syndrome. *Br J Rheumatol* 1995; **34**: 901–7.

Kachru RB, Sequire W, Mittal KK et al. A significant increase of HLA-DR3 and DR2 in SLE among blacks. *J Rheumatol* 1984; **11**: 471–4.

Kaell AT, Shetty M, Lee BCP et al. The diversity of neurologic events in systemic lupus erythematosus. *Arch Neurol* 1986; **43**: 273–6.

Kalunian K, Panosian-Sahakian N, Ebling F et al. Idiotypic characteristics of immunoglobulins associated with systemic lupus erythematosus. *Arthritis Rheum* 1989; **32**: 513–22.

Kammer GM, Stein RL. T lymphocyte dysfunctions in systemic lupus erythematosus. *J Lab Clin Med* 1990; **115**: 273–82.

Kanai Y, Kawaminami Y, Miwa M et al. Naturally occurring antibodies to poly (ADP-ribose) in patients with systemic lupus erythematosus. *Nature* 1977; **205**: 175–7.

Kanai Y, Tokano Y, Tsuda H et al. HLA-DP positive T cells in patients with polymyositis/dermatomyositis. *J Rheumatol* 1993; **20**: 77–9.

Kaneko F, Tanji O, Hasegawa T et al. Neonatal lupus erythematosus in Japan. *J Am Acad Dermatol* 1992; **26**: 397–403.

Keeling D, Isenberg DA. Haematological manifestations of systemic lupus erythematosus. *Blood Rev* 1993; 7: 199–207.

Khamashta MA, Cervera R, Asherson RA et al. Association of antibodies against phospholipids with heart valve disease in systemic lupus erythematosus. *Lancet* 1990; **335**: 1541–4.

Kiberd BA. Interleukin-6 receptor blockage ameliorates murine lupus nephritis. *J Am Soc Nephrol* 1993; **4**: 58–61.

Koffler D, Schur PH, Kunkel HG. Immunological studies concerning the nephritis of systemic lupus erythematosus. *J Exp Med* 1967; **126**: 607–24.

Kohler PF, Ten Bensel R. Serial complement alterations in acute glomerulonephritis and systemic lupus erythematosus. *Clin Exp Immunol* 1969; **4**: 191–102.

Kong NCT, Nasruruddin BA, Murad S *et al*. HLA antigens in Malay patients with systemic lupus erythematosus. *Lupus* 1994; **3**: 393–5.

Laasonen L, Gripenberg M, Leskinen R *et al*. A subset of systemic lupus erythematosus with progressive cystic bone lesions. *Ann Rheum Dis* 1990; **49**: 118–20.

Labowitz R, Schumacher AR. Articular manifestations of systemic lupus erythematosus. *Ann Intern Med* 1971; **74**: 911–21.

Lauter SA, Espinoza LR, Osterland CK. The relationship between C-reactive protein and systemic lupus erythematosus. *Arthritis Rheum* 1979; **22**: 1421.

Lee LA, Bias WB, Arnett FC *et al*. Immunogenetics of the neonatal lupus syndrome. *Ann Intern Med* 1983; **99**: 592–6.

Liang MH, Karlson EW. *Neurologic manifestations of lupus. The Clinical Management of Lupus*. 2nd ed. Schur PH. Lipponcott-Raven, Philadelphia, 1996; 141–54.

Liang MH, Sacher SA, Roberts WN *et al*. Measurement of systemic lupus erythematosus activity in clinical research. *Arthritis Rheum* 1988; **31**: 817–25.

Libman E, Sacks B. A hitherto undescribed form of valvular and mural endocarditis. *Arch Intern Med* 1924; **33**: 701–38.

Llorente L, Zou W, Levy Y *et al*. Role of interleukin 10 in the B lymphocyte hyperactivity and autoantibody production of human systemic lupus erythematosus. *J Exp Med* 1995; **181**: 839–44.

Lloyd W, Schur PH. Immune complexes, complement and anti-DNA in exacerbations of systemic lupus erythematosus (SLE). *Medicine* 1981; **60**: 208–17.

Love PE, Santoro SA. Anti-phospholipid antibodies: anti-cardiolipin and the lupus anticoagulant in systemic lupus erythematosus (SLE) and in non-SLE disorders. *Am Intern Med* 1990; **112**: 682–98.

Lu LY, Ding WZ, Fici D *et al*. Molecular analysis of major histocompatibilty complex alleleic associations with systemic lupus erythematosus in Taiwain. *Arthritis Rheum* 1997; **40**: 1138–45.

Machold KP, Smolen JS. Interferon g induced exacerbation of systemic lupus erythematosus. *J Rheumatol* 1990; **17**: 831–2.

Mackay IR, Taft LI, Cowling DC. Lupoid hepatitis and the hepatic lesions of systemic lupus erythematosus. *Lancet* 1959; **1**: 65–9.

Maddison PJ, Reichlin M. Deposition of antibodies to soluble cytoplasmic antigens in the kidneys of patients with systemic lupus erythematosus. *Arthritis Rheum* 1979; **22**: 858–63

Maddison PJ, Provost TT, Reichlin M. Serological findings in patients with 'ANA-negative' systemic lupus erythematosus. *Medicine* 1981; **60**: 87–94.

Maddison PJ, Isenberg DA, Goulding N *et al*. Anti-La (SSB) identifies a distinctive subgroup of SLE. *Br J Rheumatol* 1988; **17**: 27–31.

Mandell B. Cardiovascular involvement in systemic lupus erythematosus. *Sem Arthritis Rheum* 1987; **17**: 120–41.

Manger K, Kalden JR, Manger B. Cyclosporin A in the treatment of systemic lupus erythematosus: results of an open clinical study. *Br J Rheumatol* 1996; **35**: 669–75.

Martens J, Demedts MD, Vanmeenan MT *et al*. Respiratory dysfunction in systemic lupus erythematosus. *Chest* 1983; **84**: 170–5.

Matsukawa Y, Sawada S, Hayma T *et al*. Suicide in patients with systemic lupus erythematosus: a clinical analysis of seven suicide patients. *Lupus* 1994; **3**: 31–5.

McLaughlin J, Gladman DP, Urowitz MB *et al*. Kidney biopsy in systemic lupus erythematosus. *Arthritis Rheum* 1991; **34**: 1268–73.

McLure CE, Isenberg DA. Does plasma exchange have any part to play in the management of SLE? *Controversies in Rheumatology*, eds. Isenberg DA, Tucker LB. Martin Dunitz Ltd, London, 1997: 75–85.

Mellenkjaer L, Andersen V, Linet MS *et al*. Non-Hodgkin's lymphoma and other cancers among a cohort of patients with systemic lupus erythematosus. *Arthritis Rheum* 1997; **40**: 761–8.

Mendelovic S, Brocke S, Shoenfeld Y *et al*. Induction of a SLE-like disease in mice by a common anti-DNA idiotype. *Proc Natl Acad Sci USA* 1988; **85**: 2260–4.

Miescher P, Straessle R. New serological methods for the detection of LE factor. *Vox Surg* 1957; **2**: 283–7.

Miyagawa S, Fukumoto T, Hashimoto K, Yoshioka A, Shirai T, *et al*. Neonatal lupus erythematosus: haplotypic analysis of HLA class II alleles in child/mother pairs. *Arthritis Rheum* 1997; **40**: 982–3.

Morse JH, Muller-Eberhard HJ, Hunkel HG. Antinuclear factors and serum complement in systemic lupus erythematosus. *Bull NY Acad Med* 1962; **38**: 641–52.

Morrow WJW, Isenberg DA, Parry HF *et al*. Studies on autoantibodies to poly (adenosine diphosphate ribose) in SLE and other autoimmune diseases. *Ann Rheum Dis* 1982; **41**: 396–402.

Morrow WJW, Isenberg DA, Parry HF, Snaith ML. C-reactive protein in sera from patients with systemic lupus erythematosus. *J Rheumatol* 1981; **8**: 599–604.

Murakami M, Kumagi S, Sugita M *et al*. In vitro induction of IgG anti-DNA antibody from high density B cells of systemic lupus erythematosus patients by an HLA-DR restricted T cell clone. *Clin Exp Immunol* 1992; **90**: 245–50.

Murphy ED, Roths JB. Autoimmunity and lymphoproliferation: induction by mutant gene lpr, and acceleration by a male-associated in strain BXSB mice. In: *Genetic Control of Autoimmune Disease* (Rose NR *et al* eds.) Elsevier/North Holland Amsterdam, 1978.

Nelson JL. Microchimerism and autoimmune disease. *N Engl J Med* 1998; **338**: 1224–25.

Ng TC, Kanner SB, Humphries MJ *et al*. Integrin signalling defects in T lymphocytes in systemic lupus erythematosus. *Lupus* 1998; In press.

Nived O, Sturfeldt G. Does the black population in Africa get SLE? If not, why not? In: *Controversies in Rheumatology*, eds. Isenberg DA, Tucker LB, Martin Dunitz Ltd, London, 1997; 65–74.

Okamura M, Kanayama Y, Amastu K *et al*. Significance of enzyme linked immunosorbent assay (ELISA) for antibodies to double stranded and single stranded DNA in patients with lupus nephritis: correlation with severity of renal histology. *Ann Rheum Dis* 1993; **52**: 19–20.

Okolie EE, Shall S. The significance of antibodies to poly (ADP-ribose) in patients with systemic lupus erythematosus. *Clin Exp Immunol* 1979; **36**: 151–64.

Orens JB, Martinez FJ, Lynch JP. Pleuropulmonary manifestations of systemic lupus erythematosus. In *Rheum Dis*

Clin N Am, ed. McCune WJ. WB Saunders Co, Philadelphia, 1994; 20: 159–93.

Ozmen L, Roman D, Fountoulakis M, Schmid G, Ryffel B, Garotta G. Experimental therapy of systemic lupus erythematosus: the treatment of NZB/W mice with mouse soluble interferon gamma receptor inhibits the onset of glomerulnephritis. *Eur J Immunol* 1995; **25**: 6–12.

Pankewycz OG, Migliorini P, Madaio MP. Polyreactive autoantibodies are nephritogenic in murine lupus nephritis. *J Immunol* 1987; **139**: 3287–94.

Perry HM Jr, Tan EM, Carmody S *et al*. Relationship of acetyl transferase activity to antinuclear antibodies and toxic symptoms in hypertensive patients treated with hydralazine. *J Lab Clin Med* 1970; **76**: 114–25.

Petri M. Anti ribosomal P antibodies in SLE. A prospective cohort study. *Arthritis Rheum* 1996; **39**: S292.

Petri M, Howard D, Repke J. Frequency of lupus flare in pregnancy: the Hopkins Lupus Pregnancy Centre Experience. *Arthritis Rheum* 1991; **34**: 1538–45.

Petri M, Watson R, Winkelstein JA *et al*. Clinical expression of systemic lupus erythematosus in patients with C4A deficiency. *Medicine* 1993; **72**: 236–44.

Pistiner M, Wallace DJ, Nessim S *et al*. Lupus erythematosus in the 1980s: a survey of 570 patients. *Sem Arthritis Rheum* 1991; **21**: 55–64,

Pryor BD, Bologna SG, Kahl LE. Risk factors for serious infection during treatment with cyclophosphamide and high dose corticosteroids for systemic lupus erythematosus. *Arthritis Rheum* 1996; **39**: 1475–82.

Quimby FW, Jensen C, Nawrocki D *et al*. Selected autoimmune disease in the dog. *Vet Clin North Am* 1978; **8**: 665–82.

Rajagopalan S, Zordan T, Tsokos GC *et al*. Pathogenic anti-DNA antibody-inducing T helper cell lines from patients with active lupus nephritis: isolation of CD4-8 Y helper cell lines that express the gd T-cell antigen receptor. *Proc Natl Acad Sci (USA)* 1990; **87**: 7020–4.

Ramsay-Goldman R, Schilling E. Immunosuppressive drug use during pregnancy. *Rheum Dis Clin North Am* 1997; **23**: 149–67.

Rauch J, Murphy B, Roth JB *et al*. A high frequency idiotypic marker of anti-DNA autoantibodies in MRL/lpr mice. *J Immunol* 1982; **129**: 236–41.

Ravirajan CT, Rahman MA, Papadaki L et al. Genetic, structural and functional properties of an IgG DNA-binding monoclonal antibody from a lupus patient with nephritis. *Eur J Immunol* 1998; **28**: 339–50.

Raz E, Dudler J, Lotz M *et al*. Modulation of disease activity in murine systemic lupus erythematosus by cytokine gene delivery. *Lupus* 1995; **4**: 285–92.

Reed JC. Double identity for proteins of the Bcl-2 family. *Nature* 1997; **387**: 773–6.

Reinertsen JL, Klippel JH, Johnson AH *et al*. B-lymphocyte alloantigens associated with systemic lupus erythematosus. *N Eng J Med* 1978; **299**: 515–8.

Reveille JD, Macleod MJ, Whittington K *et al*. Specific amino acid residues in the second hypervariable region of HLA-DQA1 and DQB1 chain genes promote the Ro (SS-A)/La (SS-B) autoantibody responses. *J Immunol* 1991; **146**: 3871–6.

Richter Cohen M, Isenberg DA. Ultraviolet irradiation in SLE-friend or foe? *Brit J Rheum* 1996; **35**: 1002–8.

Richter Cohen M, Steiner G, Smollen JS. *et al*. Enzyme arthritis in systemic lupus erythematosus in analysis of a distinct clinical and serological subset. *Brit J Rheum* 1998; **37**: 421–4.

Rieux-Laucat F, Le Deist F, Hivroz C *et al*. Mutations in Fas associated with human lymphoproliferative syndrome and autoimmunity. *Science* 1995; **268**: 1347–9.

Robbins WC, Holman HR, Deicher H *et al*. Complement fixation with cell nuclei and DNA in lupus erythematosus. *Proc Soc Exp Biol Med* 1957; **9**: 575–9.

Rose LM, Latchman DS, Isenberg DA. Apoptosis in peripheral lymphocytes in systemic lupus erythematosus: a review. *Br J Rheumatol* 1997; **36**: 158–63.

Rothfield N, Ross HA, Minta JO, *et al*. Glomerular and dermal deposition of properdin in systemic lupus erythematosus. *N Engl J Med* 1972; **287**: 681–5.

Ruddy S, Everson LK, Schur P *et al*. Hemolytic assay of the ninth complement component: elevation and depletion in rheumatic disease. *J Exp Med* 1971; **134**: 259–75.

Santoro TJ, Portanova JP, Kotzin BL. The contribution of L3T4+ T cells to lymphoproliferation and autoantibody production in MRL-*lpr/lpr* mice. *J Exp Med* 1988; **167**: 1713–8.

Sasaki T, Muryoi T, Takai O *et al*. Selective elimination of anti-DNA antibody producing cells by antiidiotypic antibody conjugate to neocarzinostatin. *J Clin Invest* 1986; **77**: 1382–6.

Schreider M, Bering T, Waldendorf H *et al*. Immunoadsorbent plasma perfusion in patients systemic lupus erythematosus. *J Rheumatol* 1990; **17**: 900–7.

Schifferli JA, Peters DK. Complement, the immune-complex lattice, and the pathophysiology of complement-deficiency syndromes. *Lancet* 1983; 957–9.

Schroder JO, Euler H, Loffler H. Synchronisation of plasmapheresis and pulse cyclophosphamide in severe systemic lupus erythematosus. *Ann Intern Med* 1987; **107**: 344–6.

Schroeder JO, Scwab U, Zeuner R *et al*. Plasmapheresis and subsequent pulse cyclophosphamide in severe systemic lupus erythematosus. Preliminary results of the LPSG-trial. *Arthritis Rheum* 1997; **40**: S325

Schultz LD, Zurier RS. 'Motheaten'; a single gene model for stem cell dysfunction and early onset autoimmunity. In: Genetic Control of Autoimmune Disease (eds Rose NR, Warner N.) Elsevier, Amsterdam, 1978.

Schur PH, Monroe M. Antibodies to ribonucleic acid in systemic lupus erythematosus. *Proc Natl Acad Sci USA*. 1969; **63**: 1108–12.

Schur PH, Marcus-Bagley D, Awdeh Z *et al*. The effect of ethnicity on major histocompatibility complex complement allotypes and extended haplotypes in patients with systemic lupus erythematosus. *Arthritis Rheum* 1990; **33**: 985–92.

Schur PH, Sandson J. Immunologic factors and clinical activity in systemic lupus erythematosus. *N Engl J Med* 1968; **278**: 533–8.

Schwartz MM, Lan SP, Bernstein J *et al*. Role of pathology indices in the management of severe lupus glomerulonephritis. *Kidney Int* 1992; **42**: 743–8.

Seligmann M. Evidence in the serum of patients with systemic lupus erythematosus of a substance producing a precipitation reaction with DNA (original in French). *CR Soc Biol* (Paris) 1957; **245**: 328–33.

Sfikakis PP, Charalambopoulos D, Vayiopoulos G *et al.* Increased levels of intercellular adhesion molecule-1 in the serum of patients with systemic lupus erythematosus. *Clin Exp Rheum* 1994; **12**: 5–9.

Shoenfeld Y. Idiotypic induction of autoimmunity: a new aspect of the idiotypic network. *FASEB J* 1994; **8**: 1296–301.

Shoenfeld Y, Krause I, Blank M. New methods of treatment in an experimental murine model of systemic lupus erythematosus induced by idiotypic manipulation. *Ann Rheum Dis* 1997; **56**: 5–11.

Shortall E, Isenberg DA, Newman S. Factors associated with mood and mood disorders in SLE. *Lupus* 1995; **4**: 272–9.

Sibley JT, Braun RP, Lee JS. The production of antibodies to DNA in normal mice following immunization with poly (ADP-ribose). *Clin Exp Immunol* 1986; B: 563–9.

Sibley JT, Olszynski WP, Decoteau WE *et al.* The incidence and prognosis of central nervous system disease in systemic lupus erythematosus. *J Rheumatol* 1992; **19**: 47–52.

Silverman ED, Eddy A. Systemic lupus erythematosus in childhood and adolescence. In: *Oxford Textbook of Rheumatology*, 2nd edn, eds Maddison PJ, Isenberg DA, Woo P, Glass DN. Oxford University Press, Oxford, 1998, 1180–1202.

Silverman ED, Lang B. An overview of the treatment of childhood SLE. *Scand J Rheumatol* 1997; **26**: 241–6.

Silvestris F, D'Amore O, Cafforio P *et al.* Intravenous immunoglobulin therapy of lupus nephritis: use of pathogenic anti-DNA-reactive IgG. *Clin Exp Immunol* 1996; **104** (Suppl. 1): 91–7.

Skarsväg S, Hansen KE, Holst A *et al.* Distribution of HLA class II alleles among Scandinavian patients with systemic lupus erythematosus (SLE): an increase risk of SLE among non [DRB1*03,DQA1*0501,DQB1*0201] Class II homozygotes? *Tissue Antigens* 1992; **40**: 128–33.

Sontheimer RD, Stastny P, Gilliam JN. Human histocompatibility antigen associations in subacute cutaneous lupus erythematosus. *J Clin Invest* 1981; **67**: 312–16.

Spronk PE, ter Borg EJ, Kallenberg CGM. Patients with systemic lupus erythematosus and Jaccoud's arthropathy: a clinical subset with an increased C reactive protein response. *Ann Rheum Dis* 1992; **51**: 358–61.

Stafford FJ, Fleischer RA, Lee G *et al.* A pilot study of anti-CD5 ricin a chain immunoconjugate in systemic lupus erythematosus. *J Rheumatol* 1994; **21**: 2068–70.

Steiner G, Hartmuth K, Skriner K *et al.* Purification and partial sequencing of the nuclear autoantigen RA33 shows that it is indistinguishable from the AZ protein of the heterogenous nuclear ribonucleoprotein complex. *J Clin Invest* 1992; **90**: 106–6.

Staines N. Idiotypes of DNA-binding antibodies: recent advances. *Lupus* 1992; **1**: 313–6.

Steward MW, Hay FC. Changes in immunoglobulin class and subclass of anti-DNA antibodies with increasing age in NZB-W F$_1$ hybrid mice. *Clin Exp Immunol* 1976; **26**: 363–70.

Stoll T, Gordon C, Seifert B *et al.* Consistency and validity of patient administered assessment of quality of life by the MOS SF-36; its association with disease activity and damage in patients with systemic lupus erythematosus. *J Rheumatol* 1997a; **24**: 1608–14.

Stoll T, Stucki G, Malik J *et al.* Association of the SLICC/ACR damage index with measures of disease activity and health status in patients with systemic lupus erythematosus. *J Rheumatol* 1997b; **24**: 309–13.

Strasser A, Whittingham S, Vaux DL *et al.* Enforced bcl-2 expression in B lymphoid cells prolongs antibody responses and elicits autoimmune disease. *Proc Natl Acad Sci USA* 1991; **88**: 8661–5.

Swaak AJG, Aarden LA, Statius van Eps LW *et al.* Anti-dsDNA and complement profiles as prognostic guides in systemic lupus erythematosus. *Arthritis Rheum* 1979; **22**: 226–35.

Tam LS, Cohen MG, Li EK. Hemiballismus in systemic lupus erythematosus: possible association with antiphospholipid antibodies. *Lupus* 1995; **4**: 67–9.

Tan EM, Cohen AS, Fries JF *et al.* The 1982 revised criteria for the classification of systemic lupus erythematosus. *Arthritis Rheum* 1982; **25**: 1271–7.

Teh LS, Isenberg DA. Antiribosomal P protein antibodies in systemic lupus erythematosus. A reappraisal. *Arthritis Rheum* 1994; **37**: 307–15.

Teitlebaum D, Rauch J, Stollar BD *et al.* In vitro effects of antibodies against a high frequency idiotype of antiDNA antibodies in MRL mice. *J Immunol* 1984; **132**: 1282–5.

Ter Borg EJ, Horst G, Hemmel EJ *et al.* Measurements of increases in anti-double-stranded DNA antibody levels as a predictor of disease exacerbation in systemic lupus erythematosus. *Arthritis Rheum* 1990; **33**: 634–43.

Trenthem DV, Townes AS, Kang AH *et al.* Humeral and cellular sensitivity to collagen in type II collagen-induced arthritis in rats. *J Clin Invest* 1978; **61**: 89–96.

Tseng C-E, Buyon JP. Neonatal lupus syndrome. *Rheum Dis Clin North Am* 1997; **23**: 31–54.

Tsuji K, Aizawa M, Sasazuki T (eds) In: *HLA 1991. Proceedings of the Eleventh International Histocompatibility Workshop and conference*, Vol 1. Oxford University Press, New York, 1992; 1065–220.

Tucker LB, Menon S, Schaller J *et al.* Adult and childhood onset systemic lupus erythematosus: a comparison of onset, clinical features, serology and outcome. *Br J Rheumatol* 1995; **34**: 866–72.

Twomey BN, Dhillon VB, Latchman DS *et al.* Lupus and heat shock proteins. In: *Stress Proteins in Medicine*, eds.Van Eden W, Young DB. Marcel Dekker Inc., New York, 1996; 345–57.

Urowitz MB, Gladman DD, Farewell VT. Lupus and pregnancy studies. *Arthritis Rheum* 1993; **36**: 1392–7.

Vaishnaw AK, Walport MJ. Systemic lupus erythematosus. In: *Connective Tissues Diseases*. Belch JF, Zurier RB eds. Chapman and Hall,. London, pp 17–50.

van Vollenhoven RF, Engleman EG, McGuire Jl. Dehydroepiandrosterone in systemic lupus erythematosus. Results of a double-blind, placebo controlled, randomised clinical trial. *Arthritis Rheum* 1995; **38**: 1826–31.

Walton AJE, Snaith ML, Locniskar M *et al.* Dietary fish oil reduces the severity of symptoms in patients with SLE. *Ann Rheum Dis* 1991; **33**: 463–6.

Wang Y, Hu Q, Madri JA *et al.* Amelioration of lupus-like autoimmune disease in NZB/WF1 mice after treatment with a blocking monoclonal antibody specific for complement component C5. *Proc Natl Acad Sci USA* 1996; **93**: 8563–8.

Ware JE, Brook RH, Williams KN *et al.* A conceptualisation and measurement of health for adults in the health insur-

ance study. Vol. 1, *Model of health and methodology*. Santa Monica Rand Corp 1980.

Warner LM, Adams LM, Sehgal SN. Rapamycin prolongs survival and arrests pathophysiological changes in murine systemic lupus erythematosus. *Arthritis Rheum* 1994; **37**: 289–97.

Watson R, Scheel JN, Petri M *et al*. Neonatal lupus erythematosus syndrome: analysis of C4 allotypes and C4 genes in 18 families. Medicine 1992; **71**: 84–95.

Watson RM, Lane AT, Barnett NK *et al*. Neonatal lupus erythematosus. A clinical, serological and immunogenetic study with review of the literature. *Medicine* 1984; **63**: 362–78.

Watts R, Isenberg DA. Pancreatic complications of the autoimmune rheumatic diseases. *Sem Arthritis Rheum* 1989; **19**: 158–65.

Watts R, Isenberg DA. DNA antibody idiotypes: an analysis of their clinical connections and origins. *Int Rev Immunol* 1990; **5**: 279–93.

Wei N, Klippel JH, Husto DP. Randomised trial of plasma exchange in mild SLE. *Lancet* 1991; i: 17–22.

Wellicome SM, Kapchi P, Mason JC *et al*. Detection of a circulating form of vascular cell adhesion molecule-1: raised levels in rheumatoid arthritis and systemic lupus erythematosus. *Clin Exp Immunol* 1993; **92**: 412–8.

West SG. Neuropsychiatric lupus. In: *Systemic Lupus Erythematosus, Rheumatic Disease Clinics of North America*. WB Saunders, Philadelphia 1994; **20**: 129–58.

Wigley RD, Couchman HG. Polyarteritis nodosa-like disease in outbred mice. *Nature* 1966; **211**: 319–20.

Williams W, Isenberg DA. Idiotypes and autologous anti-idiotype types in human autoimmune disease—some theoretical and practical observations. *Autoimmunity* 1994; **17**: 343–52.

Wise CM, Vuyyuru S, Roberts WN. Methotrexate in non-renal lupus and undifferentiated connective tissue disease — a review of 36 patients. *J Rheumatol* 1996; **23**: 1005–10.

Wofsy D, Seaman WE. Reversal of advanced lupus in NZB/NZW F1 mice by treatment with monoclonal antibody to L3T4. *J Immunol* 1987; **138**: 3247–53.

Wu J, Zhou T, Zhang J, Mountz J. Correction of autoimmune disease in CD2-fas transgenic mice. *Proc Natl Acad Sci USA* 1994; **91**: 2344–8.

Wuthrich RP. Vascular cell adhesion molecule-1 (VCAM-1) expression in murine lupus nephritis. *Kidney Int* 1992; **42**: 903–14.

Wuthrich RP, Jevnikar AM, Takei F *et al*. Intercellular adhesion molecule-1 (ICAM-1) expression is upregulated in autoimmune murine lupus nephritis. *Am J Pathol* 1990; **136**: 441–50.

Yamada A, Minota S, Nojima Y *et al*. Changes in subset specificity of anti-T cell autoantibodies in systemic lupus erythematosus. *Autoimmunity* 1993; **14**: 269–73.

Yao Z, Kimura A, Hartung K *et al*. Polymorphism of the DQA1 promoter region (QAP) and DRB1, QAP, DQA1, DQB1 haplotypes in systemic lupus erythematosus. *Immunogenetics* 1993; **38**: 421–9.

Zhang W, Reichlin M. Some Autoantibodies to Ro/SS-A and La/SS-B are antiidiotypes to anti-double-stranded DNA. *Arthritis Rheum* 1996; **39**: 522–31.

5 | *Rheumatoid arthritis*

Introduction

Rheumatoid arthritis (RA) is probably the best known of the autoimmune rheumatic diseases. Most studies of point prevalence (the number of cases at a given time in a particular population) have indicated that between 0.5 and 1% of the population have RA. Its incidence is higher in women and the aetiology is unknown. However, the past decade has seen a great increase in our understanding of its immunopathology. Rheumatoid arthritis is a chronic inflammatory condition, principally affecting smaller synovial joints in a symmetrical fashion, leading, in most cases, to destruction of the joints. Extra-articular manifestations are common and a variety of immunological abnormalities are evident. The best known of these is the presence of rheumatoid factors, which are self-associating antibodies that bind the Fc region of IgG. Despite the relatively high incidence of RA in the general population, research into this disease has been hampered by the lack of a truly appropriate animal model.

Milestones in the history of rheumatoid arthritis

1400s	Botticelli depicted rheumatoid arthritis-like deformities in some of the subjects of his paintings.
1800	Landré Beauvais provided the first good clinical description of rheumatoid arthritis.
Mid-1800s	Charcot and Cornil independently described juvenile chronic arthritis.
1858	Sir Alfred Baring Garrod coined the term rheumatoid arthritis.
1897	Still described juvenile chronic polyarthritis.
1924	Felty noted a syndrome of rheumatoid arthritis associated with splenomegaly and leucopaenia.
1930s–1940s	Independent observations by Waaler (Norway) and Rose (USA) in which they noted that sheep erythrocytes coated with rabbit serum would agglutinate in the presence of serum from individuals with rheumatoid arthritis; led to the development of the diagnostic test for the disease.
Late 1940s	Corticosteroids introduced by Hench and colleagues for the treatment of rheumatoid arthritis at the Mayo clinic.
1956	Singer and Plotz devise the latex agglutination test.
1958	The American Rheumatism Association first devised a classification scheme for the disease.
1960s	The pioneering work of John Charnley led to the introduction of the hip and subsequently knee, elbow, and shoulder joint replacements, which have revolutionized the lives of many patients with rheumatoid arthritis.
1960s–1970s	Immunosuppressive therapy, for example azathioprine and subsequently methotrexate, introduced.

1987   The American College of
        Rheumatology introduced a revised
        classification scheme for rheumatoid
        arthritis.

1994–1995   Introduction of experimental
            immunotherapy including monoclonal
            antibodies against cytokines (especially
            TNF-α) and lymphocytes.

Classification

The revised criteria set out by the American College of
Rheumatology, are shown in Table 5.1. Rheumatoid
arthritis may be diagnosed if four out of seven criteria
are fulfilled. These criteria were developed by observing
so-called 'typical patients' thought to have rheumatoid
arthritis, by a number of experienced rheumatologists.
Some concerns have been expressed about these criteria
and it may be best to reserve them for use in clinical
trials focused on patients with well established disease.

It must, however, be recognized that patients who
meet these criteria will not have a homogeneous
outcome. Rheumatoid arthritis manifests several distinct disease patterns (Table 5.2). Although some
patients appear to have a relatively short-lived disease,
the majority of patients fall into categories 3 and 4.
Fortunately only 5–10% of all patients with rheumatoid arthritis develop the rapidly evolving, unremitting
form of disease that leads to multiple joint replacement, in some cases within five years of disease onset.

Epidemiology and outcome

Although rheumatoid arthritis has been identified in
virtually all populations studied, it appears to be gen-
uinely rare in rural African populations. The prevalence figures have ranged between 0.2% and 5.3%
(Spector 1990). Most studies, however, have suggested
a point prevalence of between 0.5 and 1.0%. Certain
North American Indian tribes (e.g. the Tlingit, Yakima,
and Pimas) have a particularly high prevalence of
rheumatoid arthritis.

A number of recent studies attempting to determine
the incidence of rheumatoid arthritis have produced
figures varying between 2.9 and 29 cases per 10 000
per year. The national UK epidemiology unit supported
by the Arthritis and Rheumatism Council have

Table 5.1   The revised classification criteria for rheumatoid arthritis (American College of Rheumatology)

	Criteria	Comment
1.	Morning stiffness	Duration > 1 hr lasting > 6 weeks
2.	Arthritis of at least three areas*	Soft tissue swelling/exudation lasting > 6 weeks
3.	Arthritis of hand joints	Wrists/metacarpophalangeal or proximal interphalangeal joints, lasting > 6 weeks
4.	Symmetrical arthritis	Lasting > 6 weeks
5.	Rheumatoid nodules	As observed by a physician
6.	Serum rheumatoid factor	As assessed by a method positive in < 5% of controls
7.	Radiographic changes	Erosions or juxta-articular osteoporosis

* Possible areas: proximal interphalangeal joints, metacarpophalangeal joints, wrist, elbow, knee, ankle, metatarsophalangeal joints.
Four out of seven criteria must be fulfilled; see Arnett *et al.* 1988).

Table 5.2   Patterns of disease in rheumatoid arthritis

1. Palindromic rheumatism; short-lived (24 → 48 hours) attacks of pain and swelling. Perhaps 50% of these patients
    evolve to patterns 3, 4, or 5.

2. Short-lived disease — within 1–2 years patients go into full remission with no significant sequelae.

3. Joint disease characterized by distinct periods of remission and relapse which may leave only mild/moderate residual
    damage.

4. Persistent disease often lasting several decades (there may remissions/relapses), invariably resulting in significant
    deformity.

5. Severe disease of rapid progression resulting in early, profound disability.

performed a sensitive population-based assessment of all new cases of arthritis in a stable population of 450 000 people in Norfolk and reported an incidence of 3.4 per 10 000 in women and 1.4 per 10 000 in men. The incidence in this study increased considerably with age in men after 45, whereas in women it increased steadily until age 45, then plateaued until 75, after which it fell (Symmons *et al.* 1994). It is generally agreed that mortality is increased in patients with rheumatoid arthritis. One Dutch study (Vandenbroucke *et al.* 1984) reported that life expectancy is reduced by approximately seven years in men and three years in women; increased mortality being due mainly to infections, renal and respiratory involvement, and rheumatoid arthritis itself. Others have suggested that stress, age, male sex, poor functional status, and restricted education are predictors of early demise (Suzuki *et al.* 1994; Wolfe *et al.* 1994).

The clinical picture

General symptoms

A variety of non-specific prodromal symptoms often antedate any overt joint disease. These symptoms include marked lethargy, anorexia, weight loss, generalized weakness, aching, and stiffness. Less frequently, pyrexia and lymphadenopathy may occur. Morning stiffness is often one of the first symptoms of rheumatoid arthritis. It may be due to oedema within inflamed tissues, while the patient is sleeping, and can last several hours in patients with active disease.

Joint disease

Any synovial joint may be affected by rheumatoid arthritis. The most commonly affected joints are the wrists, metacarpophalangeal (MCP) and proximal interphalangeal (PIP) joints in the hands, the knees, and the small joints in the feet (Fig. 5.1). It is remarkable how strikingly symmetrical the joint involvement usually is. However, notable exceptions are found in patients with a major disability affecting one side of the body, for example in patients who have had a stroke or poliomyelitis, in which case there is sparing of the joints on the paralysed side. The precise reasons why certain joints, for example the distal interphalangeal joints and to a lesser extent the ankle joints, are spared remains unknown.

Hands and wrists

Early involvement of the hands with pain and swelling in the MCP and PIP joints leads to characteristic appearances, with spindle-shaped deformity of the fingers and atrophy of the intrinsic muscles of the hands. The boggy and tender swellings of these joints are accompanied by pain, limitation of movement, and impairment in functional abilities to make a fist, squeeze small objects, and grip (Fig. 5.2). The MCP joints are characteristically subluxed (become misaligned) with ulnar deviation. As the disease progresses, chronic synovial inflammation leads to radial rotation of the carpal bones and ulnar deviation of the fingers. Depending upon the relative amounts of hyperflexion and extension at the PIP and distal interphalangeal (DIP) joints, either the 'swan-neck' (Fig. 5.1b) or 'boutonnière' deformity (Fig. 5.1e) may develop. The thumb may also acquire a Z-shape. The extensor tendons on the dorsum (back) of the hand may sublux and, on occasion, rupture. This complication may require urgent surgical repair. On the palmar side of the wrist, synovial hypertrophy may compromise the median nerve as it passes through the carpal tunnel. This leads to numbness and/or a 'pins and needles' sensation in the thumb, first, second, and, sometimes, third fingers, together with weakness of the muscles in the thenar eminence (the base of the thumb). Surgery is often required for this manifestation.

Elbow

Major elbow involvement is present in some 10–20% of patients with rheumatoid arthritis overall. Loss of the ability to extend the elbows fully may, however, be a relatively early sign in rheumatoid arthritis, which may occur without the patient's awareness. Epicondylitis and olecranon bursitis may also be present, and moving the joint may cause crepitation (a crunching noise) as the radial head moves.

Shoulders

Shoulder involvement is common in RA. Seventy per cent of patients develop erosions and the combination of disease in the glenohumeral and acromioclavicular joints and the thoracoscapular articulations, together with involvement of the rotator cuff leads to pain, reduced mobility, and local muscle weakness. Swelling at the shoulder is less frequently seen. Rotator cuff tears have been found in up to 20% of patients.

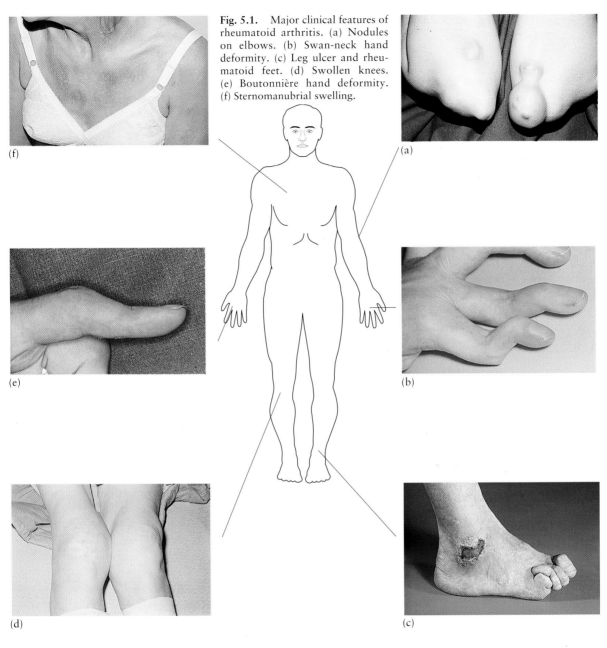

Fig. 5.1. Major clinical features of rheumatoid arthritis. (a) Nodules on elbows. (b) Swan-neck hand deformity. (c) Leg ulcer and rheumatoid feet. (d) Swollen knees. (e) Boutonnière hand deformity. (f) Sternomanubrial swelling.

Hips

Hip disease is relatively uncommon and often a relatively late manifestation. When it does occur, however, it often manifests as pain in the groin, occasionally radiating to the legs, back, or buttocks. Eberhardt *et al.* (1995) reported that 15 of 113 patients required a total hip replacement after a median disease duration of four years.

Knees

Knees are affected in over 80% of patients with rheumatoid arthritis (Fig. 5.1d). Swelling may be due to effusions, which can exceed 100 ml in volume. Synovial hypertrophy is also frequent as are a variety of deformities, including flexion contracture, ligamentous instability, and swelling of popliteal (Baker) cysts, which may rupture, leading to calf swelling that

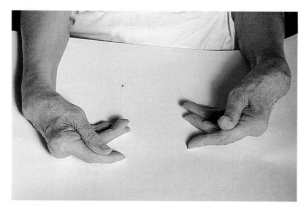

Fig. 5.2.   Severe hand and wrist involvement in RA.

needs to be distinguished from deep venous thrombosis. For long periods of time, chronic knee involvement leads to valgus instability and flexion contracture. Knee joint replacement is now much more widely used and helps to ensure the patient can continue to walk.

Ankles and feet

The ankles are usually only involved in severe disease. Apart from local swelling, the ankles may become very painful, though, as deformities such as eversion (lateral deviation) may develop. Synovitis of the metatarsophalangeal joints is common and is associated with subluxation of these joints. Patients then complain of feeling that they are 'walking on pebbles'. Bunions and clawing of the toes are additional common complaints.

Cervical spine

Generalized pain and stiffness are the most common manifestations. Subluxation of the atlantoaxial joint is

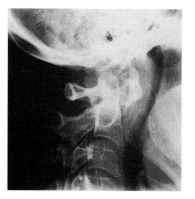

Fig. 5.3.   Gross subluxation of the atlantoaxial joint.

potentially the most serious complication (Fig. 5.3), because spinal cord compression may ensue. Symptoms of such compression may include the loss of use of arms and legs, loss of sphincter control, changes in the level of consciousness, and perhaps paraesthesiae in the hands and feet. Fortunately, such symptoms are relatively uncommon.

Temperomandibular joints

Too often no enquiry is made about involvement of these joints and yet approximately one-quarter of patients do have disease in these joints, causing pain on chewing and, less frequently, palpable synovial swelling.

Other joints

Involvement of the sternoclavicular and manubriosternal joints, sometimes leading to tender swellings, is relatively uncommon. Synovitis of the cricoarytenoid is well recognized. It causes the symptoms of a 'foreign body sensation' at the back of the throat, together with hoarseness and weakness of the voice, and occasionally stridor (harsh sound in breathing). On laryngoscopic examination, the vocal cords may appear red and swollen and hypomobile.

Extra-articular manifestations

Numerous extra-articular manifestations occur in RA. These are discussed in detail below and are summarized in Table 5.3.

Dermatological involvement

Up to one-third of patients, especially those with high titres of rheumatoid factor, develop subcutaneous nodules (Fig. 5.4a). These consist of a central necrotic zone, a middle layer of palisading fibroblasts, an outer collagenous cover containing chronic inflammatory cells (mainly lymphocytes), and plasma cells (Fig. 5.4b). These nodules are commonly found on the extensor surface of the forearm, especially round the elbow, and adjacent to the Achilles tendon. Less frequently they may be found adjacent to the sacrum, in the larynx, the heart, the lungs, or, very rarely, within the central nervous system.

Small splinter haemorrhages localized to the nail folds may come and go spontaneously. Occasionally,

Table 5.3 Extra-articular manifestations of rheumatoid arthritis

Dermatological	Nodules
	Atrophic skin and ulceration
	Vasculitis
Ocular	Sjögren's syndrome
	Scleritis/episcleritis
	Uveitis
	Cataract
Pulmonary	Pleural effusions
	Interstitial fibrosis
	Nodular lung disease
Cardiac	Pericarditis
	Myocarditis
Neurological	Entrapment neuropathy
	Peripheral neuropathy
	Spinal cord compression
Renal	Amyloid deposits
	(Drug-related damage)
Muscle	'Simple' myopathy
	Myositis
Bone	Osteopaenia
	Erosions
Haematological	Chronic normocytic anaemia
	Monocytopaenia
Vasculitis	Ulcers
	Rash
	Neuropathy

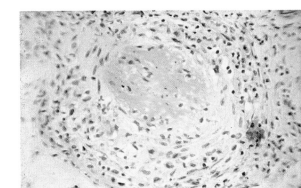

a

b

Fig. 5.4. (a) Rheumatoid nodules on elbows. (b) Histology of a rheumatoid nodule — central necrotic zone, middle layer of palisading fibroblasts, outer collagenous layer of chronic inflammatory cells (mainly lymphocytes with some plasma cells).

there may be ischaemic ulceration in the fingers, but palmar erythema is more common. The skin is often rather thin in patients with rheumatoid arthritis and prone to ulceration (Fig. 5.5).

Ocular involvement

Dryness of the eyes and mouth (secondary Sjögren's syndrome) is a frequent complaint. Primary Sjögren's syndrome is described in detail in Chapter 6. The symptoms and signs of Sjögren's syndrome in patients with rheumatoid arthritis are no different from those with primary disease. Up to 25% of patients with rheumatoid arthritis have some degree of dryness of the eyes and mouth though only 10–15% are likely to meet the criteria for Sjögren's syndrome.

The sclera (a fibrous membrane forming the outer envelope of the eye) becomes inflamed in a few patients with rheumatoid arthritis. Episcleritis is usually a benign, self-limiting condition that causes redness and discomfort. It begins acutely and settles in a few weeks. In contrast, scleritis is a more sinister condition, being slowly progressive, sometimes causing ocular pain and/or major visual loss. Oedema occurs, and nodular lesions histologically similar to rheumatoid nodules are found mainly in the upper part of the sclerae. They are surrounded by hyperaemia of the deep scleral blood vessels. Chronic scleritis leads to thinning of the tissue and a blue discoloration, actually the colour of the underlying choroid. Scleritis usually requires local and/or systemic corticosteroid therapy.

Drug-induced disease may occur in the eyes of patients with rheumatoid arthritis. For example, corticosteroids may cause subcapsular cataracts and retinal damage has (extremely rarely) been described following chloroquine therapy.

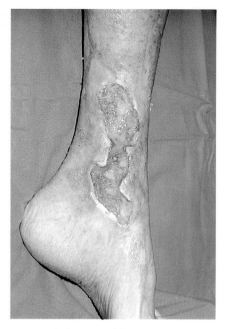

Fig. 5.5. Typical rheumatoid leg ulcer — adjacent to the medial malleolus.

Pulmonary involvement

Small pleural effusions, often asymptomatic, are a well-known complication of the disease. Analysis of the pleural fluid usually reveals a strikingly low glucose level, the cause of which is uncertain. Rheumatoid nodules may be found in the lungs, either in isolation or in association with pneumoconiosis (fibrous induration of the lungs due to an inhalation irritant). This variation of rheumatoid arthritis has been described among Welsh miners and bears the name Caplan's syndrome (Caplan 1953). A diffuse interstitial fibrosis, giving rise to a honeycomb radiological appearance, is also recognized in patients with rheumatoid arthritis. Jurick *et al.* (1982) found diffuse fibrosis in 11% of 309 patients studied. This complication is usually chronic, gradually progressing over many years. On lung function testing, a reduced pulmonary diffusion capacity is the most frequently observed finding (Oxenholm *et al.* 1982).

Cardiac involvement

Although a wide variety of cardiac lesions have been described in patients with rheumatoid arthritis, including pericarditis, myocarditis, endocarditis, conduction defects, and arteritis, they rarely cause symptomatic problems. Acute pericarditis is perhaps the most common symptomatic manifestation. Like pleural effusions, pericardial effusions often have a low glucose content.

Granulomatous lesions, histologically resembling rheumatoid nodules, may occur in the epicardium, myocardium, or valves. A myocardial infarction occasionally results from coronary arteritis.

Neurological involvement

The most common type of peripheral nervous entrapment, carpal tunnel syndrome, results from pressure on the median nerve at the wrist. Direct pressure from an overgrowth of synovial tissue may compromise a number of other peripheral nerves, including the ulnar nerve (at the elbow/wrist) and the anterior tibial nerve (which causes carpal tunnel syndrome, characterized by pain and numbness at the heel and medial aspect of the foot).

Peripheral nerve function may also be compromised by vasculitis of the blood vessels supplying the nerves. This inflammation may give rise to a mild distal sensory and/or motor neuropathy.

Involvement of the autonomic nervous system may also occur in patients with rheumatoid arthritis (Bekkelund *et al.* 1996). This involvement, manifested notably by changes in deep breathing ratios, Valsalva ratio, and variation in blood pressure on standing, is more commonly mild and of little concern to the patient.

Spinal cord compression as a result of cervical subluxation at the atlanto-axial joint is a serious complication usually requiring surgical intervention. Much less frequently, cord compression and other neurological manifestations are induced by the presence of nodules in the central nervous system.

Renal involvement

Renal involvement in patients with RA is rare, quite unlike the situation in SLE. Amyloidosis may complicate RA after many years, because of the deposition of amyloid protein in the glomerular and intrarenal blood vessels. This leads to significant proteinuria and, ultimately, to chronic renal failure. Much more frequently, drug therapy, notably gold salts and D-penicillamine, can induce a membranous nephropathy.

Muscle involvement

Muscle weakness is a common complaint in patients with RA. In many cases it is due to disuse, as painful

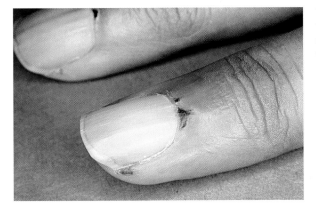

Fig. 5.6. Fingernail vasculitis.

Table 5.4   Core set of measurements in rheumatoid arthritis

Joint pain/tenderness (28 joints)
Joint swelling (28 joints)
Acute phase response
Pain
Patient's global assessment of disease activity
Physician's global assessment of disease activity
Physical disability
Radiographs

joints are generally moved much less frequently. However, a variety of other possible causes exist, including steroid myopathy, which seems to cause a selective atrophy of the type II (fast twitch) fibres, a vasculitis, and an associated myositis.

Vasculitis

Vasculitis is an uncommon but potentially serious complication of RA, typically affecting males with long-standing seropositive erosive disease (Watts *et al.* 1994). The spectrum of involvement ranges from trivial nail fold lesions (Fig. 5.6) to life-threatening, multi-organ disease. Cutaneous lesions occur in the overwhelming majority of patients with rheumatoid vasculitis, with infarcts and ulcers as the most common lesions. Neurological involvement with peripheral neuropathy and mononeuritis multiplex is the next most common feature. Other major associated features include pulmonary disease, ophthalmic, and cardio-vascular involvement. Renal vasculitis is rare.

Bone involvement

Juxta-articular osteoporosis affects bone prior to the development of erosions. Generalized osteoporosis is a particular concern in female patients following the menopause, notably in those who have been prescribed corticosteroids for long periods of time.

Clinical assessment of patients

The complete assessment of a patient with RA not only includes determination of disease activity but also of the effect on function. A number of measurement schemes have been proposed but, recently, consensus has been achieved on a core set of measurements necessary to assess a patient fully (Table 5.4). Global assessments of disease activity are usually based on a visual analogue scale. Disability can be assessed using a standardized questionnaire (e.g. Health Assessment Questionnaire). A number of joint scores have been proposed, but a 28-joint count provides as much information and correlates as well with other measures as do the more extensive counts, such as the Ritchie counts (65 joints) (Prevoo *et al.* 1993).

Complications and associated disorders

Felty's syndrome

In 1924, Felty reported the development of splenomegaly and neutropaenia in five patients with rheumatoid arthritis (Felty 1924). As a complication it is seen in probably less than 1% of patients with rheumatoid arthritis. It is most commonly found in women, notably in those between 50 and 70 years of age. It is also associated with an increased frequency of other extra-articular complications, including rheumatoid nodules and Sjögren's syndrome (Campion *et al.* 1990). It seems to be largely confined to Caucasians and both hepatomegaly and lymphadenopathy are common. In addition, fever, skin pigmentation, and leg ulcers are well recognized.

The leucopaenia observed in patients with Felty's syndrome is due to a combination of impaired production and increased removal of neutrophils. These patients are more prone to Gram-positive bacterial infections — recurrence of which may be an indication for a splenectomy. A possible pathogenic role for granulocyte-macrophage colony stimulating factor (GM-CSF) was suggested when its administration corrected the neutropaenia in a patient (Hazenberg *et al.* 1989).

Rheumatoid arthritis and cancer

Although mild lymph node enlargement is relatively common in rheumatoid arthritis, and splenomegaly has been detected in up to 10% of these patients, there has been much debate as to whether or not tumours of the lymphoreticular system have a significant association with the disease. A possible confounder in many studies is the widespread use of cytotoxic drugs in the treatment of rheumatoid arthritis. Jones *et al.* (1996), in a case-controlled study of patients with RA treated with or without immunosuppressives ($n = 259$ in each group), reported that such therapy increases the malignancy risk [relative risk = 1.5 (95% CI 0.9–2.3)] but not the mortality from other causes.

Rheumatoid arthritis and autoimmune endocrine disease

Patients with rheumatoid arthritis are more likely to have autoimmune thyroid disease and/or anti-thyroid antibodies. In addition, there is a weaker association with diabetes mellitus. This topic has been reviewed in detail elsewhere (Gordon and Isenberg 1987).

Psoriatic arthritis

Psoriatic arthritis (PA) is an inflammatory arthritis that occurs in up to 20% of psoriasis patients and it has been suggested that 0.1–1% of the population may suffer from this rheumatic disorder (Moll and Wright 1973; Gladman 1993). Although it was initially defined as a benign arthropathy, recent studies have established that in many cases PA is progressively deforming in spite of treatment that effectively reduces joint inflammation (Gladman *et al.* 1990). In the majority of cases, psoriasis precedes the development of arthritis, which can include asymmetric oligoarthritis, distal arthritis, arthritis mutilans, symmetric polyarthritis, and spondyloarthropathy (Gladman *et al.* 1987). PA is usually easy to distinguish from RA but there is a paucity of information regarding the mechanisms of pathogenesis. The disorder is seronegative in the context of rheumatoid factor or other autoantibodies, although certain immunopathological aspects of lesional tissue, such as cytokine and chemokine production as well as TCR usage, indicate that not only is the immune system involved directly in the inflammation, but also the response is antigen driven (for review see D'Cruz *et al.* 1998; Ross *et al.* 1998). However, until PA is more closely defined, it can for now be considered as a complication of psoriasis and it is important to discriminate it from rheumatoid arthritis.

Rheumatoid arthritis in childhood

For many years a nomenclature battle has raged between North American authors, who tend to refer to juvenile rheumatoid arthritis, and European paediatric rheumatologists, who prefer the term juvenile chronic arthritis. An international committee is working to get the 'neutral' juvenile idiopathic arthritis to be the preferred term. Four main forms exist.

1. Systemic-onset juvenile chronic arthritis (Still's disease).

2. Pauciarticular-onset juvenile chronic arthritis.

3. Juvenile rheumatoid arthritis (rheumatoid factor-positive polyarthritis).

4. Rheumatoid factor-negative polyarthritis (seronegative polyarthritis).

The prevalence of juvenile chronic arthritis in its various forms is probably about 50 cases per 100 000. Of the various forms, the systemic onset form is marked particularly by its extra-articular features. It is thus characterized by a high-spiking fever, evanescent rash, and myalgias, as well as arthralgias and arthritis. In addition, generalized lymphadenopathy, including hepatosplenomegaly and polyserositis, are very common. Myocarditis, uveitis, and involvement of the lungs and kidneys are occasionally seen. Amyloidosis is a rare but recognized complication. From the time of its original description the tendency of this condition to retard growth has been noted. Thus Still (1897) noted, 'A general arrested growth from the disease begins in early childhood.' This tendency may be exacerbated by the use of steroids to treat these patients. There are no specific diagnostic laboratory features of systemic onset juvenile chronic arthritis but, characteristically, these patients have the anaemia of chronic disease and/or an iron deficiency anaemia with a neutrophilic leucocytosis, a very high ESR, and a polyclonal hypergammaglobulinaemia. Approximately 25% of these patients may have an anti-nuclear antibody, but only 5% are rheumatoid factor-positive by conventional testing. This subject has recently been reviewed in detail elsewhere (Laxer and Schneider 1998).

Pauciarticular-onset juvenile chronic (rheumatoid) arthritis is the most common of the childhood arthritides, which by definition occurs before the age of 16 and involves a total of four or fewer joints during the first six months of the disease. It has a marked predilection for girls (female to male ratio is approximately 4:1) under the age of 5. Although there are no pathognomonic clinical features or laboratory investigations, the usual pattern is of a young child with arthritis usually affecting a knee, ankle, or elbow. Much less frequently a hand joint, wrist, or, very rarely, a shoulder and hip can be involved. These patients usually have only marginal elevation of their acute phase reactants, but anti-nuclear antibodies are present in up to 75% of these children, although in low titres, and they are not associated with antibodies to DNA or the extractable nuclear antigens. Rheumatoid factor is extremely rare, occurring in less than 5% of these children. In most patients with this form of pauci-articular-onset arthritis, although synovitis may develop in other joints over time, the total number of affected joints generally remains below five. However, some 20% of these patients will develop poly-articular arthritis, though this progression becomes increasingly less likely if it has not occured within five years of the onset of the disease. Among the complications of pauciarticular-onset arthritis are juxta-articular muscle atrophy, bony enlargement of the affected joints, and inequality of leg length. Chronic uveitis can be particularly important in the ANA-positive group as chronic iridocyclitis may be asymptomatic and lead to blindness, thus ophthalmological assessment is mandatory. As with other forms of arthritis, effective treatment demands a team approach utilizing a variety of specialists, including paediatric rheumatologists, ophthalmologists, and physiotherapists.

Juvenile (rheumatoid factor-positive) polyarthritis is very similar in both its clinical features and genetics from adult-onset RA. There is a female preponderance and the disease usually starts in children over the age of 10 years. Although weight loss and general malaise are present in over half of these patients, unlike systemic-onset (Still's) disease, fever and generalized lymphadenopathy are rare, and the polyarthritis is a predominant feature. The joint involvement principally involves the hands and feet, but the large joints, especially the knees and ankles, can become involved very early on. Over a 15-year follow-up period, at least a one-third of these patients do rather badly, with marked limitation of functional capacity. Among the complications of this condition are amyloidosis, aortic regurgitation, pericarditis, pleurisy, and diffuse interstitial lung disease. As in adults, the majority of these patients are HLA-DR4-positive. The management of these patients is the same as for adults, though to date there are no good studies on the more experimental forms of therapy currently being investigated extensively in adults (see later in this chapter).

Investigations in RA

Serological

Patients with rheumatoid arthritis are often anaemic. This may be due to a normochromic, normocytic anaemia of chronic disease or may be iron deficient, invariably associated with gastrointestinal bleeding linked to the use of non-steroidal anti-inflammatory drugs. As a general rule (Isenberg *et al.* 1986) a haemoglobin down to 10 g/dl may be a result of active disease alone, but below that it is very likely to have some secondary cause. With the rare exception of the neutropaenia associated with Felty's syndrome (see above) the white cell count in patients with rheumatoid arthritis is invariably normal, but both the erythrocyte sedimentation rate (ESR) and C-reactive protein (C-RP) are useful indicators of disease activity. There have been endless debates about which of these two parameters is the better marker of active disease (see, for example, Banks *et al.* 1998). The former is probably the most widely used and the cheapest.

Other serological abnormalities often observed in patients with rheumatoid arthritis include a high platelet count, a raised alkaline phosphatase, and an increased complement C3 level.

In the occasional patient whose RA is complicated by amyloidosis, close monitoring of renal function tests is required, given its predilection for involving the kidney. Careful monitoring of renal function is also mandatory in patients being treated with gold, D-penicillamine, or cyclosporin (Neoral). Cyclosporin (Neoral) is known to be particularly nephrotoxic especially in doses above 4 mg per kg (see section on Management of RA). Gold, D-penicillamine, methotrexate, and azathioprine require mandatory haematological and biochemical testing. Methotrexate and azathioprine may, in particular, affect liver function.

Immunologically, rheumatoid factor remains the most important guide to establishing the diagnosis of the disease, although it is of no value in monitoring patients with rheumatoid arthritis. The standard

Rose–Waaler test, which uses sheep cells sensitized with rabbit gammaglobulin, is still widely available and shows moderate specificity with reasonable sensitivity. Most modern laboratories use WHO standard serum to check the validity of the results and in some cases to replace the expression of the results in titres by international units. The introduction of enzyme-linked immunosorbent assays (ELISA) for the detection of subclasses of rheumatoid factor, notably IgG (up to 50%) and IgM (up to 80%) have also proved to be very popular. If IgA rheumatoid factors are included, over 90% of patients clinically thought to have rheumatoid arthritis can be shown to be rheumatoid factor-positive.

Approximately 30% of patients with RA have anti-nuclear antibodies. Although this may, on occasion, reflect some overlap with systemic lupus erythematosus, the targets of these anti-nuclear antibodies are more obscure. They are not usually directed against double-stranded DNA but are more likely to be directed against various subcomponents of histone proteins. In the past decade, Smolen and colleagues have identified an antibody known as RA33 which recognizes another, soluble, nuclear antigen (an hn-RNP). This antibody was shown to be detectable early in the course of disease in approximately one-third of patients with RA, but is no longer believed to be as specific as was originally thought (as discussed in Chapter 4).

Anti-perinuclear factors, although hindered by methodological problems, also appear to be of use in the early diagnosis of rheumatoid arthritis. Thus, in a study of 60 patients presenting with polyarthritis of recent onset during a three-year follow-up, out of 40 individuals deemed to have developed rheumatoid arthritis, 31 were shown to have had the anti-perinuclear factor at some time (Berthelot *et al.* 1997). However, it should be noted that this antibody is not disease specific. Anti-keratin antibodies have also been reported in patients with RA. The sensitivity of the presence of the antibody has been variously reported as between 36 and 59%, with a specificity of between 88 and 99% (reviewed by Hoet and Van Verooij 1992).

Problems with the antigenic substrate have meant that neither anti-perinuclear nor anti-keratin antibodies are measured on a routine basis. Furthermore, until recently the precise nature of the antigen recognized by these antibodies has been unclear. Investigations have now shown that these antibodies are both recognizing some (and possibly the same) component of filaggrin (filament-aggregating protein) (Sebbag *et al.* 1995). Filaggrin is formed during the late stages of epithelial

cell differentiation in mammals. It is synthesized as a phosphorylated precursor protein. Profilaggrin is released by proteolytic cleavage during cell differentiation. During this process the protein is dephosphorylated and about 20% of the arginine residues are converted into citrulline by an enzyme, peptidylarginine deiminase. Schellekens *et al.* (1998) explored the possibility that citrulline residues might be present in the epitopes recognized by anti-perinuclear/keratin antibody-positive sera. They synthesized a variety of peptides in which arginine residues present in the cDNA profilaggrin sequence were substituted with citrulline, and assessed the frequency with which the sera from patients with RA and control diseases reacted against them. In a study of 154 patients with RA and over 350 controls, antibodies were detected in 76% of sera from the patients with RA, with a specificity of 99%. Affinity-purified anti-peptide antibodies were found to give a positive result in tests for anti-perinuclear and anti-keratin antibodies.

Anti-neutrophil cytoplasmic antibodies (ANCA), as discussed in Chapter 2, are directed against lysozymal enzymes of human neutrophils and monocytes. A recent study of 246 patients with rheumatoid arthritis (Mustila *et al.* 1997) reported that they were present in 21% of patients, notably those with long-standing disease and severe disease associated with rheumatoid factor and anti-nuclear antibody positivity. There was a particular link between pANCA and histologically proven nephropathy, although no clear-cut association between pANCA and disease activity could be found.

Most patients with active rheumatoid arthritis have an increased percentage of IgG molecules which lack the terminal galactose moieties [Gal(0)] on the bi-antennary oligosaccharide chains attached to the Cγ2 domain (Parekh *et al.* 1988, 1989). Young *et al.* (1991) demonstrated that a combination of the Gal(0) level and rheumatoid factor titre in patients presenting with early-onset synovitis, could provide a simple and useful prognostic indicator of whether patients were likely to develop rheumatoid arthritis. These observations were extended recently (Bodman-Smith *et al.* 1996) and in a four-year prospective study of newly diagnosed rheumatoid arthritis a combination of Gal(0), grip strength, age at onset, and gender predicted the course of rheumatoid arthritis in up to 95% cases. Similar utility for Gal(0) was suggested by a study of Van Zeben *et al.* (1994). In this latter study a raised Gal(0) at first available bleed identified a group of patients more likely to have erosions or active disease and a requirement for more second-line drugs.

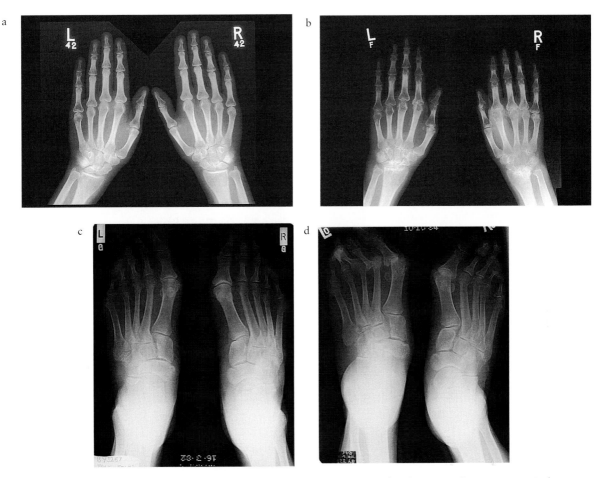

Fig. 5.7. (a) Radiological appearance of the hands in a patient with RA shortly after diagnosis. There is juxta-articular osteo-porosis and early erosive change at the metacarpophalangeal joints and at the wrist. (b) The same patient 18 months later. There is now extensive erosive change at the metacarpophalangeal joints and at the wrist. (c) Radiological appearance of the feet at diagnosis in an RA patient. (d) Two-and-a-half years later there are multiple bony erosions and subluxations of several joints.

Imaging

Regular radiological examination of the affected joints is of value in monitoring patients with rheumatoid arthritis. The use of serial studies is indicated in Fig. 5.7, where it is evident that the drug therapy has failed to prevent a dramatic increase in erosions in both hands and feet. It is worth emphasizing the importance of studying the atlantoaxial joint radiologically (see Fig. 5.3); an increase in the distance between the anterior edge of the odontoid peg and the posterior rim of the anterior arch of the atlas bone is a sign of impending pressure on the cervical cord. Surgical inter-vention is sometimes necessary to remove the harmful overgrowth of synovial tissue in this region.

The introduction of computerized tomography (CT) and magnetic resonance imaging (MRI) has provided a means of demonstrating the early changes in the rheumatoid joint far more accurately than conventional radiography. These means are available, however, at a considerable price, and certainly regular CT or MRI examination is unlikely to be financially possible in most countries for the foreseeable future. A more detailed discussion of the optimal method of imaging different aspects of rheumatoid arthritis has appeared recently (Renton 1998).

Immunogenetics

HLA-DR4 and the cellularly defined 'Dw' specificities in RA patients

Stastny and Fink (1977) first reported an increase of Dw4 in rheumatoid arthritis patients in 1977. Dw4 is an HLA-typing specificity that is cellularly defined. Irradiated homozygous-typing cells are used as stimulator cells in a modified mixed lymphocyte culture to assess a test cell of interest as a responder cell (see Chapter 2). However, the mainstay of HLA-typing techniques prior to 1990 was serological techniques and, following Stastny's report, the serological specificity DR4 was shown to be increased in RA patients (Panayi and Wooley 1977; Winchester 1977). The extent to which risk of RA is increased with HLA-DR4 varies depending on the population studied. For example, among Native American Chippewas the relative risk was 13.4 and among Southern Spaniards 1.8 (Harvey *et al.* 1983; Sanchez *et al.* 1990).

It is now known that DR4 is actually a family of more than 20 different molecules. As information evolved it became clear that only some DR4 variants are associated with risk of RA. Dw4 is the most common DR4 allelic variant in most Caucasian populations and early reports also confirmed Stastny's observation that Dw4 is increased in RA patients (McMichael *et al.* 1977; Thomsen *et al.* 1979). The other cellularly defined 'subtypes' of DR4 are Dw10, Dw13, Dw14, Dw15, and DwKT2. It was soon discovered that Dw10 was not associated with RA (Zoschke and Segall 1986; Ollier *et al.* 1988; Pawelec *et al.* 1988). At least within Caucasian populations, Dw13 was also not associated with RA (Ollier *et al.* 1988; Pawelec *et al.* 1988). Studies in Japanese also found no association with Dw10 or Dw13. However, Dw4 was also not increased and, instead, RA was significantly associated with Dw15 in this population (Ohta *et al.* 1982). The picture was less clear for Dw14. While some investigators found a significant increase of Dw14 (Ollier *et al.* 1988; Pawlec *et al.* 1988), others did not (Hakala *et al.* 1986; Zoscke and Segall 1986). It is now known that 'subtypes' of DR4 that are defined by cellular techniques are a population with further heterogeneity that can be detected using DNA-based typing techniques, and these are discussed further below.

DR4, DR1, DR14 Shared Amino Acid Sequence Associated with RA

Fig. 5.8. The DRβ1 amino acid sequences 'QKRAA' and 'QRRAA' are present on some DR4, DR1, and DR14 molecules. The sequence 'RRRAA' is present on DR10 molecules (see text).

Other HLA-DR specificities associated with RA: the shared epitope hypothesis

In some populations a significant increase of HLA-DR1 was found in RA patients (Woodrow *et al.* 1981; Schiff *et al.* 1982). The association of particular subtypes of DR4 and of DR1, and an evolving knowledge of the amino acid sequences of these molecules, led Gregersen *et al.* (1987) to propose a model for understanding the genetics of HLA associations with RA. The model was based on the observation that HLA molecules associated with RA have similarity of the amino acid sequence in the third hypervariable region of the DRβ1 chain, from positions 70 to 74, where the sequence of DRB1*0401 (Dw4) is QKRAA and of Dw14 and Dw15 is QRRAA, differing only for a conservative substitution at position 71. The model is referred to as the shared epitope hypothesis and proposes that the third hypervariable region shared amino acid sequence of DRβ1 is the underlying 'unit' of susceptibility to RA (Fig. 5.8). Further data lending support to this model were forthcoming in studies that identified a variant of DR14 and DR10 in association with RA.

DNA-typing and specific DRB1 alleles associated with RA

Beginning early in the 1990s DNA-typing techniques have been applied to the study of HLA associations with RA. The application of DNA-typing resulted in the finding that cellularly defined HLA specificities are also heterogeneous and can be further subdivided into additional variants. When DNA-typing was used to study Native American populations, in which both

DR4 and DR1 are uncommon, investigators found that a specific allelic variant of DR14 was highly prevalent. Interestingly, this allelic variant, DRB1*1402, has a similar third hypervariable region amino acid sequence as that described above for DR4 and DR1 alleles associated with RA. One study investigated Yakima Indians who were at least one-quarter Native American (Willkens *et al.* 1991) and another study Tlingit Native Americans most of whom were full quantum (100%) Tlingit (Nelson *et al.* 1992a). Both studies found a predominance of DRB1*1402 in RA patients; however, the frequency in control populations was also very high so that the difference between RA patients and controls was not statistically significant in either study. Williams *et al.* (1995) reported similar findings from Pima and Tohono O'odham Indians and was able to demonstrate statistical significance in a meta-analysis.

An extension of the shared epitope hypothesis includes the sequence RRRAA which is encoded by DRB1*1001 (DR10). In this sequence a positively charged arginine replaces the uncharged polar amino acid glutamine at position 70. A number of studies have found an increase of DR10 in RA in selected populations, including Asian Indians (Ollier *et al.* 1991), Greeks (Carthy *et al.* 1993), Spaniards (Sanchez *et al.* 1990) and Zimbabweans (Cutbush *et al.* 1993).

Limitations of the shared epitope hypothesis

Although the shared epitope hypothesis has gained considerable support a number of limitations are worth noting. First, the DR1 association with RA has not been uniformly observed even in larger studies of similar racial/ethnic populations to those originally described (Mehra *et al.* 1982; Brautbar *et al.* 1986) and the relative risk associated with DR1 has generally been lower than that observed with DR4. Secondly, although it is appealing to presume (based on the shared epitope hypothesis) that both DRB1*0101 and DRB1*0102 are associated with RA, to date, a statistically significant increase of DRB1*0102 has not been demonstrated in any study. Using DNA-typing techniques, four allelic variants of DR1 can be distinguished and are designated DRB1*0101, *0102, *0103 and *0104. In a case–control study by Gao *et al.* (1990), the DR1 association with RA was found to be owing exclusively to DRB1*0101. Thirdly, the shared epitope hypothesis also fails to explain the synergistic effect of particular combinations of alleles now reported by numerous investigators.

Hierarchies of risk and synergy associated with particular HLA-DR combinations

Nepom *et al.* (1984) first reported an unexpectedly high frequency of patients with a particular combination of DR4 variants, Dw4 and Dw14. Dw14 actually consists of two different molecules encoded by DRB1*0404 and another by DRB1*0408. Nelson *et al.* (1991), in studies limited to women with RA, described a marked synergistic increase of risk when DRB1*0404 was present along with DRB1*0401, but did not find that DRB1*0404 conferred risk in the absence of DRB1*0401. A thorough assessment of hierarchies of risk associated with particular combinations of DRB1 alleles was presented in a report by Wordsworth *et al.* (1992). The spectrum of risk spanned a range from a high of 49 to a low of 3, with the highest risk associated with Dw4, Dw14 and the lowest with DR1, X (heterozygote). In a report by MacGregor *et al.* (1995) the odds ratio associated with the high risk combination of alleles in women was 16.7, and in men was 90.0. Meyer *et al.* (1996) also described a particularly marked increase of DRB1*0401 and *0404 in male patients with RA.

The synergism associated with particular combinations of alleles adds some complexity to the analysis of HLA associations with RA. To address appropriately whether an allele that is found in synergistic combinations is also an independent risk factor it is necessary to conduct an analysis in which individuals with the other allele are removed from patient and control populations. This principle is exemplified in the evolving description of the role of Dw14 in RA. As previously discussed, initial studies were conflicting as to whether Dw14 is increased in RA patients. The cellularly defined specificity Dw14 consists of DRB1*0404 and DRB1*0408, both of which type as 'Dw14', and differ at position 86, where the former has a valine and the latter a glycine. In a prior study it was suggested that glycine at position 86 might also contribute to the shared epitope sequence (Gao *et al.* 1990). DRB1*0404 represents a good test of this possibility since it differs from DRB1*0408 only at position 86. However, because of the well-described synergistically increased risk associated with DRB1*0404 and DRB1*0401 in combination, it was necessary to conduct an analysis in which DRB1*0404 is assessed after exclusion of DRB1*0401, and other alleles encoding the shared epitope sequence with glycine at position 86. Until recently, this analysis had not been employed and a significant independent effect shown for the DRB1*0404 allele. However, in a large study (201 RA patients, 139 controls) reported by MacGregor *et al.*

(1995), this analysis showed DRB1*0404 to be significantly independently associated with RA. Thus, for DRB1*0404 there appears to be both a DRB1*0401-dependent effect in which risk is increased more than eightfold over either DR4 variant alone, and also, at least in some populations, an independent effect.

Susceptibility, protection, or both?

A number of studies have reported a protective effect of specific HLA-DR molecules on risk of RA. A frequently reported observation among Caucasian populations, is a protective effect of DR2 (Panayi *et al.* 1977; Larsen *et al.* 1989) and Dw2 (Nuotio *et al.* 1986), a cellularly defined subtype of DR2. In addition, as summarized in the RA component of the *XIth International HLA Workshop* (Nelson *et al.* 1992b) a protective effect of DR8 was reported in Japanese. A report of the study in Japanese by Tsuchiya *et al.* (1992) described one of the largest and most complete studies of RA in which alleles of DRB1, DQA1, DQB1, DPA1, and DPB1 were determined in 204 Japanese patients and 293 controls. Interestingly, a strong protective effect was found for the DR8 allele DRB1*0803 which was actually dominant over that of the DRB1*0405 susceptibility allele in this population.

Susceptibility or progression and/or severity?

It has been proposed that the HLA contribution to RA may have more to do with disease progression and/or

severity than with susceptibility. Supporting this concept, in a community-based study, Thomsen *et al.* (1993) found no association of early RA with DR4 or with the shared epitope sequence. A number of studies have examined HLA antigens in relation to disease severity. Although the term 'severity' has been used descriptively for many different outcome measures, no single measure can be equated with it. A diagram depicting various measures of severity is shown in Fig. 5.9, and is grouped into finite measures and time-dependent measures. An additional category (not shown) includes observations that are not themselves measures of severity but that suggest severity by inference, i.e. nodules and rheumatoid factor positivity.

When functional capacity is used as the measure of severity, reports are conflicting as to whether there is an association with DR4 (Vullo *et al.* 1987) or not (Gran *et al.* 1983; Silman *et al.* 1986). Similarly, when need for second-line therapy is used as the measure of severity, some studies found an association with DR4 (Jaraquemada *et al.* 1979) and others did not (Silman *et al.* 1986).

When radiographic changes are analysed, some reports describe no association of severity with DR4 (Scherak *et al.* 1980; Queiros *et al.* 1982; Walton *et al.* 1985; Westedt *et al.* 1986). However, in two studies that analysed female and male patients separately, both found an association with DR4 only in female patients (Young *et al.* 1984; Jaraquemada *et al.* 1986). In one of these studies (Young *et al.* 1984), DR4 correlated most strongly with severity of erosions in females with onset under the age of 50. Additionally, DR2 was negatively associated with severity of erosions. DR4

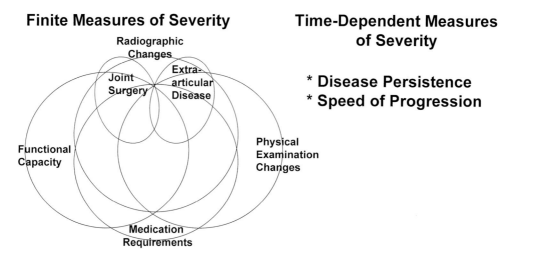

Fig. 5.9. The term 'severity' has been used to refer to a number of different outcome measures of rheumatoid arthritis and include both measures that can be quantitated at a specific point in time and time-dependent measures such as the speed of progression of joint damage.

correlated with a poor and DR2 with a good outcome with respect to radiographic changes at follow-up in another study from the Netherlands (van der Hejde *et al.* 1992a).

A number of studies have evaluated extra-articular disease as the measure of disease severity. Ollier *et al.* (1984) found an association of DR4 with extra-articular disease. Others have described an association of DR4 with Felty's and with leucocytoclastic vasculitis (Wedsedt *et al.* 1986; Hillarby *et al.* 1991).

In two reports by Weyand and colleagues extra-articular disease, history of joint surgery and nodulosis were evaluated as measures of severity (Weyand *et al.* 1992a,b). The results of these studies have often been interpreted as showing that two copies of the shared epitope sequence are associated with disease severity. However, the authors state that the association with extra-articular disease was not seen unless both copies of the shared epitope sequence were on DR4-containing haplotypes. A correlation was observed for history of joint surgery according to the number of copies of the shared epitope sequence, irrespective of whether the haplotype was one with DR4. However, for nodulosis, the correlation again was exclusively seen among those who were DRB1*04,*04. Thus two of three measures of severity correlated with homozygosity for DRB1*04, rather than with the shared epitope sequence *per se* (on non-DR4-containing haplotypes).

HLA-DQ and RA

It has been difficult to determine the role of HLA-DQ in susceptibility to RA owing in significant part to the linkage disequilibrium patterns of class II genes. Some have argued that DQ is not relevant to RA susceptibility since the same DQ molecules are observed in linkage disequilibrium with RA-associated and non RA-associated DRB1 alleles (for example DRB1*0401 and DRB1*0402 are both in linkage disequilibrium with DQ7 and DQ8). However, this is not necessarily a valid conclusion since another possibility is that particular DQ molecules may be contributory when accompanied by a primary DRB1 susceptibility allele but have no independent effect. An argument can be made against the requirement for a specific DQ molecule based on two observations. First, the DQ molecule found in linkage disequilibrium with DRB1*0405 in Japanese patients with RA has a differing DQβ chain from that which is found on haplotypes with DR4 and DQ7 in Caucasian populations, although the DQα

chain is identical. Secondly, among Native American patients with RA, the DQ molecule on haplotypes with DRB1*1402, differs in its DQα chain, although it has the same DQβ chain as DQ7 that is on DR4 containing haplotypes (even though both molecules type as 'DQ7' by serological techniques, see Fig. 2.16 in Chapter 2).

Although the role of DQ in susceptibility remains controversial, some studies suggest that DQ molecules can affect disease manifestations of RA. A number of studies describe associations of DQ with measures of disease severity (primarily DQ7 with severity). These include disability as measured by HAQ (Sansom *et al.* 1989), radiographic erosions and response to medications (Singal *et al.* 1990), IgM rheumatoid factor and higher titres of rheumatoid factor (Stephens *et al.* 1989; Sansom *et al.* 1989), and extra-articular disease, notably Felty's syndrome (Clarkson *et al.* 1990; So *et al.* 1988; Sansom *et al.* 1987).

An interpretation that is consistent with all of these observations is that DQ is not a primary susceptibility factor, but that particular DQ molecules may affect disease manifestations and/or severity. A different DQ molecule is in linkage disequilibrium with DR1 (DQ1) so that this interpretation is also consistent with observations by other investigators that patients with DR1 have less severe disease (Singal *et al.* 1990).

Mechanisms for association

How the HLA molecules associated with RA contribute to disease pathogenesis remains unknown. A number of mechanisms have been proposed, many of which focus on a particular role for the shared epitope sequence of the DRβ1 molecule. One possibility is that DR molecules that encode these sequences specifically, or preferentially, bind particular arthritogenic peptides. This explanation appears unlikely given the wide array of peptides that can be bound by various HLA molecules. A second possibility is that particular HLA molecules result in predisposition to RA because of the way in which they have shaped the TCR receptor repertoire. A third possibility is that the shared epitope sequence is a site of cross-reactivity with the peptide sequence of, for example, an invading microorganism. Yet another possibility is that specific DRB1 alleles could affect antigen processing. With respect to this possibility, in studies reported from Auger *et al.* (1996), QKRAA and RRRAA peptides were examined for binding with bacterial and human heat shock proteins, the results of which suggested that particular DRβ1 molecules might specifically affect intracellular trafficking.

A model that incorporates both the second and third possibilities above has been proposed by Albani and colleagues and termed 'multi-step molecular mimicry' (Albani *et al.* 1995). The model focuses on studies of RA patients with the QKRAA sequence (DRB1*0401). In this model, T cells with low affinity for self-DR peptides are positively selected, resulting in positive selection of T cells with low affinity for the QKRAA sequence. The QKRAA amino acid sequence is also found on the bacterial heat shock protein dnaJ, and on the GP110 protein of Epstein–Barr virus. In the next step, exposure to such bacterial proteins results in expansion of the T cells. Immune response could continue in the joints because of expression of heat shock proteins resembling dnaJ, mechanical stress, and epitope spreading. In this model human dnaJ homologues become the eventual target of T lymphocytes that have been positively selected by a self peptide (QKRAA), later triggered by exogenous antigens.

A final model that has been proposed is based on studies of collagen-induced arthritis in a murine model. Numerous studies in which peptides have been eluted and sequenced from HLA molecules have found that many peptides derive from self proteins, and include peptides derived from other HLA molecules (Englehard *et al.* 1994). In the model proposed by Zanelli *et al.* (1995), a DQ molecule presents a peptide derived from a self-DRβ1 molecule. A model in which DQ presents peptides derived from DRβ1 is also appealing in light of studies that examined the fetal–maternal HLA relationship and the pregnancy-induced remission of rheumatoid arthritis. In these studies, correlation between remission and fetal disparity for HLA class II antigens was observed, and was particularly marked for DQ (Nelson *et al.* 1993).

Genes in linkage disequilibrium

Genes encoding TNF-α are located in the MHC complex and have been of particular interest for investigation because ample evidence supports a pro-inflammatory role for TNF. In a recent study by Mulcahy *et al.* (1996) TNF microsatellite markers were determined in 50 multiplex families and the TNFc1 allele was found to increase risk of RA independent of HLA-DR genes. Polymorphisms in TAP2 genes, have also been described but are thought to be secondary to the those at DRB1 (Marshal *et al.* 1994).

Immunogenetics of juvenile idiopathic arthritis (JIA)

Just as there are distinct clinical subgroups of juvenile chronic arthritis (JCA), HLA associations are also distinct for each subgroup of disease. Much investigative work has focused on HLA associations with pauci-articular JCA. Polyarticular rheumatoid factor negative and systemic onset JCA are also discussed. The immunogenetics of rheumatoid factor positive poly-articular JRA (Nepom *et al.* 1984) is similar to that of adult RA previously discussed.

The problems with nomenclature in children with arthritis have been discussed (p. 112). Although there is a growing acceptance of the term JIA, most of the literature refers either to juvenile rheumatoid arthritis (JRA) or juvenile chronic arthritis. We have tended to follow the original author's usage.

A number of studies have provided substantial evidence indicating that there are HLA associations at multiple HLA loci with persistent pauciarticular JCA. The first of these is an association with HLA-DR/DQ. Increases of DR5, DR8/DQ4, and DR6/DQ1 have been reported (Stastny *et al.* 1979; Glass *et al.* 1980; Barron *et al.* 1991; Hall *et al.* 1986). The increase of DR6 has been reported primarily in studies from North America, and has not been found in many European populations. The association with DR6 can be attributed to the DRB1*1301 allele (Fernandez-Vina *et al.* 1990; Ploski *et al.* 1993). The alleles associated with pauciarticular JCA in patients with DR8 are DRB1*0801 and the DQ alleles that are in linkage disequilibrium, DQA1*0401 and DQB1*0402 (Fernandez-Vina *et al.* 1990; Van Kerckhove *et al.* 1990). Among patients who have pauciarticular JCA, but who go on to develop a polyarticular course, an association with DQA1*0101 has been reported (Ploski *et al.* 1993; Van Kerckhove *et al.* 1991).

Another HLA locus that is involved in susceptibility to pauciarticular JCA is HLA-DP. HLA-DPw2 was initially identified, with subsequent application of DNA-typing techniques identifying the allelic variant as DPB1*0201 (Hoffman *et al.* 1986; Odum *et al.* 1986; Begovich *et al.* 1989). Finally, the class I locus HLA-A also contributes to susceptibility to pauciarticular JCA. HLA-A2 is increased in patients with pauciarticular JCA (Oen *et al.* 1982). Using DNA-typing techniques, the A2 allelic variant was determined to be A*0201 (Fernandez-Vina *et al.* 1992).

Associations at the various HLA loci are not explained by linkage disequilibrium and different loci have been shown to contribute independently to susceptibility. However, an interesting aspect of the multiple HLA associations with pauciarticular JCA is that definite interactive effects have also been demonstrated (Morling *et al.* 1991; Paul *et al.* 1993; Ploski *et al.* 1995). In particular, a greater than additive effect has been observed with combinations of DRB1*1301 and DPB1*0201, and also with the combination of DRB1*0801 with DPB1*0201. Of final note, some HLA antigens are thought to contribute to resistance to pauciarticular JCA. Notable among these is a decrease of DR53 (encoded by a gene at the DRB4 locus) which has been reported from several groups (Fernandez-Vina *et al.* 1990; Paul *et al.* 1993; Ploski *et al.* 1993).

The number of patients with any specific HLA associated antigen or allele has generally been a relatively low proportion of the whole population of patients. In part, because of this observation, genes in the MHC class III region have been investigated. Results of some studies have suggested an independent contribution for genes for tumour necrosis factor and proteosomal genes, while others have concluded associations were due to linkage disequilibrium with HLA class II genes (Donn *et al.* 1994; Ploski *et al.* 1994; Epplen *et al.* 1995; Pryhuber *et al.* 1996).

Systemic onset JRA is relatively less common, fewer studies have investigated this subgroup, and results have been heterogeneous. Associations with DR4, DR7, DR5, and DR8 have been reported in Caucasian populations (Stastny *et al.* 1979; Miller *et al.* 1985; Morling *et al.* 1985), whereas only a negative association with DR4 was found in a Japanese study (Okubo *et al.* 1993). Recently, a protective effect of DPB1*0401 was reported (Paul *et al.* 1995), although a prior study found no association (positive or negative) with any DPB1 allele (Ploski *et al.* 1993).

DRB1*0801 is associated with rheumatoid factor negative polyarticular JCA (Fernandez-Vina *et al.* 1990; Barron *et al.* 1992; Ploski *et al.* 1993). DPB1*0301 is also significantly increased in this subgroup (Fernandez-Vina *et al.* 1990). An interaction between DPB1*0301 and DRB1*0801 has been described, as has resistance associated with DR7 and DR4 (Paul *et al.* 1993; Ploski *et al.* 1993).

As discussed above, an interesting aspect of the HLA associations with JIA, is clear interactive effects of alleles from different HLA loci. A potential explanation for this observation is that alleles from different HLA loci act at separate steps in the disease pathogenesis; for example a synergistic effect of particular class I and class II genes might be explained by an interaction of two cell populations (Fernandez-Vina *et al.* 1990). Another possible explanation is if the HLA molecule encoded by one locus presented a peptide from an HLA molecule encoded by another locus. For example, a peptide from DP could be presented by an HLA-DR molecule.

Animal models

Although a wide variety of animal models of RA are used in studies of experimental therapies and in order to understand inflammatory mechanisms, none truly reflect the diversity of the clinical disease. The main examples of animal models are shown in Table 5.5 and are summarized below.

Spontaneous model

The MRL/*lpr* mouse strain is most commonly studied as a model of SLE (see Chapter 4). Although there is notable interlaboratory variation, up to 75% of the animals develop histological evidence of synovitis (Hang *et al.* 1985). O'Sullivan *et al.* (1985) reported that the disease progressed through three distinct phases. In the first phase, between the ages of seven and thirteen weeks, synovial cell proliferation in the joint recesses occurs. In the second stage, there is continued proliferation of synovial cells, which take on the appearance of transformed and mesenchymal cells; also the first signs of damage are evident and marginal erosions followed by cartilage destruction can be observed. The final stage of the disease is characterized by extensive cartilage destruction and formation of scar tissue with only limited infiltration of macrophages and neutrophils into the synovial stroma.

The MRL/*lpr* arthropathy is similar to the pathology of human RA in that:

- the histological appearance of the proliferating synovial cells resembles transformed mesenchymal cells;
- the proliferating synovial cells tend to adhere to articular and subchondral bone, where they are associated with the destruction of this tissue; and
- formation of scar tissue occurs in areas of extensive damage.

However, proliferation of synovial stroma cells and pannus formation, which are invariably found in human disease, are rarely seen in the mouse.

Table 5.5 The main animal models of rheumatoid arthritis

Species	Features	Reference
Spontaneous model		
MRL/*lpr* mouse	Usually studied as a model of SLE, a variable number of these animals (there is marked laboratory to laboratory variation) also develop a significant synovitis.	Hang *et al.* (1982) O'Sullivan *et al.* (1985)
Induced models		
a. Adjuvant arthritis		
Rat	Following a single injection of FCA a severe polyarthropathy develops within 2 weeks which dissipates within 1–2 months. Only develops in certain susceptible strains, e.g. Lewis.	Stoerk *et al.* (1954) Pearson (1956)
Mouse	Approximately 2 months after FCA injection, clinically overt arthritis was apparent in BALB/c, SJL, CBA/c, and C57 Bl/10 mice. There was no accompanying RF.	Knight *et al.* (1992)
b. Collagen-induced arthritis		
Rat	Type II collagen emulsified in FIA given to susceptible strains causes a polyarthritis with RF production.	Steffen and Wicks (1971) Trentham *et al.* (1978)
Rabbit Mouse Monkey		Steffen *et al.* (1978) Courtenay *et al.* (1980) Cathcart *et al.* (1986)
c. Streptococcal cell wall arthritis		
Rat	A single peritoneal injection of an aqueous suspension of group A streptococcal cell wall components leads to a polyarthritis involving peripheral joints; maximum at 3 days followed by a chronic arthritis 2–4 weeks later. Lewis female rats are particularly susceptible. Low titres of RF are produced.	Cromartie *et al.* (1977)
d. Serum sickness		
Rabbit	A variety of reagents, including bovine serum albumin, bovine serum, or homologous aggregated IgG can induce a chronic arthritis when injected in previously sensitized animals.	Reviewed by Heymer *et al.* (1982)
e. Trangenic models		
Mice	(i) Introduction of a modified human TNF-α gene into fertilized ova leads to dysregulated TNF-α production and a progressive arthritis by 4 weeks of age.	Keffer *et al.* (1991)
	(ii) HTLV-1 genome introduction lead to a chronic erosive arthritis in approximately one-third of these mice Low levels of RF identified.	Iwakura *et al.* (1991)

FCA = Freund's complete adjuvant; FIA = Freund's incomplete adjuvant; RF = rheumatoid factor.

Induced models

Adjuvant arthritis

It was initially demonstrated in susceptible strains of rats, that a parenteral injection of Freund's complete adjuvant (FCA), a water-in-oil emulsion containing *Mycobacterium*, causes a chronic polyarthritis (Stoerk *et al.* 1954; Pearson 1956). Since these initial observations numerous other reports describing the adjuvant arthritis model of rheumatoid arthritis have been published (see, for example, the review by Heymer *et al.* 1982). The single intradermal injection of the adjuvant into the footpad or tail of the rat induces a severe arthropathy which begins within 2 weeks involving the wrists, ankles, paws, and caudal part of the spine and tail. The arthropathy ultimately consists of synovitis with villus formation, pannus eroding cartilage and bone, periostitis with new bone formation, and an accompanying inflammation and fibrosis of the periarticular tissues. The susceptibility is believed to be due to multiple genes, with no convincing role

for the MHC genes. The major inflammatory arthritis has usually subsided within one to two months.

Cohen *et al.* (1985) demonstrated that the disease is mediated by T lymphocytes that recognize mycobacterial peptides. Further studies have shown evidence of molecular mimicry between cartilage antigens and a mycobacterial antigen which is believed to be a nonapeptide present in the heat shock family, hsp65 (van Eden *et al.* 1985, 1988). These authors showed that different T cell clones, designated A2b and A2c, derived from a parent line A2, developed from a rat with adjuvant arthritis, had very different effects when inoculated into irradiated syngeneic Lewis rats. The A2b clone induced a severe arthritis whereas, paradoxically, A2c for unknown reasons protected from disease induction (and indeed caused a rapid remission of disease).

When hsp65 or a nonapeptide (amino acids 180–188) were given before the complete Freund's adjuvant, the rats were found to be protected from the disease. It is now approximately 10 years since these studies were performed and it is disappointing that

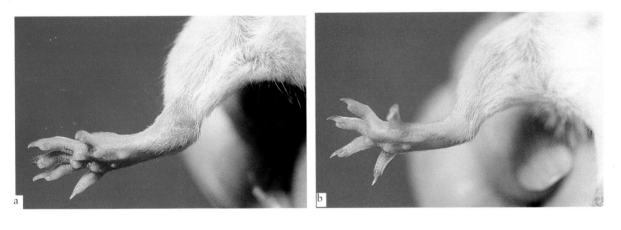

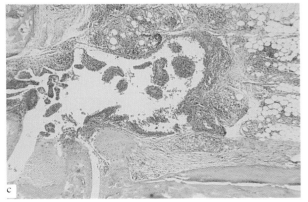

Fig. 5.10. (a) Hind limb of a BALB/c mouse injected with Freund's complete adjuvant showing severe swelling of both footpad and ankle joint (8 weeks after injection) (× 4). (b) Control hind limb injected with phosphate buffered saline only shows no swelling (× 4). (c) Representative histology from ankle joint injected with Freund's complete adjuvant showing synovial thickening, proliferation of surface lining cells, some villus formation, chronic inflammation, and erosion of articular cartilage.

although some attempts were made to develop ideas about therapy of patients with rheumatoid arthritis, no significant progress has been made. Furthermore, there has been a paucity of supporting data to confirm these interesting findings.

For many years it proved difficult to reproduce the adjuvant model in species other than the rat. Thus Glenn *et al.* (1977) failed to reproduce it in dogs, monkeys, chickens, hamsters, guinea pigs, rabbits, gerbils, pigs, or horses! Their comment that the 'probable reason for the lack of success is failure to wait longer than 2–3 months' was borne out by a study showing that adjuvant arthritis would develop in a number of normal mouse strains approximately two months after the injection of FCA (Knight *et al.* 1992, Fig. 5.10). This condition persists for several months.

Collagen-induced arthritis

When type II collagen, a major component of joint cartilage, is emulsified in Freund's incomplete adjuvant and administered to rats, a polyarthritis results (Steffen and Wicks 1971; Trentham *et al.* 1993). This effect is clearly not confined to rats having been identified in mice (Courtenay *et al.* 1980), rabbits (Steffen *et al.* 1978), and monkeys (Cathcart *et al.* 1986).

Streptococcal cell wall arthritis

Several groups have described the arthritogenic properties of bacterial preparations. The best studied are the peptidoglycan–carbohydrate polymers of group A streptococcal cell wall. This fragment induces a peripheral arthritis, particular in Lewis female rats. Histologically, it is characterized by a villus synovial thickening, with surface fibrin, thickening of the synovial lining layer, polymorphonuclear leucocyte exudation into joint fluid, and a predominantly CD4+ T cell mononuclear cell infiltrate. Ultimately, there is erosion of both cartilage and bone, so that the clinical features of this model do give a reasonable approximation to the histopathological appearance of rheumatoid arthritis. Interestingly, hsp65 protects against streptococcal cell-wall-induced arthritis (Van den Broek *et al.* 1989) and this has led to a suggestion that this heat shock protein may be the target for a T cell response that is thought to be important in the pathogenesis of the disease.

Serum sickness

Dixon *et al.* (1958) first described a transient inflammatory arthritis of serum sickness in rabbits induced by

antigen and mediated by antigen–antibody complexes. Subsequently, it was shown that allergic arthritis can be induced by multiple injections into a sensitized host. Many variations of this approach have been described and the antigens used in these studies include bovine gammaglobulin, bovine serum albumin, bovine serum, homologous aggregated IgG, and autologous IgG-F(ab')$_2$ (see Heijmer *et al.* 1982 for review). In many cases the resulting disease closely resembles RA although the pathogenesis is again unclear. In some instances, classical antigen excess immune complex disease has been described and deposition of the complexes has occurred in the joints. In the cases in which homologous/autologous antigens were employed, true autoimmune reactions may have been observed, although the use of Freund's complete adjuvant (once referred to as 'the immunologists' dirty secret!') in many of these experiments raises the possibility that the disease induced was merely adjuvant arthritis.

Transgenic models of arthritis

A modified human TNF-α gene under its own promoter was introduced into fertilized ova of a mouse. The gene was modified by replacement of the TNF-α 3′-untranslated region, which confers mRNA instability, with the 3′-untranslated region of β globin, which has very stable mRNA. Within four weeks the mice had developed progressive arthritis, which was shown to be preventable by injecting anti-human TNF-α monoclonal antibodies from birth onwards. The arthritis was characterized by subchondral erosions, but it remains to be clarified how closely the disease approximates to human rheumatoid arthritis (Keffer *et al.* 1991).

A transgenic mouse was produced carrying the human T cell leukaemia virus-1 (HTLV-1) genome. These transgenic mice develop a chronic erosive arthritis, notably in those animals that highly express the transgene. There is synovial inflammation and cartilage erosion which closely resembles pannus. Low levels of rheumatoid factor have been recorded. Iwakura *et al.* (1991) showed that IL-1σ mRNA is expressed in the joints of these mice, analogous to the situation in the joints of patients with rheumatoid arthritis. The clear implication is that this transgene in some way influences the overexpression of interleukin-1, which is in turn associated with the development of arthritis.

Other models

Intriguingly, a diet of cows milk can elicit an RA-like syndrome in Old English rabbits. These rabbits develop synovitis as well as antibodies to proteins found in milk, including anti-C1q, conglutinin, β-lactoglobulin, and IgG (Hanglow *et al.* 1985). Although it has been postulated that the pathology observed in these animals is due to the formation and deposition of immune complexes, it may well be that the dietary change induced in the animals may alter gut flora and allow the proliferation of arthritogenic bacteria.

Carrageenin is a polysaccharide isolated from seaweed and has inflammatory properties. Intra-articular injection in rabbits causes histological evidence of synovitis within 24 hours. However, the resultant pathology, chondrocyte destruction, and inhibition of proteoglycan synthesis bears little resemblance to autoimmune disorders. This model is thus of limited usefulness in experimental studies of rheumatoid arthritis.

Infective agents as a potential cause of arthritis have been analysed for over 20 years. Thus, infection with mycoplasma (Decker and Barden 1975) and *Eryispelothrix* have both been identified as causes of chronic arthritis in swine. In the former, the arthritis persists long after viable organisms can be cultured from the joints. In the latter, a chronic disease in experimental animals is induced which responds to anti-inflammatory drugs in the initial stages. The arthritis is characterized by the destruction of cartilage owing to pannus formation, with plasma cells, lymphocytes, and sometimes polymorphonuclear cells being observed in the synovial lining (Schultz *et al.* 1977).

Immunopathogenesis of rheumatoid arthritis

The immunopathogenesis of RA is multifactorial, highly complex, and development of disease is dependent upon genetic susceptibility, infection, and other environmental factors. Current knowledge suggests that inflammation and damage in the rheumatoid joint is the result of interaction between antigen presenting cells (APC) and CD4+ T helper cells, macrophage activation and the secretion of proinflammatory cytokines. Cytokine release mediates tissue destruction by the activation of synovial fibroblasts and chondrocytes that disperse enzymes leading to joint damage. In addition, the production of rheumatoid factor and other autoantibodies, the formation of immune complexes and the release of reactive oxygen species play a part in disease progression.

The development of RA can be summarized as involving many aspects of the immune response, including an initiating factor (or factors) and pathologic cell-cell interactions leading to the evolution of a self perpetuating inflammatory response (Fig 5.11a). This results in conversion of the synovium to resemble a component of the lymphoid system leading to joint damage and systemic features of the disease. Key areas of active interest include the role of APC, T cells, synoviocytes, cytokines, immune complexes and rheumatoid factor. These areas are under intense investigation, they influence the initiation, perpetuation and chronicity of RA and are discussed below in more detail.

Cellular abnormalities

Antigen presenting cells

The concept that exogenous antigen, possibly from an infectious agent(s), is responsible for initiating disease in RA, is an area of controversy. An exogenous arthritogenic antigen(s) has not been recognized and it may be possible that endogenous antigen is capable of initiating and driving disease processes. Dendritic cells (DC) are termed 'professional APCs' and have been shown to accumulate in rheumatoid synovial tissue (Zvaifler *et al.* 1985), where they differentiate under the influence of abundant monocyte and fibroblast derived cytokines and express high levels of MHC class I and II molecules and costimulatory molecules. Presentation of endogenous, DC derived antigen, including MHC derived peptides, to low affinity, self reactive CD4+ T cells under the influence of tumour necrosis factor (TNFα) and granulocyte monocyte colony stimulating factor (GM-CSF) has been demonstrated (Thomas *et al.* 1994). This event provides a model by which RA could be initiated and also accounts for the strong association between RA and MHC class II alleles (for review see Thomas and Lipsky 1996).

Repeated non specific stimulation culminating in TNFα and GM-CSF production in the joint, may result in DC differentiation and autoreactive T cell activation. This response could be perpetuated by activated T cells that would stimulate cytokine secretion and provide help for B lymphocytes. The chronic phase of RA involving effector cell recruitment and tissue damage, could result in a polyclonal, self perpetuating response.

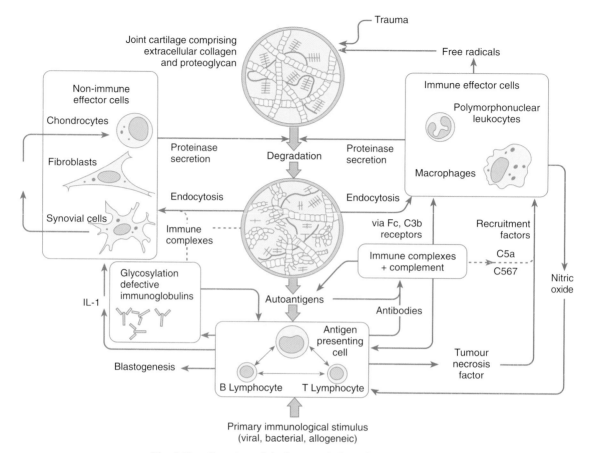

Fig. 5.11. Overview of the immopathological processes in RA.

T cells

The concept that T cells play a central role in the pathogenesis of RA became prominent in the 1980s (Janossy *et al.* 1981). Evidence supporting this hypothesis included the linkage of RA to specific MHC class II alleles, the abundance of T cells found in synovial tissue and fluid, the selective accumulation of specific T cell subsets in the joint, and observations from animal models of disease. It was expected that T cell directed therapeutic strategies would lead to an improvement in patients with disease, however, this has not been born out in clinical trials. The central role of the T cell and its contribution to rheumatoid inflammation is now under intense debate (Fox 1997; Stamenkovec *et al.* 1988, Duby *et al.* 1989).

RA is strongly associated with MHC class II alleles (DR4/1) and this observation suggests that antigen specific CD4 T helper cells are necessary for disease development. Possible pathological mechanisms include presentation of self MHC class II derived antigens to T

cells; defects in the antigen processing mechanism by APC which affect the ability of these cells to present specific exogenous antigen to T helper cells; and molecular mimicry involving cross reactivity between self peptides, MHC and exogenous antigen (Baum *et al.* 1996; Albani and Carson 1996). The immunogenetics of RA has been reviewed elsewhere in this chapter.

No disease specific autoantigen has been isolated in patients with RA and demonstration of monoclonal or oligoclonal T cell clones has been difficult with different clones isolated in different patients (Stamenkovec *et al.* 1988; Duby *et al.* 1989). It has been suggested that in chronic disease the T cell response becomes polyclonal due to bystander activation effects (Thomas and Lipsky 1996).

Many studies have analyzed T cell populations in synovial tissue aiming to identify antigen specific T cell receptors (TCRs). Most studies have been directed at the Vβ chain repertoire (for review see Struyk *et al.* 1995). This work has not been conclusive, although it has been demonstrated that T cell repertoires are skewed in both the joint and peripheral blood in RA, with various TCR Vβ families being over-represented in CD4 and CD8 T cell populations (Goronzy *et al.* 1994; Gonzalez-Quintial *et al.* 1996; Hingorani *et al.* 1996). This could be due to selective outgrowth of a subset of T cell clones stimulated by antigen or superantigen or to the non-specific effects of local or systemic inflammation. The expansion of T (and B) cell clones may be the result of non specific defects in immunoregulation, and suggests that subclinical or overt infection may affect the lymphocyte repertoire expressed in RA patients. This could explain why a single clone common to all patients cannot be identified (Fox and Smith 1986; McGee *et al.* 1996). However it does not exclude the possibility that an antigen specific T cell clone is responsible for the initiation or progression of RA as the frequency of antigen specific cells in an autoimmune lesion can be very low (<1%) (Fox 1997).

Synovial T cells from RA patients display a number of differentiation and activation markers. Isoforms of CD45 can distinguish between naive and memory cells and memory cell types are expressed more extensively in the RA synovium (Morimoto *et al.* 1988; Kohem *et al.* 1996). It has also been reported that $\delta\gamma$ T cells, normally a rare subset, have increased representation in the RA joint (Lunardi *et al.* 1992; Bucht *et al.* 1992) and their possible role in pathogenesis is supported by animal models for inflammatory arthritis where they serve a pathogenic or regulatory function (Peterman *et al.* 1993; Pelegri *et al.* 1996).

Experimental and clinical evidence seems to suggest that although T cells play a role in the initiation of the inflammatory response in RA, they are not primary to mechanisms of chronic disease processes. Other areas of the immune response need to be fully explored to permit complete understanding of the pathogenesis of RA.

B cells

Synovitis, the major lesion in RA, is characterized by the formation of ectopic lymphoid tissue regions consisting of follicular B cell areas. This process is enhanced by molecules expressed by synovial fibroblasts which favour B cell survival and differentiation in the joint. B cell follicular formation and local plasma cell differentiation is promoted by VCAM-1, delay accelerating factor (DAF) and complement receptor 2 (CR2). A significant proportion of B cell clones in the RA synovium generate rheumatoid factor (Rf), these can aggregate into small and large immune complexes

and perpetuate inflammation in the joint (Edwards and Cambridge 1998).

The production of Rf is a normal physiological process but in RA patients Rf formation has been shown to be defective. It has been recognized that the variable heavy genes used in Rfs are restricted to those expressed in fetal development (Huang *et al.* 1998) and that there is a mechanism controlling the affinity of Rfs, ensuring that only low affinity autoantibodies are produced. This mechanism is dysfunctional in RA patients and B cells are able to produce Rf that has undergone affinity maturation, this may be significant in the pathology of the disease (Thompson *et al.* 1995; Borretzen *et al.* 1997).

Costimulation and accessory molecules

The investigation of T cell costimulation is an important area for the consideration of RA pathogenesis, especially as signal transduction through the TCR is believed to be defective in these patients (Allen *et al.* 1995). Many cells in the RA synovium are able to act as APCs or accessory cells including, monocytes, macrophages, B lymphocytes, dendritic cells, fibroblasts, and synoviocytes type A (macrophage like) and type B (fibroblastic). These cells must provide both specific activation for T helper cells, via TCR binding to specific peptide presented by MHC class II molecules, and a second costimulatory signal, via molecules such as CD28 and CD15 on T cells binding to CD80/CD86 on APCs. Other molecules and their ligands have been shown to perform a costimulatory function in the RA synovium, including CD6 and its ligand ALCAM expressed strongly on keratinocytes and synoviocytes, and CD60 identified on synovial T cells and believed to have a role in T cell homing (Semnani *et al.* 1994). Different APCs are concentrated in different areas of the synovial tissue and have restricted expression of specific costimulatory molecules which effectively control T cell differentiation, for example type B synoviocytes express CD2 ligand (LFA3) and ICAM1 but not CD80/86 (CD28 ligand). Synoviocytes also strongly express VCAM1. Soluble VCAM1 promotes angiogenesis in the synovial membrane (Koch *et al.* 1995). Activation and costimulation are both enhanced by the upregulation of adhesion molecules that direct cell migration and interaction and animal models have aided the study of these molecules and their use as potential therapeutic targets is under investigation. (for review see Liao and Haynes 1995). Integrins and their ligands and CD44 (hyluronic acid binding) are important molecules in recruiting T cells to the synovial tissue and their expression is cytokine mediated.

Apoptosis

Cell death by apoptosis has been recognized in the rheumatoid synovium and study of the regulation of this process may facilitate understanding of the disease mechanism. Initial investigations have revealed that apoptosis mediated by the Fas/Fas ligand pathway are important in cells of the RA joint including synoviocytes and T cells (Hashimoto *et al.* 1998; see Nishioka *et al.* 1998 for review). Defects in the cell survival molecule bcl-2 have been reported in subsets of T cells, which may favour the outgrowth of autoreactive T cell clones and influence disease pathogenesis (Schirmer *et al.* 1998; Sfikakis *et al.* 1998).

Macrophages

Macrophages play a central role in the amplification of stimulatory signals and tissue destruction in RA. Activated macrophages are found in the synovium, destructive pannus tissue and rheumatoid nodules (Palmer 1995). Both circulating and synovial macrophages produce large quantities of prostanoids and proinflammatory cytokines and they are able to act as APCs. In the RA synovial environment, they are induced to upregulate Fcγ RI and FcγRIII, important in the capture of immune complexes, and MHC II together with many costimulatory and accessory molecules, possibly leading to T cell activation by presentation of (auto)antigens (for review see Burmester *et al.* 1997). It has recently been highlighted that FcγRIIIa receptors may play an important role in the stimulation of macrophages and perpetuation of the inflammatory response in the synovium and extra-articular areas affected in RA (Edwards *et al.* 1997a).

Macrophages constitute a major part of the synovial lining where they act as scavengers and protect against infection, in RA they are activated and mediate inflammation by the production of TNFα and IL1 (Firestein *et al.* 1990) and may carry micro-organisms into the joint. The hyperplastic rheumatoid synovium is characterized by pronounced macrophage infiltration that correlates with radiological assessment of joint damage (Mulherin *et al.* 1996). However, the destruction of cartilage and bone in RA is the result of complex cellular interactions and although macrophages amplify the pathogenic cascade they are not necessarily the primary effector cell.

A model describing the contribution of macrophages to the process of tissue damage and inflammation in RA involves T cell activation of macrophages by direct cell contact or by soluble means (cytokines) (Lacraz *et al.* 1994). Cytokine production by macrophages, including IL1, TNFα, platelet derived growth factor (PDGF) and transforming growth factor (TGFβ), activates synovial fibroblasts, which in turn maintain macrophage activation by secretion of GM-CSF, IL8 and others. Synovial fibroblasts invade bone and cartilage, chondrocytes are activated to produce further proinflammatory cytokines and the cascade develops its own momentum. Macrophages are also a source of proteolytic enzymes which directly degrade synovial matrix material.

Demonstration of the importance of macrophages in the pathogenesis of RA can be seen by the relative success of therapies directed against cytokines such as TNFα. Neutralization and blockade of monocyte recruitment is also under investigation as a possible immunotherapeutic strategy and has had some success in animal models.

Synoviocytes

There are two types of synoviocytes, type A (macrophage like) and type B (fibroblast-like or FLS). Macrophages and fibroblasts, by secreting a series of proinflammatory cytokines, play an essential part in the initiation, perpetuation and joint destruction observed in RA. The synovial membrane becomes hyperplastic, oedematous and infiltrated with inflammatory cells leading to the formation of villous projections. The mechanism of villous hyperplasia is not understood but may be due to defects in apoptosis and not due to increased cell division (Firestein *et al.* 1995).

Under normal conditions, the synovial lining provides nutrients for the maintenance of healthy cartilage, and proteoglycans in the synovial fluid providing lubrication for articular surfaces. In RA, the lining is responsible for much of the deformative tissue destruction seen. Under the influence of inflammatory cytokines many classes of enzyme are released, the most important being the matrix metalloproteinases (MMP) produced by FLS (Woessner 1991).

The FLS secrete a large number of products intimately involved in tissue destruction, including cytokines, proteoglycans, arachidonic acid metabolites and MMPs and in addition express a number of adhesion molecules. Exposure of FLS to IL-1 or TNFα rapidly induces MMP production, TGFβ and IFNγ have been shown to protect against MMP production. This shows that FLS can be induced to protect or digest synovial matrix depending on the cytokine network. The paracrine and autocrine interaction of cytokines secreted by neighbouring type A and B synoviocytes is central to tissue damaging mechanisms in RA and leads to perpetuation of the inflammatory response in the joint. There is also evidence however, that some FLS become transformed and continue to migrate and invade tissue causing damage without the need of further stimulation (for review see Firestein 1996).

Cytokines

Cytokines are dominant players in the pathogenesis of RA, however, their interaction is complex and poorly understood. Distinct Th1/Th2 cytokine profiles are not observed in RA synovial tissue. The T cell cytokine IL2 is not found in the RA joint, this may be due to the presence of IL10 which is anti-inflammatory and suppresses Th1 cytokine production. However, IL15, which has similar functions to IL2 and is produced by non T cells, is present and may attract and activate T cells in the rheumatoid synovium (McInnes 1997).

Most cytokines present in the synovial tissue and fluid are derived from non lymphocyte cells mainly macrophages and fibroblasts which have been activated non specifically. These cytokines in-turn activate T cells and other leucocytes, endothelium, synoviocytes and chondrocytes to secrete further cytokines, proteolytic enzymes and oxygen free radicals and induce the expression of cell surface molecules such as adhesion molecules. All these factors contribute to the inflammatory environment in the synovium.

The initiating factor(s) inducing cytokine production is unknown but could be non specific due to trauma, infection, allergic or vaccination reactions or deposition of immune complexes. This could account for the often non specific nature of events preceding onset or exacerbation of RA.

Many cells in the RA synovium are activated to produce cytokines, synovial macrophages are responsible for production of IL1, TNFα, GM-CSF, TGFβ, PDGF and chemokines as well as proteolytic enzymes. FLS produce IL6, angiogenic factors such as fibroblast growth factor (FGF) and vascular endothelial growth factor. Cytokines such as IL1 and TNFα stimulate FLS to produce GM-CSF and IL8 together with proteases and small molecule mediators of inflammation. Chemokines, IL8 and monocyte chemoattractant protein (MCP-1), perpetuate inflammation by recruiting additional macrophages to the synovium. In addition, IL8 is a powerful promoter of angiogenesis. The cytokine cascade is a complex network of paracrine and autocrine interaction leading to perpetuation of the inflammatory response in the joint and tissue destruction (for review see Burmester *et al.* 1997; Feldmann *et al.* 1996).

Cytokine antagonists that serve to down regulate inflammation are produced but their secretion or action may be defective, for example IL1 receptor agonist (IL1ra), is secreted by FLS and macrophages, however the balance between IL1 and IL1ra is shifted in the favour of IL1 in RA (Firestein *et al.* 1994).

The central role of cytokines is confirmed by the success of cytokine directed immunotherapy. The use of anti TNFα monoclonal antibodies is described in this chapter. Other candidates for immunotherapy in RA are IL10 and IL11 (Hermann *et al.* 1998), however, understanding of the biology of many cytokines is not sufficiently complete to predict their therapeutic value.

Serology

Rheumatoid factors

For nearly six decades it has been recognized that the serum of RA patients contains antibodies which react with both autologous and heterologous immunoglobulins. These autoantibodies have been termed rheumatoid factor (Rf) or antiglobulins. This phenomenon was first recognized by Waaler (1940) and later by Rose *et al.* (1948) and then characterized by Franklin *et al.* (1957). The dominant Rf class is IgM, detected by agglutination assays, although IgG, IgA and even IgE antiglobulins have been detected using solid-phase assays. IgG Rf has been detected in both the serum and synovial fluid of the majority of patients with RA. The suggestion that these antiglobulins, in the form of self-associated immune complexes, play a major pathological role in RA is under debate. IgA and IgE Rf are less well understood and little is known about their significance.

Rfs have a wide range of specificities but in general, react preferentially with aggregated immunoglobulin. The antigenic binding site can be on the F(ab')$_2$ fraction of the Ig molecule but is most usually located on the Fc portion and can be a genetic or structural determinant. IgG autosensitization, possibly to an altered molecule, has been suggested as a primary immunological lesion in RA (for review see Soltys *et al.* 1995). IgG molecules from patients with RA are glycosylated in a different way to IgG from normal subjects. This abnormality could lead to immune complex formation in a number of ways; either by: (1) exposing previously masked protein determinants or by creating novel protein-oligosaccharide specificities that may be immunogenic; (2) the increase in the level of certain IgG subpopulations could lead to the exposure of certain Fc determinants at much higher concentrations than before, resulting in a new (pathogenic) immune response. Finally (3) oligosaccharide binding sites on the Cγ2 domain lose their polysaccharide determinants and this characteristic could make them 'sticky' by creating a lectin-like activity.

Other autoantibodies identified and studied in RA patients over that last 20 years include anti-collagen antibodies, anti-keratin antibodies, antibodies to smooth muscle antigens and intermediate filaments, anti-nuclear antibodies, EBV-associated antibodies and anti-lymphocyte antibodies, although it is not thought that they play an important role in disease pathogenesis. Most autoantibodies demonstrated in RA are believed to be present as a result of tissue damage and inflammation.

Immune complexes

Immune complexes have been detected in both the serum and synovial fluid of RA patients by a variety of techniques and can be present in high levels (Elkon, 1984; for review). Immune complexes in the joint can initiate inflammation either via the complement system or by interacting with immunoglobulin Fc receptors (van de Winkel and Capel, 1993) and in RA, this leads to a series of pathological events giving rise to joint damage and eventual destruction. The possible pathogenic role of immune complexes has remained controversial. It is believed that small IgG Rf self associating immune complexes may be significant in the immunopathogenesis of RA (Edwards and Cambridge 1998). IgG Rf self associating dimers produce small immune complexes which fix complement poorly and are able to gain access to extra vascular space where they interact with tissue macrophages. High local concentration of IgG Rf can initiate the formation of larger complexes capable of fixing complement and thereby contributing to local inflammation. Immune complexes that are IgM Rf based, will be large and speedily cleared from the circulation by complement receptors.

Complement and acute phase proteins

Although abnormalities in the levels of various components have been noted on occasions (Franco and Schur 1971; Schur 1977) no major perturbations of serum complement are evident, probably because the majority of autoimmune pathology occurs in the region of the joints and not systemically. This observation is in contrast to SLE where pronounced hypo-comlementemia, reflecting complement fixation, con-

sumption by immune complexes and complement component deficiency is frequently seen (for review see Davies 1996). Plasma levels of C3 component are elevated, sometimes as much as four times the mean normal value in RA and this may be due to C3 behaving as an acute phase protein produced in response to inflammation, however this hypothesis remains to be confirmed. Other acute phase proteins of note include the P and A components of serum amyloid (SAP and SAA respectively) and C reactive protein.

Free radicals

Free radicals are chemical species with an unpaired electron. They are unstable, highly reactive and intermediates in chemical reactions. Oxygen free radicals are of special interest. The generation of oxygen-derived free radicals such as singlet oxygen, superoxide, the hydroxyl radical and hydrogen peroxide (this latter molecule is not a free radical but may derive and contribute to free radical radical reactions) occurs after inflammatory cell activity (see Blake *et al*, 1984 for review), their inappropriate production leads to tissue damage and the release of proteoltic enzymes in the joint.

Nitric oxide (NO) plays a vital role in modulation of inflammatory responses and excessive NO is produced in rheumatic diseases including RA. NO is synthesized with the aid of nitric oxide synthases (iNOS) which are produced by many cells including macrophages and chondrocytes when stimulated by cytokines such as IL1 and TNFα. The balance of cytokines in the microenvironment will regulate the expression of iNOS and it has been recognized that TGFβ, IL4, and IL10 all inhibit iNOS expression in macrophages. The excessive cytokine production seen in the RA joint will non-specifically induce iNOS production in many cell types, this will lead to increased NO levels and promotion of tissue injury.

The amount of NO produced can exert different effects. A small quantity can have an anti-inflammatory effect by relaxing endothelial smooth muscle and protecting against leucocyte and platelet adhesion to blood vessel walls. Large quantities will cause tissue damage and impair cellular responses and may act as an immunomodulator affecting the course of diseases such as RA. NO has been shown to promote apoptosis in many cell types.

The importance of NO in the development of RA is being increasingly recognized. Increased concentrations have been demonstrated in the synovial fluid of RA patients and this has been linked to the high levels of TNFα present in the joint. The proinflammatory actions of NO are many and include increased vasodilation and permeability, potentiation of IL1 and TNFα release, the stimulation of angiogenic activity by macrophages and activation of chondrocytes to degrade articular material (for review see Clancy *et al.* 1998).

Hypothesis

It can be seen that the pathogenesis of RA is highly complex and may in fact represent multiple diseases defined by some common clinical manifestations. Edwards and colleagues (Edwards and Cambridge, 1998; Edwards *et al*, 1997b) have recently advanced an hypothesis that incorporates many of the mechanisms outlined in the above review and which can account for the varied clinical manifestations of the disease.

This hypothesis emphasizes the importance of small immune complexes consisting mainly of self associating IgG Rf, the expression of FcγRIIIa receptors which preferentially bind such complexes and the effect of cytokines such as TNFα which facilitate local ectopic lymphoid tissue formation in the joint (Fig 15.12).

Management of RA

The management and treatment of RA requires a multidisciplinary approach and provides a challenge both to

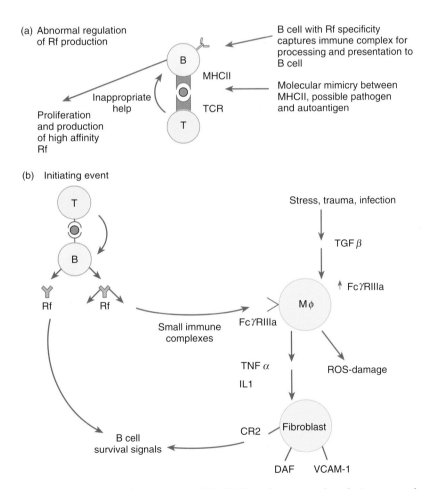

Fig. 5.12. (a) Initiating events leading to tissue dyregulation in RA. (b) Hypothesis to explain the immunopathogenesis of RA (Edwards *et al.* 1998).
DAF – decay accelerating factor; ROS – reactive oxygen species.

Table 5.6   Predictors of poor outcome in new-onset inflammatory arthritis

Abnormal HAQ
Elevation of acute phase response (ESR/C-RP)
Rheumatoid factor positivity
Early involvement of large joints
Persistence of symptoms for more than 12 weeks
Presence of HUR3 (disease epitope)
Elevated Gal(0) level

HAQ = health assessment questionnaire; HUR3 = disease-associated epitope.

physicians and other therapists. The physical and psychological consequences of RA diminish both life expectancy and quality of life. The aim of treatment is to control the symptoms of the disease (pain and disability) and to prevent permanent joint damage and so one of the major changes in the management of patients with RA over the last decade has been the realization that treatment needs to be started early in the disease. Patients with persistent inflammation (determined by the acute phase response) inevitably lose bone from both the axial skeleton (Gough *et al.* 1994) and the hands (Deodhar *et al.* 1995), develop bony erosion on X-ray (van Leuwen *et al.* 1993), and deteriorate functionally (Devlin *et al.* 1997). Furthermore, two-thirds of patients develop joint destruction in the first year of disease (van der Heijde *et al.* 1992). At present, it is difficult to predict which patients presenting with new onset inflammatory arthritis have a risk of developing destructive disease: however, a number of potentially predictive factors have been identified (Table 5.6). The role of genetic typing, particularly for the conserved HVR3 epitope, is controversial. Over the next few years it should become possible to anticipate which patients will require early aggressive therapy to control disease.

Monitoring the patient

As with all the autoimmune rheumatic diseases, no single immunological assay completely reflects clinical activity. The most useful laboratory test is measurement of acute

Table 5.7   ARA preliminary criteria for clinical remission in RA

Morning stiffness < 15 minutes
No fatigue
No joint pain
No joint tenderness or pain on motion
No soft tissue swelling of joint or tendon sheath
ESR < 20 mm/h in males and < 30 mm/h in females

phase response (ESR or C-RP). There is evidence that continued elevation of C-RP is associated with functional deterioration, thus monitoring of C-RP may give a useful guide to progress (Devlin *et al.* 1997). Radiological assessment is only repeated to investigate specific complications or for detection of new erosions. This should not be done on a routine basis. Other clinical assessments should include joint score and functional assessment. Criteria for disease remission have been described by the ARA but these are stringent and few patients ever achieve full remission (Table 5.7) (Pinals *et al.* 1981).

Drug therapy

Drugs used to treat RA fall into three main groups, the non-steroidal anti-inflammatory drugs (NSAIDs) ('first-line drugs'), and the second-line agents, alternatively known as disease-modifying anti-rheumatic drugs (DMARDs) or slow-acting anti-rheumatic drugs (SAARDs). The third-line agents, include other immunosuppressive drugs (chlorambucil, cyclophosphamide) and experimental therapies. The position of corticosteroids is controversial!

Non-steroidal anti-inflammatory drugs

The NSAIDs are used as the first line of treatment of RA, reducing pain, swelling, and inflammation, but having no influence on the progression of disease. To obtain maximum efficacy they should be used in full doses and it may be necessary to try several different agents. Unfortunately, as well as minor side effects such as nausea, dyspepsia, anorexia, and flatulence, serious upper gastrointestinal bleeding may occur in up to 4% of patients who take NSAIDs for one year. Various agents have been used to reduce the incidence of NSAID-induced lesions. These include antacids, cimetidine, ranitidine, and, in particular, misoprostol (Silverstein *et al.* 1995). A combination of diclofenac and misoprostol (Arthrotec) has proved very practical for many patients. Recently, interest has developed in the use of selective COX-2 inhibitor NSAIDs, which are believed to cause fever, gastrointestinal, or renal side-effects (Wojtulewski *et al.* 1996).

Second-line treatment

Several SAARDs are used in the treatment of RA including gold, sulphasalazine, hydroxychloroquine, D-penicillamine (Tables 5.8 and 5.9) and immunosuppressive agents such as methotrexate and cyclo-

Table 5.8 Drugs commonly used in rheumatoid arthritis

Drug	Standard dose	Monitoring	Toxicity
Intramuscular gold	50 mg (weekly to monthly)	FBC and urinalysis	Cutaneous, renal
D-Penicillamine	250–500 mg/day occasionally up to 1 g/day	FBC and urinalysis	Cutaneous, renal, autoimmune disorders
Sulphasalazine	0.5–2.0 g/day	FBC and LFT	Mucocutaneous, bone marrow suppression, dyspepsia
Methotrexate	7.5–20 mg/week	FBC and LFT	Hepatic, bone marrow suppression, pulmonary
Azathioprine	50–150 mg/day	FBC	Bone marrow suppression, hepatic
Oral gold (auranofin)	6–9 mg/day	FBC and urinalysis	Cutaneous, renal
Chloroquine	125–250 mg/day	Ophthalmic assessment	Retinal toxicity (very rare)
Hydroxychloroquine	200–400 mg/day	Ophthalmic assessment	Retinal toxicity (very rare)
Cyclosporin	2.5–5.0 mg/kg/day	Blood pressure, U&E	Renal

FBC = full blood count (complete blood count = CBC in N. America); LFT = liver function tests; U & E = urea and electrolytes.

134

Table 5.9 Slow-acting drugs used in RA

Drug	Mechanism	Comment
Sulphasalazine	Uncertain	Synthetic combination of sulphapyridine and salicylic acid first synthesized in the 1940s (Svartz 1948). Efficacy similar to intramuscular gold, DP, and MTX. Slows development and progression of erosions (van der Heijde et al. 1990). Relatively few side-effects.
Gold	Uncertain ? inhibition of macrophage function	Gold has been used to treat RA since the 1920s (Forrestier 1935). Equal efficacy to SZP, MTX, or DP, superior to placebo. Slows erosions but does not reverse existing joint damage (Jones and Brooks 1996). Skin rash, nephrotoxicity, and bone marrow toxicity are well-recognized side-effects.
D-Penicillamine	Uncertain. Inhibits fibroblast proliferation	First described by Jaffe in the mid-1950s (reviewed by Jaffe 1963). Equal efficacy to intramuscular gold and SZP, superior to placebo (reviewed in Munro and Capell 1997). Little evidence that it reduces erosion rate or useful in extra-articular disease. Similar side-effect profile to gold and may induce a number of drug-induced conditions, e.g. lupus and myasthenia gravis-like disease.
Antimalarials	Uncertain	Used since 1950s. Weaker than gold or D-Penicillamine. Very few side-effects.

SZP = sulphasalazine; DP = D-penicillamine; MTX = methotrexate.

Table 5.10 Immunosuppressive drugs used in RA

Drug	Mechanism	Comment
Methotrexate	Folate antagonist but this is probably not its mechanism of action in RA	Increasingly used since 1980s. Effective in comparison to placebo and as effective as gold, DP, and SZP. Quicker onset of action (6 weeks).
Cyclosporin	Inhibits T cell function	Shows benefit versus placebo and reduces rate of bone erosion (Tugwell *et al.* 1995; Ferraccioli *et al.* 1996).
Cyclophosphamide	Prevents DNA cross-linking	Now mainly used to treat extra-articular disease such as vasculitis
Chlorambucil	Prevents DNA cross-linking	Too toxic for routine use
Azathioprine	Inhibits cell cycle	Effective in treating refractory RA, main use is as 'steroid sparing' agent in treatment of extra-articular disease

SZP = sulphasalazine; DP = D-Penicillamine; MTX = methotrexate.

sporin (Neoral) (Table 5.10). As their names imply, these drugs are considered to modify the progression of RA but also act slowly. Drugs should be considered truly disease modifying if there is, over the course of one year or more: (i) sustained improvement in physical function; (ii) decrease in inflammatory synovitis; and (iii) slowing or prevention of structural damage. Overall, SAARDs are more effective than NSAIDs and placebo in suppressing inflammatory arthritis and in short-term studies may slow the progression of radiographic erosion. The choice of SAARD in early disease is difficult. In the UK the most frequently used drugs are sulphasalazine (which causes relatively few side-effects) and intramuscular gold, but in the USA methotrexate is a popular first choice and it is becoming more commonly used in the UK.

Corticosteroids where first introduced into the treatment of RA shortly after their discovery (Hench *et al.* 1949). The use of oral corticosteroids has remained controversial ever since (Morrison and Capell 1996). High doses of oral steroids are associated with significant side effects (see Table 3.2). Recently, low dose (7.5 mg/day) prednisolone has been claimed to slow erosive rate in newly diagnosed patients, but at two years not to confer any other clinical benefit (Kirwan 1995). However this claim remains controversial. For uncomplicated RA, prednisolone should not be used in doses > 10 mg/day and every effort should be made to limit its use to a short course or, if maintenance treatment is required, to the smallest possible dose. Corticosteroids may also be given by intravenous, intramuscular, and intra-articular routes. Intra-articular steroids are particularly useful when only a limited number of large joints are active. Intramuscular methylprednisolone is a useful means of providing symptomatic relief during the induction phase of SAARD therapy and improves the efficacy of gold therapy (Choy *et al.* 1993).

Combination therapy

Slow-acting antirheumatic drugs have traditionally been used in a sequential pyramid approach; however, this has been questioned (Wilske and Healey 1989). The rationale for combination therapy is that a combination may have synergistic effects without increasing toxicity (reviewed in Vorhoeven *et al.* 1998). Most possible combinations have been tried. Combinations can either be used in an additive fashion, adding a second or third agent to existing partially successful therapy, or in a step down approach, in which several agents are started simultaneously and treatment is reduced when disease control is obtained. A combination of cyclosporin (Neoral) and methotrexate showed promise when cyclosporin (Neoral) was added to methotrexate in patients in whom methotrexate had already produced a partial response (Tugwell *et al.* 1995). Recently, a combination of sulphasalazine, hydroxychloroquine, and methotrexate has been shown to be useful (O'Dell *et al.* 1996).

While effective, cyclosporin (Neoral) (renal toxicity, increased hair growth) and methotrexate (liver toxicity, increased rheumatoid nodules, lung fibrosis — see Fig. 5.13) may both cause side-effects. Gold and D-penicillamine are well known to be nephrotoxic and may cause skin rashes and bone marrow suppression. Gold salts rarely deposit on the skin causing a condition known as chrysiasis (Fig. 5.14).

a
b

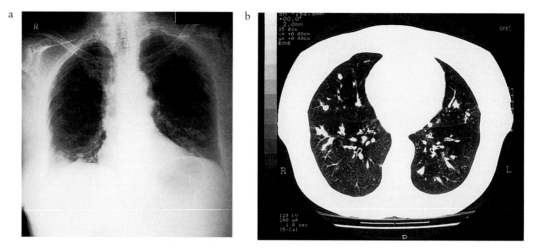

Fig. 5.13.   (a) Chest X-ray showing lung fibrosis which developed following the use of methotrexate. (b) CT cross-section of the chest from patient shown in Fig. 5.11a.

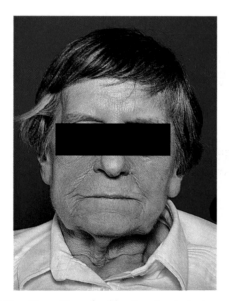

Fig. 5.14.   Deposition of gold salts, chrysiasis, in a patient with long-standing rheumatoid arthritis.

Experimental therapies

Many novel therapies for RA are being developed. The principles of these have been described in Chapter 3. Potential targets include T cells, cytokines (e.g. TNF-α), and the MHC–TCR interaction (Table 5.11).

T cells as targets

Early attempts at biological treatments were directed against the T cell, based on the notion that the T cell is a key player in the disease process. Several different murine anti-CD4 Mabs have been used to treat refractory RA, all with apparent clinical benefit in open trials. Murine CD4 MAbs-induced transient CD4 lymphopaenia. Human anti-mouse antibody (HAMA) responses occurred in the majority of patients. A chimeric CD4 (cM-T412) produced encouraging results in open trials, but two placebo-controlled trials failed to show any significant benefit compared with placebo (Moreland *et al.* 1995a; van der Lubbe *et al.* 1995). Similarly CAMPATH-1H (a humanized monoclonal antibody directed against the glycoprotein CD52 which depletes B and T lymphocytes) produced encouraging results in open trials but clinical improvement was not maintained (Isaacs *et al.* 1992). Other agents, including anti-CD5 (an immunotoxin formed by the combination of a murine anti-CD5 Mab conjugated to the ricin A chain), reversibly reduced CD5+ T cells and T cell proliferative responses failed to show any clinical benefit in a large placebo-controlled trial (Olsen *et al.* 1996).

IL-2-DAB is an immunotoxin comprising human IL-2 and diphtheria toxin. IL-2 binds to its receptor and the diphtheria toxin is internalized, killing the cell. In an open label, short duration placebo-controlled trial, the IL-2 fusion protein DAB486 IL-2 caused modest clinical improvement (Moreland *et al.* 1995b). A shortened version, DAB389 IL-2 has also been used in refractory RA (Sewell *et al.* 1993). Toxicity included elevation of liver transaminases.

Interleukin-1 receptor antagonist (IL-Ra) is a naturally occurring inhibitor of IL-1. It blocks the binding of IL-1 to its receptor but does not possess agonist activity.

Table 5.11 Biological agents that have been used experimentally in RA

Biological agent	Target antigen
T cell function	
Murine anti-CD4 Mab	CD4[+] T cell
Chimeric anti-CD4 (depleting) Mab	CD4[+] T cell
Humanized anti-CD4 (non-depleting) Mab	CD4[+] T cell
Primatized anti-CD4	CD4[+] T cell
Murine anti-CD5 ricin toxin	CD5
Anti-CD7 Mab	CD7
CAMPATH-1H Mab	CD52
Anti-IL-2 Mab	IL-2 receptor
Diphtheria IL-2 fusion protein	IL-2 receptor
MHC–TCR interaction	
TCR peptide vaccine	TCR-α/β
Autologous T cell vaccine	TCR-α/β
Placenta eluted gammaglobulin	MHC
Murine anti-idiotype Mab	MHC
Allogeneic mononuclear cell vaccination	MHC
DR4/DR1 peptide vaccine	MHC
Cytokine targets	
IL-1 receptor antagonist	IL-1
Soluble IL-1 receptor	IL-1
Chimeric anti-TNF-α Mab	TNF-α
Humanized anti-TNF-α Mab	TNF-α
TNF-α (p75 and p80) fusion proteins)	TNF-α
Recombinant IFN-γ	Multiple
IL-6 Mab	IL-6
Recombinant IL-10	Multiple
Recombinant IL-4	Multiple
Adhesion molecules	
Murine anti-ICAM-1 Mab	ICAM-1

Recombinant IL-1Ra has been used in double-blind, placebo-controlled trials in RA with encouraging results; there was a significant reduction in disease activity and a reduction in the rate of erosion (Bresnihan *et al.* 1996).

Total lymphoid irradiation

Total lymphoid irradiation was considered to be an effective method of T cell depletion in the 1980s and was associated with some clinical benefit. However, long-term follow-up has shown a worse outcome for patients who received total lymphoid irradiation compared with conventional chemotherapy (Westhovens *et al.* 1997). This study emphasizes the importance of long-term follow-up of patients receiving novel immunosuppressive therapy.

TNF-α

Chimeric and humanized Mabs against TNF-α have been used in both open and controlled trials alone and in combination with methotrexate with encouraging results (Elliot *et al.* 1994; Rankin *et al.* 1995; Maini *et al.*, 1998). Retreatment may be effective but the development of antibodies against murine components may limit the length of response. It was also observed that several patients developed autoantibodies against cell nuclei, DNA, and cardiolipin. However, to date, one patient treated with the chimerized antibody has developed clinical evidence of SLE (M. Feldman, personal communication).

Recombinant human TNFR p75-Fc fusion protein will neutralize TNF-α. A recent three-month, double-blind-controlled trial showed that this protein was associated with improvement in the inflammatory symptoms of RA (Moreland *et al.* 1997). Inhibition of TNF-α by either Mab or a fusion protein is a promising treatment for RA but further studies, in particular looking at the effect on joint damage, are awaited.

Diet therapy

Many patients are attracted to the idea of treating chronic diseases with some form of dietary manipulation, either by adding 'health promoting supplements' or by eliminating dietary components believed to be harmful. This form of treatment is perceived as 'natural' and non-toxic compared with conventional medical treatment.

The efficacy of dietary fish oil supplements (containing omega 2 fatty acids) has been studied in a number of trials, suggesting that there is a consistent but modest effect (reviewed in Cleland *et al.* 1995). Gamma-linolenic acid, a plant seed derived unsaturated fatty acid with anti-inflammatory properties, is effective when compared with placebo (Zurier *et al.* 1996). A number of elimination diets have been proposed, the 'Dong' diet is popular and this involves removal of red meat, dairy products, fruit, herbs, additives, and preservatives. A placebo-controlled trial showed no difference between the groups but some patients responded well (Panush *et al.* 1983). Artificial elemental diets in which free amino acids or oligopeptides of low allergenicity are used, followed by reintroduction of food, have been used in several randomized trials. Elemental diet can cause improvement in disease activity but this is not sustained by an individualized diet following food reintroduction. Many patients do not identify foods that exacerbate their disease (Kavanagh *et al.* 1995).

Mucosal tolerance is a novel approach to manipulate the TCR–MHC interaction (see Chapter 3). In a randomized, placebo-controlled trial of type II chicken collagen in 60 RA patients there was a reduction in disease activity in the treated group, but this was only of short duration (Trentham *et al.* 1993). A second study using bovine type II collagen showed no difference between placebo and the treated group (Sieper *et al.* 1996).

Antibiotics

There has been long-standing interest in the use of antibiotics to treat RA, because infection has been considered by some to be important, either in the initiation of the disease or in its maintenance. Tetracyclines such as minocycline or doxycycline provide modest clinical benefit in RA compared with placebo (reviewed in Paulus 1995). Whether the mechanism of action is antibacterial or some other mechanism such as inhibition of metalloproteinases is unclear.

Treatment of extra-articular disease

Extra-articular disease occurs predominately in patients with long-standing seropositive erosive disease. Second-line agents such as gold, D-penicillamine, and sulphasalazine do not control extra-articular disease and immunosuppressive therapy (azathioprine or cyclophosphamide) together with corticosteroids is often required. Pleuritis, pericarditis, and vasculitis may respond to high dose corticosteroids (up to 1 mg/kg/day prednisolone or pulse intravenous methylprednisolone). Because these complications are relatively infrequent there are few controlled data. Pulse cyclophosphamide and oral azathioprine are both effective in controlling systemic rheumatoid vasculitis (Scott and Bacon 1984; Heurkins *et al.* 1991).

Role of surgery in the management of RA

Joint replacement has been one of the great advances in the management of patients with RA, permitting many with severely destroyed joints to have greatly reduced levels of pain, improved mobility, and consequently much better quality of life. Other surgical procedures that are often beneficial include tendon transfers, particularly in the hand where function may be greatly improved after these procedures, and synovectomy, although less frequently practised, can usefully debulk a synovial mass with improvement in pain. Whether synovectomy stops further joint damage is debatable.

Treatment of juvenile chronic arthritis

Juvenile chronic arthritis is treated in a similar fashion to adult onset disease. Initial management is with a NSAID if disease is not resolved then methotrexate is becoming the drug of choice (Giannini *et al.* 1992). Methotrexate has a more anti-inflammatory action than immunosuppression of the doses used for treatment of arthritis. Sulphasalazine is also used. Intra-articular steroids are widely used and are effective in squelching inflammation in injected joints. Oral steroids are avoided if possible because of the toxicity, but when used are given in the least possible dose to minimize toxicity (particularly growth retardation) (Cassidy and Petty 1995). However, treatment of children with arthritis is very much a team effort and the role of physiotherapy and hydrotherapy cannot be underestimated. Careful attention must also be paid to the child's social needs and education.

Summary

In conclusion, RA is a chronic autoimmune condition affecting as many as 3% of the population, a statistic that makes it the most commonly occurring auto-immune rheumatic disease. Although various organs can be involved, the disease manifests primarily in the joints, causing inflammation and damage. The natural history of RA is variable, but it may persist for many years, causing a significant decrease in the quality of life for the patient.

The aetiology of RA is uncertain, although experimental evidence has suggested that several microoganisms (bacterial peptidoglycans and parvoviruses seem to be the best candidates) may act as a triggering mechanism, perhaps in association with a genetic predisposition. In the latter regard, both HLA-Dw4 and HLA-DR4 have been associated with the disease or rheumatoid factors, although these lymphocyte phenotypes are not a *sine qua non* for developing RA and, like all the other disorders discussed in this text, other factors (i.e. environmental and hormonal) will determine its appearance and course.

The immunopathology of RA has been partially elucidated and as with SLE, numerous immunological defects have been found, although most are evident in the synovial fluid rather than the circulation. Serologically, the most remarkable abnormality is the presence of autoantibodies directed against other immunoglobulins. As with SLE, the nature of the sensitizing antigen is controversial but there is good experimental evidence to suggest that the autoimmune attack is targeted at immunoglobulin molecules. Some recent evidence has indicated that immunoglobulins from RA patients are abnormally glycosylated and thus may present as novel antigenic structures which initiate the disease process. Other autoantibodies may be detected, including anti-collagen, anti-keratin, anti-proteoglycan, and ANA, although these may be epiphenomenal. High levels of immune complexes can be found in the synovial fluid and the fact that antiglobulins, or rheumatoid factors, appear to be manufactured by plasma cells residing in the synovial tissue also suggests that the joint is the site of immune complex formation. Joint damage most likely occurs as a result of the inflammatory effects of complement-fixing immune complexes, which can recruit polymorphonuclear leucocytes into the joint, where they may release lysosomal enzymes. Free radicals may also be generated by the respiratory burst from these neutrophils and may also contribute further to tissue damage. Overall, this onslaught on the joint tissue may cause new antigens to be exposed and thus the autoimmune cascade is amplified as new autoantibodies are produced.

Although many defects have been described at the cellular level, most of the abnormalities reported in the circulating lymphocyte populations are trivial and it is clear that the joint fluid and tissue contain cells with both unusal functional and phenotypic characteristics.

No satisfactory animal model exists for RA. To date most studies have been carried out on animals in which arthropathies have been induced by a variety of materials (including infectious agents, protein antigens, chemical irritants, *etc.*). Some of the conditions produced have borne only the most superficial resemblance to the human disease: probably the best studied and most useful of these models are the diseases elicited by the administration of adjuvant and type II collagen. The MRL/*lpr* mouse strain, which has been used extensively in experimental studies of SLE, spontaneously develops a synovitis similar to human RA although it has been virtually ignored as a model for this latter disease.

Clinical treatment for RA conventionally progresses through three lines of therapy. The first comprises nonsteroidal anti-inflammatory drugs, used alone or in combination. If the disease should remain unresponsive to this treatment, the second line is instigated. This comprises the so-called 'disease modifying' drugs, D-penacillamine and gold. The third line of therapy, used in cases of severely active disease, is major immunosuppressive intervention. Several trials of apheretic procedures have been conducted, but all appear to be of limited benefit. The use of fractionated lymphoid irradiation has been used for cases of intractable RA, and although this has appeared to give some promising results, it needs further evaluation before being used as a general procedure. Control of RA by dietary manipulation has long been an attractive prospect and although some clinical findings do not support the claims of certain diets popular in the lay press, there is both clinical and experimental evidence to suggest that a diet rich in fish oil may partially control the disease. The use of monoclonal antibodies to TNFα has shown considerable short term benefit. Long term outcome studies are eagerly awaited.

References

Albani S, Carson DA. A multiple molecular mimicry hypothesis for the pathogenesis of rheumatoid arthritis. *Immunology Today* 1996; **17**: 466–70.

Albani S, Keystone EC, Nelson JL *et al.* Positive selection in autoimmunity: abnormal immune responses to a bacterial dnaJ antigenic determinant in patients with early rheumatoid arthritis. *Nature Med* 1995; **1**: 448–52.

Allen ME, Young SP, Michell RH, Bacon PA. Altered T lymphocyte signalling in rheumatoid arthritis. *Eur J Immunol* 1995; **25**: 1547–54.

Arnett FC, Edworthy SM, Bloch DA *et al.* The American Rheumatism Association 1987 revised criteria for the classification of rheumatoid arthritis. *Arthritis Rheum* 1988; **31**: 315–24.

Auger I, Escola J, Gorvel JP *et al.* HLA-DR4 and HLA-DR10 motifs that carry susceptibility to rheumatoid arthritis bind 70-kD heat shock proteins. *Nature Med* 1996; **2**: 306–10.

Banks RF, Whicher JT, Thompson D *et al.* Acute phase response. In: *Oxford Textbook of Rheumatology*, 2nd Edn, eds Maddison PJ, Isenberg DA, Woo P, Glass DN. Oxford University Press, Oxford, 1998; 623–32.

Barron K, Joseph A, McLeon M *et al.* DNA analysis of HLA-DR, DQ and DP genes in pauciarticular juvenile arthritis. *J Rheumatol* 1991; **18**: 1723–9.

Barron KS, Silverman ED, Gonzales JC *et al.* DNA analysis of HLA-DR, DQ and DP alleles in children with polyarticular juvenile rheumatoid arthritis. *J Rheumatol* 1992; **19**: 1611–6.

Baum H, Davies H, Peakman M. Molecular mimicry in the MHC: hidden clues to autoimmunity? *Immunology Today* 1996; **17**: 64–70.

Begovich A, Bugawant T, Nepom BS *et al.* A specific HLA-DPB allele is associated with pauciarticular juvenile rheumatoid arthritis but not adult rheumatoid arthritis. *Proc Natl Acad Sci USA* 1989; **86**: 9489–93.

Bekkelund SI, Jorde R, Husby G *et al.* Autonomic nervous system function in rheumatoid arthritis. A controlled study. *J Rheumatol* 1996; **23**: 1710–4.

Berthelot JM, Maugars Y, Castagne A *et al.* Antiperinuclear factors are present in polyarthritis before ACR criteria for rheumatoid arthritis are fulfilled. *Ann Rheum Dis* 1997; **56**: 123–5.

Blake DR, Lunec J, Brailsford S, Winyard PG, Bacon PA. Oxygen free radicals and inflammatory joint disease. *Perspectives in Rheumatology*. Current Medical Literature 1984; 19–33.

Bodman-Smith K, Sumar N, Sinclair H *et al.* Agalactosyl IgG [Gal(0)] — an analysis of its clinical utility in the long term follow up of patients with rheumatoid arthritis. *Br J Rheumatol* 1996; **35**: 1063–6.

Borretzen M, Chapman C, Natvig JB *et al.* Differences in mutational patterns between rheumatoid factors in health and disease are related to variable heavy chain and germline gene usage. *Eur J Immunol* 1997; **27**: 735–41.

Brautbar C, Naparstek Y, Yaron M *et al.* Immunogenetics of rheumatoid arthritis in Israel. *Tissue Antigens* 1986; **28**: 8–14.

Bresnihan B, on behalf of the collaborating investigators *et al.* Treatment with recombinant human interleukin-1 receptor antagonist (rhu-1ra) in rheumatoid arthritis: results of a randomised double blind placebo controlled multicenter trial. *Arthritis Rheum* 1996; **39** (suppl.); S73.

Bucht A, Soderstrom K, Hultman T *et al.* T cell receptor diversity and activation markers in the Vd1 subset of rheumatoid syniovial fluid and peripheral blood T lymphocytes. *Eur J Immunol* 1992; **22**: 567–74.

Burmester GR, Stuhlmuller B, Keyszer G *et al.* Mononuclear phagocytes and rheumatoid synovitis: Mastermind or workhorse in arthritis? *Arthritis Rheum* 1997; **40**: 5–18.

Clancy RM, Amin AR, Abramson SB. The role of nitric oxide in inflammation and immunity. *Arthritis Rheum* 1998; **41**: 1141–51.

Campion G, Maddison PJ, Goulding N *et al.* The Felty syndrome: a case-matched study of clinical manifestations and outcome, serologic features and immunogenetic associations. *Medicine* 1990; **69**; 69–80.

Caplan A. Certain unusual radiological appearances in the chest of coal miners suffering from rheumatoid arthritis. *Thorax* 1953; **8**: 29–37.

Carthy D, Ollier W, Papasteriades C *et al.* A shared HLA-DRB1 sequence confers RA susceptibility in Greeks. *Eur J Immunogenetics* 1993; **20**: 391–8.

Cassidy JT. *Textbook of pediatric rheumatology*, 3rd ed. 1995; WB Saunders, Philadelphia.

Cathcart ES, Hayes KC, Gonnerman WA *et al.* Experimental arthritis in a non-human primate. I. Induction by bovine type II collagen. *Lab Invest* 1986; **54**: 26–31.

Choy EH, Kingsley GH, Corkhill MM *et al.* Intramuscular methylprednisolone is superior to pulse oral methylprednisolone during the induction phase of chrysotherapy. *Br J Rheumatol* 1993; **32**: 734–9.

Clancy RM, Amin AR, Abramson SB. The role of nitric oxide in inflammation and immunity. *Arthritis Rheum* 1998; **41**: 1141–51.

Clarkson R, Bate A, Grennan D *et al.* DQw7 and the C4B null allele in rheumatoid arthritis and Felty's syndrome. *Ann Rheum Dis* 1990; **49**: 976–79.

Cleland LG, Hill CL, James MJ. Diet and arthritis. *Bailliere's Clin Rheumatol* 1995; **9**: 771–85.

Cohen IR, Holoshitz J, van Eden W *et al.* T lymphocyte clones illuminate pathogenesis and effect therapy of experimental arthritis. *Arthritis Rheum* 1985; **28**: 841–5.

Courtenay JS, Dallman MJ, Dayan AD *et al.* Immunisation against heterologous type II collagen induces arthritis in mice. *Nature* 1980; **283**: 666–8.

Cromartie WJ. Craddock JC, Schwab JH *et al.* Arthritis in rats after systemic injection of streptococcal cells or cell walls. *J Exp Med* 1977; **146**: 1585–1602.

Cutbush SD, Chikanza IC, Lutalo S *et al.* Sequence-specific oligonucleotide typing in Shona patients with rheumatoid arthritis and healthy controls from Zimbabwe. *Tissue Antigens* 1993; **41**: 169–72.

D'Cruz D, Ross EL, Morrow WJW. Psoriatic arthritis: identifying and controlling an insidious killer. *J Musculoskeletal Med* 1998; **15**: 17–35.

Davies KA. Complement, immune complexes and systemic lupus erythematosus. *Br J Rheumatol* 1996; **35**: 5–23.

Decker JL, Barden JA. Mycoplasma hortinis of swine: a model for rheumatoid arthritis? *Rheumatology* 1975; **6**: 338–45.

Deodhar AA, Brabyn J, Jones PW *et al.* Longitudinal study of hand bone densitometry in rheumatoid arthritis. *Arthritis Rheum* 1995; **38**: 1204–10.

Devlin J, Gough AK, Huissoon A *et al.* The acute phase and function in early rheumatoid arthritis. CRP levels correlate with functional outcome. *J Rheumatol* 1997; **24**: 9–13.

Dixon FJ, Vasquez JJ, Weigle WD *et al.* Pathogenesis of serum sickness. *Arch Pathol* 1958; **65**: 18–22.

Donn RP, Davies EJ, Holt PJ *et al*. Increased frequency of TAP2B in early onset pauciarticular juvenile chronic arthritis. *Ann Rheum Dis* 1994; **53**: 261–264.

Duby AD, Sinclair AK, Osbourne-Lawrence SL *et al*. Clonal heterogeneity of synovial fluid T lymphocytes from patients with rheumatoid arthritis. *Proc Natl Acad Sci USA* 1989; **86**: 6206–10.

Eberhardt KB, Fex E, Johnsson K *et al*. Hip involvement in early rheumatoid arthritis. *Ann Rheum Dis* 1995; **54**: 45–8.

Edwards JC, Cambridge G. Rheumatoid arthritis: The predictable effect of small immune complexes in which antibody is also antigen. *Br J Rheumatol* 1998; **37**: 126–30.

Edwards JC, Blades S, Cambridge G. Restrricted expression of Fc GammaRIII (CD16) in synovium and dermis: implications for tissue targeting in rheumatoid arthritis (RA). *Clin Exp Immunol* 1997a; **108**: 401–6.

Edwards JC, Leigh RD, Cambridge G. Expression of molecules involved in B lymphocyte survival and differentiation by synovial fibroblasts. *Clin Exp Immunol* 1997b; **108**: 407–14.

Elkon KB. Rheumatoid factors, immune complexes and complement. *Perspectives in Rheumatology* 1984; 33–42.

Elliot MJ, Maini RN, Feldman M *et al*. Randomised double blind comparison of chimeric monoclonal antibody to tumour necrosis factor a (cA2) versus placebo in rheumatoid arthritis. *Lancet* 1994; **344**: 1104–10.

Engelhard V. Structure of peptides associated with class I and class II MHC molecules. *Annu Rev Immunol* 1994; **12**: 181–207.

Epplen C, Rumpf H, Albert E *et al*. Immunoprinting excludes many potential susceptibility genes as predisposing to early onset pauciarticular juvenile chronic arthritis expect HLA class II and TNF. *Eur J Immunogenet* 1995; **22**: 311–22.

Feldmann M, Brennan FM, Maini RN. Role of cytokines in rheumatoid arthritis. *Ann Rev Immunol* 1996; **14**: 397–440.

Felty AR. Chronic arthritis in the adult associated with splenomegaly and leucopenia; a report of five cases of an unusual clinical syndrome. *Bulletin Johns Hopkins Hospital* 1924; **35**: 16–20.

Fernandez-Vina MA, Fink CW, Stastny P. HLA antigen in juvenile arthritis. Pauciarticular and polyarticular juvenile arthritis are immunogenetically distinct. *Arthritis Rheum* 1990; **33**: 1787–94.

Fernandez-Vina MA, Falco M, Sun Y *et al*. DNA typing for HLA class I alleles: I. Subsets of HLA-A2 and of A28. *Human Immunol* 1992; **33**: 163–73.

Ferraccioli GF, Casa-Alberighi OD, Marubini E *et al*. Is the control of disease progression within our grasp? Review of the Grisar study. *Br J Rheumatol* 1996; **35**(Suppl. 2): 8–13.

Firestein GS. Invasive fibroblast-like synoviocytes in rheumatoid arthritis: passive responders or transformed aggressors? *Arthritis Rheum* 1996; **39**: 1781–90.

Firestein GS, Alvaro-Gracia JM, Maki R. Quantitative analysis of cytokine gene expression in rheumatoid arthritis. *J Immunol* 1990; **144**: 3347–53.

Firestein GS, Boyle DL, Yu C *et al*. Synovial interleukin–1 receptor antagonist and interleukin–1 balance in rheumatoid arthritis. *Arthritis Rheum* 1994; **37**: 644–52.

Firestein GS, Yeo M, Zvaifler NJ *et al*. Apoptosis in rheumatoid arthritis synovium. *J Clin Invest* 1995; **96**: 1631–38.

Forrestier J. Rheumatoid arthritis and its treatment with gold salts. *J Lab Clin Med* 1935; **20**: 827–40.

Fox D. The role of T cells in the immunopathogenesis of rheumatoid arthritis. *Arthritis Rheum* 1997; **40**: 598–609.

Fox DA, Smith BR. Evidence for oligoclonal B cell expansion in peripheral blood of patients with rheumatoid arthritis. *Ann Rheum Dis* 1986; **45**: 991–5.

Franco AR, Schur PH. Hypocomplementemia in rheumatoid arthritis. *Arthritis Rheum* 1971; **14**: 231–8.

Franklin EC, Holman HR, Muller-Eberhard HJ, Kunkel HG. An unusual protein component of high molecular weight in the serum of certain patients with rheumatoid arthritis. *J Exp Med* 1957; **105**: 425–38.

Gao X, Olsen NJ, Pincus T *et al*. HLA-DR alleles with naturally occurring amino acid substitutions and risk for development of rheumatoid arthritis. *Arthritis Rheum* 1990; **33**: 939–46.

Giannini EH, Brewer EJ, Kuzmina N *et al*. Methotrexate in resistant juvenile rheumatoid arthritis. Results of the USA-USSR double-blind, placebo-controlled trial. *N Eng J Med* 1992; **326**: 1043–9

Gladman DD. Toward unraveling the mystery of psoriatic arthritis. *Arthritis Rheum* 1993: **36**, 881–884.

Gladman DD, Shukett R, Russell ML *et al*. Psoriatic arthritis (PSA) — An analysis of 220 patients. *Q J Med* 1987; **62**: 127–41.

Gladman, DD, Stafford-Brady F, Chang C *et al*. Longitudinal study of clinical and radiological progression in psoriatic arthritis. *J Rheumatol* 1990; **17**: 809–12.

Glass D, Litvin D, Wallace K *et al*. Early onset pauciarticular juvenile rheumatoid arthritis associated with human leukocyte antigen DRw5, iritis, and antinuclear antibody. *J Clin Invest* 1980; **66**: 426–9.

Glenn EM, Bowman BJ, Rohloff NA *et al*. A major contributory cause of arthritis in adjuvant-inoculated-rats: granulocytes. *Agents Actions* 1977; **7**: 265–82.

Gononzy JJ, Bartz-Bazzanella P, Hu W *et al*. Dominant clonotypes in the repertoire of peripheral CD4+ T cells in rheumatoid arthritis. *J Clin Invest* 1994; **94**: 2068–76.

Gonzalez-Quintial R, Baccala R, Pope RM *et al*. Identification of clonally expanded T cells in rheumatoid arthritis using a sequence enrichment nuclease assay. *J Clin Invest* 1996; **97**: 1335–43.

Gordon T, Isenberg D. The endocrinologic associations of the autoimmune disease. *Sem Arthritis Rheum* 1987; **17**: 58–70.

Gough AK, Lilley J, Eyre S *et al*. Generalised bone loss in patients with early rheumatoid arthritis occurs early and relates to disease activity. *Lancet* 1994; **344**: 23–7.

Gran JT, Husby G, Thorsby E. The association between rheumatoid arthritis and the HLA antigen DR4. *Ann Rheum Dis* 1983; **42**: 292–6.

Gregersen PK, Silver J, Winchester RJ. The shared epitope hypothesis. An approach to understanding the molecular genetics of susceptibility to rheumatoid arthritis. *Arthritis Rheum* 1987; **30**: 1205–13.

Hakala M, van Assendelft AHW, Ilonen J *et al*. Association of different HLA antigens with various toxic effects of gold salts in rheumatoid arthritis. *Ann Rheum Dis* 1986; **45**: 177–82.

Hall PJ, Burman SJ, Laurent MR *et al*. Genetic susceptibility to early onset pauciarticular juvenile chronic arthritis: a study of HLA and complement markers in 158 British patients. *Ann Rheum Dis* 1986; **45**: 464–74.

Hang L, Theofilopoulos AN, Dixon FJ. A spontaneous rheumatoid-like disease in MRL/l mice. *J Exp Med* 1982; **155**: 1690–701.

Hanglow AC, Welsh CJR, Conn P *et al*. Early rheumatoid like lesions in rabbits drinking cows' milk. II. Antibody responses to bovine serum proteins. *Int Arch Allergy Appl Immunol* 1985; **78**: 152–60.

Harvey J, Lotze M, Arnett FC *et al*. Rheumatoid arthritis in a Chippewa band. II. Field study with clinical serologic and HLA-D correlations. *J Rheumatol* 1983; **10**: 28–32.

Hashimoto H, Tanaka M, Suda T, Tomita T, Hayashida K, Takeuchi E, Kaneko M, Takano H, Nagata S, Ochi T. Soluble Fas ligand in the joints of patients with rheumatoid arthritis and osteoarthritis. *Arthritis Rheum* 1998; **41**: 657–62.

Hazenberg BP, van Leewen MA, van Rijwijk MK *et al*. Correction of granulocytopenia in Felty's syndrome by granulocyte-macrophage colony-stimulating factor. Simultaneous induction of interleukin-6 release and flare-up of the arthritis. *Blood* 1989; **74**: 2769–70.

Hench PS, Kendall EC, Slocumb CH *et al*. The effect of a hormone of the adrenal cortex (17-hydroxy-11-dehydrocortisone:compound E) and of pituitary adrenocorticotrophic hormone on rheumatoid arthritis. Preliminary report. *Proc Staff Meet Mayo Clin* 1949; **24**: 181–97.

Hermann JA, Hall MA, Maini RN, Feldmann M, Brennan FM. Important immunoregulatory role of interleukin-11 in the inflammatory process in rheumatoid arthritis. The role of nitric oxide in inflammatiion and immunity. *Arthritis Rheum* 1998; **41**: 1388–97.

Heurkins AHM, Westedt ML, Breedfeld FC. Prednisolone plus azathioprine treatment in patients with rheumatoid arthritis complicated by vasculitis. *Arch Intern Med* 1991; **15**: 2249–54.

Heymer B, Spanel R, Herferkamp O. Experimental models of arthritis. *Curr Top Pathol* 1982; **71**: 123–52.

Hillarby MC, Hopkins J, Grennan DM. A re-analysis of the association between rheumatoid arthritis with and without extra-articular features, HLA-DR4, and DR4 subtypes. *Tissue Antigens* 1991; **37**: 39–41.

Hingorani R, Monteiro J, Furie R *et al*. Oligoclonality of Vβ3 TCR chains in the CD8+ T cell population of rheumatoid arthritis patients. *J Immunol* 1996; **156**: 852–8.

Hoet RM, Van Verooij WJ. The antiperinuclear and anti-keratin antibodies in rheumatoid arthrtis.In: *Rheumatoid Arthritis*, eds Smollen J, Kalden J, Maini RN. Springer Verlag, Berlin, 1992; 299–318.

Hoffman RW, Shaw S, Francis LC *et al*. HLA-DP antigens in patients with pauciarticular juvenile rheumatoid arthritis. *Arthritis Rheum* 1986; **29**: 1057–62.

Huang SC, Jiang R, Hufnagle WO *et al*. VH usage an somatic hypermutation in peripheral blood B cells of patients with rheumatoid arthritis (RA). *Clin Exp Immunol* 1998; **112**: 516–27.

Isaacs JD, Watts RA, Hazleman BL *et al*. Humanised monoclonal antibody therapy for rheumatoid arthritis. *Lancet* 1992; **340**: 748–52.

Isenberg DA, Martin P, Hajiroussou V *et al*. Haematological reassessment of rheumatoid arthritis using an automated method. *Br J Rheumatol* 1986; **25**: 152–7.

Iwakura Y, Yosu M, Yoshida *et al*. Induction of inflammatory arthropathy resembling rheumatoid arthritis in mice transgenic for HTLV. *Science* 1991; **253**: 1026–8.

Jaffe IA. Comparison of the effect of plasmapheresis and penicillamine on the level of circulating rheumatoid factor. *Ann Rheum Dis* 1963; **22**: 71–6.

Janossy G, Panayi GS, Duke O, BofillM, Poulter LW, Goldstein G. Rheumatoid arthritis: a disease of T lymphocyte/macrophage immunoregulation. *Lancet* 1981; **2**: 839–42.

Jaraquemada D, Pachoula-Papasteriadis C, Festenstein H *et al*. HLA-D and DR determinants in rheumatoid arthritis. *Transplant Proc* 1979; **9**: 1306.

Jaraquemada D, Ollier W, Awad A *et al*. HLA and rheumatoid arthritis: susceptibility or severity? *Dis Markers* 1986; **4**: 43–53.

Jones G, Brooks PM. Injectable gold compounds: an overview. *Br J Rheumatol* 1996; **35**: 1154–8.

Jones M, Symmons D, Finn J *et al*. Does exposure to immunosuppressive therapy increase the 10 year malignancy and mortality risk in rheumatoid arthritis? A matched cohort study. *Br J Rheumatol* 1996; **35**: 738–40.

Jurick AG, Davidson D, Gvardal KH. Prevalence of pulmonary involvement in rheumatoid arthritis and its relationship to some characteristics of the patients: arthritis radiological and clinical study. *Scand J Rheumatol* 1982; **11**: 217–24.

Kavanagh R, Workman E, Nash P *et al*. The effects of elemental diet and subsequent food reintroduction on rheumatoid arthritis. *Br J Rheumatol* 1995; **34**: 270–3.

Keffer J, Lesley P, Cuzlaris H *et al*. Transgenic mice expressing human tumour necrosis factor: a predictive gene model of arthritis. *EMBO J* 1991; **10**: 4025–31.

Kirwan JR. The effect of glucocorticoids on the joint destruction in rheumatoid arthritis. *N Eng J Med* 1995; **333**: 142–6.

Knight B, Katz DR, Isenberg DA *et al*. Induction of adjuvant arthritis in mice. *Clin Exp Immunol* 1992; **90**: 459–65.

Koch AE, Halloran MM, Haskell CJ *et al*. Angiogenesis mediated by soluble forms of E-selectin and vascular cell adhesion molecule–1. *Nature* 1995; **376**: 517–19.

Kohem CL, Brezinschek RI, Wisbey H *et al*. Enrichment of differentiated CD45RB (dim), CD27- memory T cells in the peripheral blood, synovial fliud and synovial tissue of patients with rheumatoid arthritis. *Arthritis Rheum* 1996; **39**: 844–54.

Lacraz S, Isler P, Vey E *et al*. Direct contact between T lymphocytes and monocytes is a major pathway for induction of metalloproteinase expression. *J Biol Chem* 1994; **269**: 22027–33.

Larsen BA, Alderdice CA, Hawkins D *et al*. Protective HLA-DR phenotypes in rheumatoid arthritis. *J Rheumatol* 1989; **16**: 455–8.

Laxer R, Schneider R. Systemic-onset juvenile chronic arthritis. In: *Oxford Textbook of Rheumatology*, 2nd edn. Maddison P, Isenberg D, Woo P, Glass DN. Oxford University Press, Oxford, 1998; 1114–31.

Liao HX, Haynes BF. Role of adhesion molecules in the pathogenesis of rheumatoid arthritis. *Rheum Dis Clin North Am* 1995; **21**: 715–40.

Lunardi C, Marguerie C, Walport MJ *et al*. Tγδ cells and their subsets in blood and synovial fluid from patients with rheumatoid arthritis. *Br J Rheumatol* 1992; **31**: 527–30.

MacGregor A, Ollier W, Thomson W *et al*. HLA-DRB1*0401/0404 genotype and rheumatoid arthritis: increased association in men, young age at onset, and disease severity. *J Rheumatol* 1995; **22**: 1032–6.

Maini RN, Breedveld FC, Kalden JR *et al*. Therapeutic efficacy of multiple intravenous infusions of anti-tumour necrosis factor α monoclonal antibody combined with low dose weekly methotrexate in rheumatoid arthritis. *Arthritis Rheum* 1998; **41**: 1552–63.

Marshal S, Hall MA, Panayi GS *et al*. Association of TAP2 polymorphism with rheumatoid arthritis is secondary to allelic association with HLA-DRB1. *Arthritis Rheum* 1994; **37**: 504–13.

McGee B, Small RE, Singh R *et al*. B lymphocyte clonal expansion in rheumatoid arthritis. *J Rheumatol* 1996; **23**: 36–43.

McInnes IB, Leung BP, Sturrock RD *et al*. Interleukin-15 mediates T cell-dependent regulation of tumor necrosis factor-α production in rheumatoid arthritis. *Nature Med* 1997; **3**: 189–95.

McMichael AJ, Sasazuki T, McDevitt HO *et al*. Increased frequency of HLA-Cw3 and HLA-Dw4 in rheumatoid arthritis. *Arthritis Rheum* 1977; **20**: 1037–42.

Mehra NK, Vaidya MC, Taneja V *et al*. HLA-DR antigens in rheumatoid arthritis in North India. *Tissue Antigens* 1982; **20**: 300–2.

Meyer JM, Han J, Singh R *et al*. Sex influences on the penetrance of HLA shared-epitope genotypes for rheumatoid arthritis. *Am J Hum Genet* 1996; **58**: 371–83.

Miller ML, Aaron S, Jackson J *et al*. HLA gene frequencies in children and adults with systemic onset juvenile rheumatoid arthritis. *Arthritis Rheum* 1985; **28**: 146–50.

Moll, JMH, Wright V. Familial occurrence of psoriatic arthritis. *Ann Rheum Dis* 1973; **32**: 181–201.

Moreland LW, Pratt PW, Mayes MD *et al*. Double-blind placebo-controlled multicenter trial using chimeric monoclonal anti-CD4 antibody, cM-T412, in rheumatoid arthritis patients receiving concomitant methotrexate. *Arthritis Rheum* 1995a; **38**: 1568–80.

Moreland LW, Sewell KL, Trentham DE *et al*. Interleukin-2 diphtheria fusion protein (DAB486-IL-2) in refractory rheumatoid arthritis. *Arthritis Rheum* 1995b; **38**: 1177–86.

Moreland LW, Baumgartner SW, Schiff MH *et al*. Treament of rheumatoid arthritis with a recombinant human tumour necrosis factor receptor (p75)-Fc fusionm protein. *N Eng J Med* 1997; **337**: 141–7.

Morimoto C, Romain PL, Fox DA *et al*. Abnormalities in CD4+ T lymphocyte subsets in inflammatory rheumatic diseases. *Am J Med* 1988; **84**: 817–25.

Morling N, Friis J, Heilmann C *et al*. HLA antigen frequencies in juvenile chronic arthritis. *Scand J Rheumatol* 1985; **14**: 209–16.

Morling N, Friis J, Fugger L *et al*. DNA polymorphism of HLA class II genes in pauciarticular juvenile rheumatoid arthritis. *Tissue Antigens* 1991; **38**: 16–23.

Morrison E, Capell H. Corticosteroids in the management of rheumatoid arthritis. *Br J Rheumatol* 1996; **35**: 2–4.

Mulcahy B, Waldon-Lynch F, McDermott MF *et al*. Genetic variability in the tumor necrosis factor-lymphotoxin region influences susceptibility to rheumatoid arthritis. *Am J Hum Genet* 1996; **59**: 676–83.

Mulherin D, Fitzgerald O, Bresnihan B. Synovial tissue macrophage populations and articular damage in rheumatoid arthritis. *Arthritis Rheum* 1996; **39**: 115–24.

Munro R, Capell HA. Penicillamine. *Br J Rheumatol* 1997; **36**: 104–9.

Mustila A, Korpela M, Mustoner J *et al*. Perinuclear antineutrophil cytoplasmic antibody in rheumatoid arthritis. *Arthritis Rheum* 1997; **40**: 710–7.

Nelson JL, Mickelson EM, Masewicz SA *et al*. Dw14 (DRB1*0404) is a Dw4-dependent risk factor for rheumatoid arthritis. *Tissue Antigens* 1991; **38**: 145–51

Nelson JL, Boyer GS, Templin DW *et al*. HLA antigens in Tlingit Indians with rheumatoid arthritis. *Tissue Antigens* 1992a; **40**: 57–63.

Nelson JL, Hansen JA, Singal D *et al*. Rheumatoid Arthritis Joint Report. In: *HLA 1991* eds. Tsuji K, Aizawa M, Sasazuki T, Vol 1. Oxford University Press, New York, 1992b; 772–4.

Nelson J, Hughes K, Smith A *et al*. Fetal HLA class II allo-antigen disparity and the pregnancy induced amelioration of rheumatoid arthritis. *N Eng J Med* 1993; **329**: 466–71.

Nepom BS, Nepom GT, Mickelson EM *et al*. Specific HLA-DR4-associated histocompatibility molecules characterize patients with seropositive juvenile rheumatoid arthritis. *J Clin Invest* 1984; **74**: 287–91.

Nepom G, Byers P, Seyfried C *et al*. HLA genes associated with rheumatoid arthritis. *Arthritis Rheum* 1989; **32**: 15–21.

Nishioka K, Hasunuma T, Kato T, Sumida T, Kobata T. Apoptosis in rheumatoid arthritis. *Arthritis Rheum* 1998; **41**: No 1: 1–9.

Nuotio P, Nissila M, Ilonen J. HLA-D antigens in rheumatoid arthritis and toxicity to gold and penicillamine. *Scand J Rheumatol* 1986; **15**: 255–8.

O'Dell JR, Haire CE, Erickson N *et al*. Treatment of rheumatoid arthritis with methotrexate, sulphasazine and hydroxychloroquine, or a combination of these medications. *New Engl J Med* 1996; **334**: 1287–91.

Odum N, Morling N, Friis J *et al*. Increased frequency of HLA-DPw2 in pauciarticular onset juvenile chronic arthritis. *Tissue Antigens* 1986; **28**: 245–50.

Oen K, Petty RE, Scyroeder ML. An association between LA-A2 and juvenile rheumatoid arthritis in girls. *J Rheumatol* 1982; **9**: 916–20.

Ohta N, Nishimura YK, Tanimoto K *et al*. Association between HLA and Japanese patients with rheumatoid arthritis. *Human Immunol* 1982; **5**: 123–32.

Okubo H, Itou K, Tanaka S *et al*. Analysis of the HLA-DR gene frequencies in Japanese cases of juvenile rheumatoid arthritis and rheumatoid arthritis by oligonucleotide DNA typing. *Rheumatol Int* 1993; **13**: 65–9.

Ollier W, Carthy D, Cutbush S *et al*. HLA-DR4 associated Dw types in rheumatoid arthritis. *Tissue Antigens* 1988; **33**: 30–7.

Ollier W, Stephens C, Awad J *et al*. Is rheumatoid arthritis in Indians associated with HLA antigens sharing a DRβ1 epitope? *Ann Rheum Dis* 1991; **50**: 295–7.

Ollier W, Venables PJW, Mumford PA *et al*. HLA antigen associations with extra-articular rheumatoid arthritis. *Tissue Antigens* 1984; **24**: 279–91.

Olsen NJ, Brooks RH, Cush JJ *et al*. A double-blind placebo-controlled study of anti-CD5 immunoconjugate in patients with rheumatoid arthritis. *Arthritis Rheum* 1996; **39**: 1102–8.

O'Sullivan FX, Fassbender H, Gay S *et al.* Etiopathogenesis of the rheumatoid arthritis-like disease in MRL/l mice. I. The histomorphologic basis of joint destruction. *Arthritis Rheum* 1985; **28**: 529–36.

Oxenholm P, Madsen EB, Monthorpe R *et al.* Pulmonary function in patients with rheumatoid arthritis. *Scand J Rheumatol* 1982; **11**: 109–12.

Palmer DG. The anatomy of the rheumatoid lesion. *Br Med Bull* 1995; **51**: 286–95.

Panayi GS, Wooley PH. B lymphocyte alloantigens in the study of the genetic basis of rheumatoid arthritis. *Ann Rheum Dis* 1977; **36**: 365–8.

Panush RS, Carter RL, Katz D *et al.* Diet therapy for rheumatoid arthritis. *Arthritis Rheum* 1983; **26**: 462–71.

Parekh R, Isenberg DA, Roitt I *et al.* Galactosylation of IgG associated oligosaccharides: reduction in patients with adult and juvenile onset rheumatoid arthritis and relation to disease activity. *Lancet* 1988; **1**: 966–9.

Parekh R, Isenberg DA, Rook G *et al.* A comparative analysis of disease associated changes in the galactosylation of serum IgG. *J Autoimmun* 1989; **2**: 101–14.

Paul C, Schoenwald U, Truckenbrodt H *et al.* HLA-DP/DR interaction in early onset pauciarticular juvenile chronic arthritis. *Immunogenetics* 1993; **37**: 442–8.

Paul C, Yao Z, Nevinny-Stickel C *et al.* Immunogenetics of juvenile chronic arthritis. *Tissue Antigens* 1995; **45**: 280–3.

Paulus HE. Minocycline treatment of rheumatoid arthritis. *Ann Intern Med* 1995; **122**: 147–8.

Pawelec G, Reekers P, Brackertz D *et al.* HLA-DP in rheumatoid arthritis families. *Tissue Antigens* 1988; **31**: 83–9.

Pearson CM. Development of arthritis, periarthritis and periostitis in rats given adjuvants. *Proc Soc Exp Biol Med* 1956; **91**: 95–101.

Pelegri C, Kuhnlein P, Buchner E *et al.* Depletion of γ/δ T cells does not prevent or ameliorate, but rather aggravates, rat adjuvant arthritis. *Arthritis Rheum* 1996; **39**: 204–15.

Peterman G, Spencer C, Sperling A *et al.* Role of gdT cells in murine collagen-induced arthritis. *J Immunol* 1993; **151**: 6546–58.

Pinals RS, Masi AT, Larsen RA. Prelimary criteria for clinical remission in rheumatoid arthritis. *Arthritis Rheum* 1981; **24**: 1308–15.

Pincus T, Marcum SB, Callahan LF. Long term drug therapy for rheumatoid arthritis in seven rheumatology private practices: second line drugs and prednisolone. *J Rheumatol* 1992; **19**: 1885–94.

Ploski R, Vinje O, Ronningen KS *et al.* HLA class heterogeneity of juvenile rheumatoid arthritis. DRB1*0101 may define a novel subset of the disease. *Arthritis Rheum* 1993; **36**: 465–72.

Ploski R, Undlien DE, Vinje O *et al.* Polymorphism of human major histocompatibility complex-encoded transporter associated with antigen processing (TAP) genes and susceptibility to juvenile rheumatoid arthritis. *Human Immunol* 1994; **39**: 54–60.

Ploski R, McDowell TL, Symons JA *et al.* Interaction between HLA-DR and HLA-DP, and between HLA and interleukin 1 alpha in juvenile rheumatoid arthritis indicates heterogeneity of pathogenic mechanisms of the disease. *Human Immunol* 1995; **42**: 343–7.

Prevoo MLL, van Riel PLCM, van't Hof MA *et al.* Validity and reliability of joint indices. A longitudinal study in pa-

tients with recent onset rheumatoid arthritis. *Br J Rheumatol* 1993; **32**: 589–94.

Pryhuber KG, Murray KJ, Donnelly P *et al.* Polymorphism in the LMP2 gene influences disease susceptibility and severity in HLA-B27 associated juvenile rheumatoid arthritis. *J Rheumatol* 1996; **23**: 747–52.

Queiros MV, Sancho MR, Caetano JM. HLA-DR4 antigen and IgM rheumatoid factors. *J Rheumatol* 1982; **9**: 370–3.

Rankin ECC, Choy EHS, Kassimos D *et al.* The therapeutic effects of an engineered human anti-tumour necrosis factor a antibody CDP571 in rheumatoid arthritis. *Br J Rheumatol* 1995; **34**: 334–42.

Renton P. Radiology in adults. In: *Oxford Textbook of Rheumatology*, 2nd edn, eds Maddison PJ, Isenberg DA, Woo P, Glass DN. Oxford University Press, Oxford, 1998; 715–50.

Rose HM, Ragan C, Pearce E *et al.* Differential agglutination of normal and sensitized sheep erthrocytes by sera of patients with rheumatoid arthritis. *Proc Soc Exp Biol Med* 1948; **68**: 1–6.

Ross, EL, D'Cruz, D, Morrow, WJW. The immunopathology of psoriatic arthritis. *Hosp Med* 1998; **59**: 534–8.

Sambrook PN, Browne CD, Champion GD *et al.* Terminations of treatment with gold sodium thiomalate in rheumatoid arthritis. *J Rheumatol* 1982; **9**: 932–4.

Sanchez B, Moreno I, Magarino R *et al.* HLA-DRw10 confers the highest susceptibility to rheumatoid arthritis in a Spanish population. *Tissue Antigens* 1990; **36**: 174–6.

Sansom D, Bidwell J, Maddison P *et al.* HLA DQ alpha and DQ beta restriction fragment length polymorphisms associated with Felty's Syndrome and DR4-positive rheumatoid arthritis. *Hum Immunol* 1987; **19**: 269–78.

Sansom D, Amin S, Bidwell J *et al.* HLA-DQ-related restriction fragment length polymorphisms in rheumatoid arthritis: evidence for a link with disease expression. *Br J Rheumatol* 1989; **28**: 374–8.

Schellekens GA, de Jong BAW, van den Hoogen FHJ *et al.* Citrulline is an essential constituent of antigenic determinants recognised by rheumatoid arthritis specific autoantibodies. *J Clin Invest* 1998; **101**: 273–81.

Scherak O, Smolen J, Mayr W. Rheumatoid arthritis and B lymphocyte alloantigen HLA-DRw4. *J Rheumatol* 1980; **7**: 9–12.

Schiff B, Mizrachi Y, Orgad S *et al.* Association of HLA-Aw31 and HLA-DR1 with rheumatoid arthritis. *Ann Rheum Dis* 1982; **41**: 403–4.

Schirmer M, Vallejo AN, Weyand CM, Gorozy JJ. Resistance to apoptosis and elevated expression of Bc1-2 in clonally expanded CD4+CD28-T cells from rheumatoid arthritis patients. *J Immunol* 1998; **161**: 1018–25.

Schultz LCI, Erhard H, Hertrampf B *et al.* Hemostasis, fibrin incorporation and local mesenchymal reaction in Erysipelothrix infection as a model for rheumatism research. In: *Experimental Models of Chronic Inflammatory Disease*, eds Glynn LE, Schlumberger CHD. Springer, Berlin, 1977; 215–37.

Schur PH. Complement testing in the diagnosis of immune and autoimmune diseases. *Am J Clin Pathol* 1977; **68**: 647–58.

Scott DGI, Bacon PA. Intravenous cyclophosphamide plus methyl prednisolone in the treatment of systemic rheumatoid vasculitis. *Am J Med* 1984; **76**: 377–84.

Sebbag M, Simon M, Vincent C *et al.* The antiperinuclear factor and the so-called antikeratin antibodies are the same rheumatoid arthritis specific autoantibodies. *J Clin Invest* 1995; **95**: 2672–9.

Semnani R, Nutman T, Hochman P *et al.* Costimulation by purified intercellular adhesion molecules 1 and lymphocyte function-associated antigen3 induces distinct proliferation, cytokine and cell surface antigen profiles in human 'naive' and 'memory' CD4+ T cells. *J Exp Med* 1994; **180**: 2125–35.

Sewell KL, Moreland LW, Cush JJ *et al.* Phase I/II double-blind dose response trial of a second fusion toxin DAB389-IL-2 in rheumatoid arthritis. *Arthritis Rheum* 1993; **36**(Suppl.): S130.

Sfikakis PP, Dimopoulos MA, Souliotis VL, Charalambopoulos D, Mavrikakis M, Panayiotidis P. Effects of 2-chlorodeoxyadenosine and gold sodium thiomalate on human bcl-2 gene expression. *Immunopharmacol Immunotoxicol* 1998; **20**: 63–77.

Sieper J, Kary S, Sörensen H *et al.* Oral type II collagen treatment in early rheumatoid arthritis: double-blind placebo-controlled trial randomised trial. *Arthritis Rheum* 1996; **39**: 41–52.

Silman A, Reeback J, Jaraquemada D. HLA-DR4 as a predictor of outcome three years after onset of rheumatoid arthritis. *Rheumatol Int* 1986; **6**: 233–5.

Silverstein FE, Graham DY, Senior JR *et al.* Misoprostol reduces serious gastrointestinal complications in patients with rheumatoid arthritis receiving non-steroidal anti-inflammatory drugs. *Ann Intern Med* 1995; **123**: 241–9.

Singal D, Reid B, Green D *et al.* Polymorphism of major histocompatibility complex extended haplotypes bearing HLA-DR3 in patients with rheumatoid arthritis with gold induced thrombocytopenia or proteinuria. *Ann Rheum Dis* 1990; **49**: 582–6.

So A, Warner C, Sansom D *et al.* DQB polymorphism and genetic susceptibility to Felty's syndrome. *Arthritis Rheum* 1988; **31**: 990–4.

Soltys AJ, Bond A, Westwood OM *et al.* The effects of altered glycosylation of IgG on rheumatoid factor-binding and immune complex formation. *Adv Exp Med Biol* 1995; **376**: 155–60.

Spector TD. Rheumatoid arthritis. In: *Epidemiology of Rheumatic Diseases*, ed. Hochberg MC. Saunders, Philadelphia, 1990; 513–37.

Stamenkovic I, Stegagno M, Wright KA *et al.* Clonal dominance among T-lymphocyte infiltrates in arthritis. *Proc Natl Acad Sci USA* 1988; **85**: 1179–83.

Stastny P, Fink CW. HLA-Dw4 in adult and juvenile rheumatoid arthritis. *Transplant Proc* 1977; **9**: 1863–6.

Stastny P, Fink CW. Different HLA-D associations in adult and juvenile rheumatoid arthritis. *J Clin Invest* 1979; **63**: 124–30.

Steffen C, Wicks G. Delayed hypersensitivity reactions to collagen in rats with adjuvant-induced arthritis. *Z Immunitäts Allergieforsch* 1971; **141**: 169–80.

Steffen C, Zeitlhofer J, Zielinski C *et al.* Acute autoimmune collagen-induced arthritis in rabbits. *J Rheumatol* 1978; **37**: 275–85.

Steiner G, Hartmuth K, Skriner H *et al.* Purification and partial sequencing of the nuclear autoantigen RA33 shows that it is indistinguishable from the A2 protein of the heterogeneous nuclear ribonucleoprotein complex. *J Clin Invest* 1992; **92**: 1061–6.

Stephens H, Sakkas L, Vaughan R *et al.* HLA-DQw7 is a disease severity marker in patients with rheumatoid arthritis. *Immunogenetics* 1989; **30**: 119–22.

Still GF. On a form of chronic joint disease in children. *Med Chir Trans* 1897; **80**: 47–59.

Stoerk HC, Bielinski TC, Budzilovich T. Chronic polyarthritis in rats injected with spleen in adjuvants. *Am J Pathol* 1954; **30**: 616.

Struyk L, Hawes GE, Chatila MK *et al.* T cell receptors in rheumatoid arthritis. *Arthritis Rheum* 1995; **38**: 577–89.

Suzuki A, Ohosone Y, Obana M *et al.* Cause of death in 81 autopsied patients with rheumatoid arthritis. *J Rheumatol* 1994; **21**: 33–6.

Svartz N. The treatment of rheumatic polyarthritis with acid azo compounds. *Rheumatism* 1948; **4**: 56–60.

Symmons DP, Barrett EM, Bankhead CR *et al.* The incidence of rheumatoid arthritis in the United Kingdom: results from the Norfolk Arthritis Register. *Br J Rheumatol* 1994; **33**: 735–9.

Thomas R, Davis LS, Lipsky PE. Rheumatoid synovium is enriched in mature antigen presenting dendritic cells. *J Immunol* 1994; **152**: 2613–23.

Thomas R, Lipsky PE. Presentation of self peptides by dendritic cells: possible implications for the pathogenesis of rheumatoid arthritis. *Arthritis Rheum* 1996; **39**: 183–90.

Thompson KM, Borretzen M, Randen I *et al.* V-gene repertoire and hypermutation of rheumatoid factors produced in synovial inflammation and immunized healthy donors. *Ann N Y Acad Sci* 1995; **764**: 440–9.

Thomsen M, Morling N, Snorrason E *et al.* HLA-Dw4 and rheumatoid arthritis. *Tissue Antigens* 1979; **13**: 56–60.

Thomsen W, Pepper L, Payton A *et al.* Absence of an association between HLA-DRB1*04 and RA in newly diagnosed cases from the community. *Ann Rheum Dis* 1993; **52**: 539–41.

Trentham DE, Dynesius-Trentham RA, Orav EJ *et al.* Effects of oral administration of type II collagen on rheumatoid arthritis. *Science* 1993; **261**: 1669–70.

Tsuchiya K, Kondo M, Kimura A *et al.* The DRB1 and/or the DQB1 locus controls susceptibility and DRB1 controls resistance to RA in the Japanese. In: *HLA 1991*, eds Tsuji K, Aizawa M, Sasazuki T, Vol. 2. Oxford University Press, New York, 1992; 509–12.

Tugwell P, Pincus T, Yocum D *et al.* Combination therapy with cyclosporine and methotrexate in severe rheumatoid arthritis. *New Eng J Med* 1995; **333**: 137–41.

Van den Broek MF, Hogervast EJ, van Bruggen MC *et al.* Protection against streptococcal cell-wall induced arthritis by treatment with the 65kD mycobacterial heat shock protein. *J Exp Med* 1989; **170**: 449–66.

Vandenbroucke JP, Hazeroet HM, Cats A. Survival and cause of death in rheumatoid arthritis: a 25 year prospective follow-up. *J Rheumatol* 1984; **11**: 158–61.

van der Heijde DM, Van Riel PCLM, Nuver-Zvart HH *et al.* Sulphasalazine versus hydroxychloroquine in rheumatoid arthritis: 3 year follow up. *Lancet* 1990; **335**: 539 (letter).

van der Heijde DM, van Riel P, van Leeuwen M *et al.* Prognostic factors for radiographic damage and physical disability in early rheumatoid arthritis. A prospective follow-up study of 147 patients. *Br J Rheumatol* 1992a; **31**: 519–25.

van der Heijde DM, van Leeuwen MA, van Riel PCLM *et al*. Biannual radiographic assessments of hands and feet in a three year prospective follow up of patients with early rheumatoid arthritis. *Arthritis Rheum* 1992b; **35**: 26–34.

van der Lubbe PA, Dijkmans BAC, Markusse HM *et al*. A randomised double-blind placebo controlled trial of CD4 monoclonal antibody therapy in early rheumatoid arthritis. *Arthritis Rheum* 1995; **38**: 1097–106.

van de Winkel JG, Capel PJ. Human IgG Fc receptor heterogeneity: molecular aspects and clinical implications. *Immunol Today* 1993; **14**: 215–21.

van Eden W, Holoshitz J, Nevo Z *et al*. Arthritis induced by a T lymphocyte clone that responds to mycobacterium tuberculosis and to cartilage proteoglycans. *Proc Natl Acad Sci USA* 1985; **82**: 5117–20.

van Eden W, Thole JER, van der Zee R *et al*. Cloning of the mycobacterial epitope recognised by thymocytes in adjuvant arthritis. *Nature* 1988; **331**: 171–3.

van Kerckhove C, Melin-Aldana H, Elma M *et al*. A distinct HLA-DRw8 haplotype characterizes patients with juvenile rheumatoid arthritis. *Immunogenetics* 1990; **32**: 304–8.

van Kerckhove C, Luyrink L, Taylor J *et al*. HLA-DQA1*0101 haplotypes and disease outcome in early onset pauciarticular juvenile rheumatoid arthritis. *J Rheumatol* 1991; **18**: 874–9.

van Leeuwen MA, van Rijswijk MH, van der Heijde DMFM *et al*. The acute phase response in relation to radiographic progression in early rheumatoid arthritis: a prospective study during the first three years of the disease. *Br J Rheumatol* 1993; **32**(Suppl. 3): 3–8.

Van Zeben D, Rook GAW, Hazes MW *et al*. Early galactosylation of IgG is associated with a more progressive disease course in patients with rheumatoid arthritis: results of a follow-up study. *Br J Rheumatol* 1994; **33**: 36–43.

Verhoeven AC, Boers M, Tugwell P. Combination therapy in rheumatoid arthritis: updated systematic review. *Br J Rheumatol* 1998; **37**: 612–9.

Vullo CM, Pesoa SA, Onetti CM *et al*. Rheumatoid arthritis and its association with HLA-DR antigens. I. Cell mediated immune response against connective tissue antigens. *J Rheumatol* 1987; **14**: 221–5.

Waaler E. On the occurrence of a factor in human serum activating the specifc aggulination of sheep blood corpustles. *Acta Pathol Microbiol Scand* 1940; **17**: 172–88.

Walton K, Dyer P, Grennan D *et al*. Clinical features, autoantibodies and HLA-DR antigens in rheumatoid arthritis. *J Rheumatol* 1985; **12**: 223–6.

Watts RA, Carruthers DM, Symmons DPM *et al*. The incidence of rheumatoid vasculitis. *Br J Rheumatol* 1994; **33**: 832–3.

Westedt ML, Breedveld FC, Schreuder GM *et al*. Immunogenetic heterogeneity of rheumatoid arthritis. *Ann Rheum Dis* 1986; **45**: 534–8.

Westhovens R, Verwilghen J, Dequeker J. Total lymphoid irradiation in rheumatoid arthritis. A ten-year follow up. *Arthritis Rheum* 1997; **40**: 426–9.

Weyand C, Hicok K, Conn D *et al*. The influence of HLA-DRB1 genes on disease severity in rheumatoid arthritis. *Ann Int Med* 1992a; **117**: 801–6.

Weyand C, Xie C, Goronzy J. Homozygosity for the HLA-DRB1 allele selects for extraarticular manifestations in rheumatoid arthritis. *J Clin Invest* 1992b; **89**: 2033–9.

Williams RC, Jacobsson LTH, Knowler WC *et al*. Meta-analysis reveals association between most common class II haplotype in full-heritage Native Americans and rheumatoid arthritis. *Human Immunol* 1995; **42**: 90–4.

Willkens RF, Nepom GT, Marks CR *et al*. Association of HLA-Dw16 with rheumatoid arthritis in Yakima Indians. *Arthritis Rheum* 1991; **34**: 43–7.

Wilske KR, Healey LA. Remodelling the pyramid — a concept whose time has come. *J Rheumatol* 1989; **16**: 565–7.

Winchester RJ. B-lymphocyte allo-antigens, cellular expression, and disease significance with special reference to rheumatoid arthritis. *Arthritis Rheum* 1977; **20**: 159–63.

Woessner JF Jr. Matrix metalloproteinases and their inhibitors in connective tissue remodeling. *FASEB J* 1991; **5**:2145–54.

Wolfe F, Mitchell DM, Sibley JT *et al*. The mortality of rheumatoid arthritis. *Arthritis Rheum* 1994; **37**: 481–94.

Wollheim F. Rheumatoid arthritis — the clinical picture. In: *Oxford Textbook of Rheumatology*, 2nd edn, eds Maddison PJ, Isenberg DA, Woo P, Glass DN. Oxford University Press, Oxford, 1998, 1004–31.

Woodrow JC, Nichol FE, Zaphiropoulos G. DR antigens and rheumatoid arthritis: a study of two populations. *Br Med J* 1981; **283**: 1201–2.

Wordsworth P, Pile KD, Buckely *et al*. HLA heterozygosity contributes to susceptibility to rheumatoid arthritis. *Am J Hum Genet* 1992; **51**: 585–91

Wostulewski JA, Schottenkirchner M, Barcelo P *et al*. A six month double-blind trial to compare the efficacy and safety of meloxicam 7.5 mg daily and naproxen 750 mg daily in patients with RA. *Br J Rheumatol* 1996; **35** (Suppl. 1) 22–8.

Young A, Jaraquemada D, Awad J *et al*. Association of HLA-DR4/Dw4 and DR2/Dw2 with radiologic changes in a prospective study of patients with rheumatoid arthritis. *Arthritis Rheum* 1984; **27**: 20–5.

Young A, Sumar N, Bodman K *et al*. Agalactosyl IgG — an aid to differential diagnosis in early synovitis. *Arthritis Rheum* 1991; **34**: 1425–9.

Zanelli E, Gonzalez-Gay MA, David CS. Could HLA-DRB1 be the protective locus in rheumatoid arthritis? *Immunol Today* 1995; **16**: 274–8.

Zoschke D, Segall M. Dw Subtypes of DR4 in rheumatoid arthritis: evidence for a preferential association with Dw4. *Hum Immunol* 1986; **15**: 118–24.

Zurier RB, Rossetti RG, Jacobson EW *et al*. Gamma-linolenic acid treatment of rheumatoid arthritis. *Arthritis Rheum* 1996; **39**: 1808–17.

Zvaifler NJ, Steinman RM, Kaplan G *et al*. Identification of immunostimulatory dendritic cells in the synovial effusions of patients with rheumatoid arthritis. *J Clin Invest* 1985; **76**: 789–800.

Introduction

Sjögren's syndrome (SS) is a chronic inflammatory autoimmune disorder characterized by mixed cellular infiltration of exocrine glands, notably the lachrymal and saliva glands (autoimmune exocrinopathy). This inflammation causes dryness of the eyes (xerophthalmia), dryness of the mouth (xerostomia), and very frequently dryness of the throat, nose, and vagina. The combination of dry eyes and dry mouth alone is often referred to as the sicca syndrome. In many cases, however, these clinical features are associated with other autoimmune diseases, which are listed in Table 6.1. It is also evident that Sjögren's syndrome is associated with an increased risk of mucosa-associated lymphoid tissue (MALT) lymphoma.

Table 6.1 Other autoimmune diseases may be associated with Sjögren's syndrome

Chronic active hepatitis
Coeliac disease
Dermatitis herpetiformis
Diabetes
Graft-versus-host disease
Graves' disease
Myasthenia gravis
Polyarteritis nodosa
Polymyositis/dermatomyositis
Primary biliary cirrhosis
Rheumatoid arthritis
Scleroderma
Systemic lupus erythematosus

Milestones in the history of Sjögren's syndrome

1888   Filamentary keratitis described by Leber.

1888   Hadden described xerostomia; von Mikulicz described enlargement of lachrymal and salivary glands 'consisting of small round cells'.

1925   Stock associated filamentary keratitis with disease of lachrymal glands and reduced tear secretion.

1933   Henrik Sjögren described the association of keratoconjunctivitis sicca; dry mouth and rheumatoid arthritis.

1951   Link between Sjögren's syndrome and non-Hodgkin's lymphoma first described.

1961   Anderson and co-workers first reported the occurrence of autoantibodies in the sera of patients with Sjögren's syndrome.

1968   Chisolm and Mason reported the first histological grading system for assessing labial biopsies.

1977   First association of SS with HLA alloantigens made by Mann and colleagues.

1982–1984   Monoclonal antibodies utilized to show that the $CD4^+$ cells outnumber the $CD8^+$ cells in both primary and secondary disease in lesional tissue.

1993   European Concerted Action Study identifies a set of classification criteria that wins widespread support.

The sicca syndrome may occur following radiation therapy of the head and neck given for a variety of tumours, notably Hodgkin's lymphoma. On rare occasions, dryness of the eyes and mouth may occur with salivary gland enlargement and sarcoidosis, amyloidosis, tuberculosis, histoplasmosis, leprosy, and various tumours, including lymphomas and salivary gland tumours. Other clinical features and additional histological abnormalities invariably enable the correct diagnosis to be made. In this chapter we will focus on the form of sicca syndrome that is clearly autoimmune in origin.

Classification of Sjögren's syndrome

We propose the following working classification for patients with Sjögren's syndrome.

Primary Sjögren's syndrome

This comprises the 'sicca' syndrome without an associated autoimmune rheumatic disease. Exocrine function tends to be more severely impaired than in the secondary type. Primary Sjögren's syndrome is associated frequently with a variety of extraglandular manifestations.

Secondary Sjögren's syndrome

This describes the association of a 'sicca' complex, which may be subclinical or relatively mild, with one of the autoimmune diseases listed in Table 6.1. Although the clinical expression of Sjögren's syndrome is similar in these patients there are significant differences in the serological profile, for example, in patients whose secondary Sjögren's syndrome complicates RA as opposed to SLE. These differences are discussed later in this chapter.

Lymphoma linked with Sjögren's syndrome

Primary, occasionally secondary, Sjögren's syndrome may be associated with either low or high grade MALT lymphomas. The indolent clinical course associated with the former has led to the use of the term pseudolymphoma. It is now known that monoclonality defines the lymphoid infiltrates, especially in the parotid gland and stomach where these tumours are particularly prone to occur. Transformation to a high grade lymphoma does occur, and on occasion may disseminate widely.

Sjögren's syndrome in the elderly

Definite sicca syndrome has been found in approximately 3% of the population over the age of 80. No association with autoantibodies has been established in this group. This observation suggests that trophic changes in the secretory glands rather than an autoimmune process are responsible.

Other forms

Sjögren's syndrome rarely occurs in children but there are a handful of case reports. In a case study and literature review (39 patients with primary disease in all) Anaya *et al.* (1995) reported a mean age of onset of 7.8 years and stressed that parotitis at onset was more frequent in children than adults (62.5% vs. 13%) but articular manifestations and a positive ANA had a lower frequency. Other clinical and serological features were broadly similar to adult cases. It is of interest that many mothers whose babies have neonatal lupus (see Chapter 4) have symptoms of Sjögren's syndrome (Lee 1993).

Diagnostic criteria

In the past 20 years a number of sets of diagnostic criteria have been attempted but it seems highly likely that the criteria established by a prospective concerted action (Vitali *et al.* 1993) involving 26 centres in 12 European countries will be the most widely used. A subsequent prospective study (Vitali *et al.* 1996) confirmed the high sensitivity (97.5%) and specificity (94.2%) of these criteria. These are shown in Table 6.2.

Using these criteria, it was recently shown (H. Moutsopoulos, personal communication) that the prevalence of definite and probable Sjögren's syndrome was 0.6 and 3%, respectively. In a separate epidemiological study, of over 700 adults in Sweden, the prevalence of the disease was found to be 2.7% (Jacobsson *et al.* 1989).

The clinical picture

Sjögren's syndrome is associated with a wide variety of clinical features (Fig. 6.1). It may also arise in conjunction with other autoimmune disorders; these are considered in some detail below.

Table 6.2 Preliminary criteria for the classification of Sjögren's syndrome

1. Ocular symptoms
   A positive response to at least one of the following three questions.
   (a) Have you had daily, persistent, troublesome dry eyes for more than three months?
   (b) Do you have a recurrent sensation of sandy or gravel feeling in the eyes?
   (c) Do you use tear substitutes more than three times a day?

2. Oral symptoms
   A positive response to at least one of the following three questions.
   (a) Have you had a daily feeling of dry mouth for more than three months?
   (b) Have you had recurrent or persistently swollen salivary glands as an adult?
   (c) Do you frequently drink liquids to aid in swallowing dry foods?

3. Ocular signs
   Objective evidence of ocular involvement determined on the basis of a positive result on at least one of the following two tests.
   (a) Schirmer — one test ($\leqslant$ 5 mm in 5 minutes)
   (b) Rose Bengal score ($\geqslant$ 4, according to the van Bijsterveld scoring system)

4. Histopathological findings
   Focus score $\geqslant$ 1 on minor salivary gland biopsy (focus defined as an agglomeration of at least 50 mononuclear cells, focus score defined as the number of foci/4 mm^2 of glandular tissue).

5. Salivary gland involvement
   Objective evidence of salivary gland involvement, determined on the basis of a positive result on at least one of the following three tests.
   (a) Salivary scintigraphy
   (b) Parotid sialography
   (c) Unstimulated salivary flow ($\leqslant$ 1.5 ml in 15 minutes)

6. Autoantibodies
   Presence of at least one of the following autoantibodies in the serum.
   Antibodies to Ro/SS-A or La/SS-B antigens or anti-nuclear antibodies or rheumatoid factor.

A patient is considered as having probable SS if three of the six criteria are present and definite SS if four of the six criteria are present.

From Vitali *et al.* (1993).

Ocular involvement

Patients frequently complain of their eyes feeling dry, gritty, and sore. It may become difficult to tolerate the wearing of contact lenses (see Table 6.3). Cutting up onions may no longer induce tears. Routine examination may reveal no gross abnormality although somewhat thickened conjunctival secretions may be observed.

Confirmation of the symptoms is confirmed by taking tests to assess the quantity of tears. Schirmer's test (Fig. 6.2) is an easy to perform, though crude, estimate of tear secretion. It utilizes a thin filter strip approximately 35 mm in length, which is 'tucked in' beneath the lower eyelid with the remainder of the strip hanging out. More than 15 mm of wetting of this strip in 5 minutes is normal. Typically, a patient with severe Sjögren's syndrome will damp the strip to less than 5 mm. Many 'false-positives' are removed when

patients are challenged with a 10% ammonia solution held just below the nose. Dryness of the eyes may be confirmed by the instillation of a 1% aqueous solution of Rose Bengal stain. This is an aniline dye that stains the devitalized or damaged epithelium of both the cornea and conjunctiva (Fig. 6.3). Slit lamp examination may demonstrate the presence of filamentary keratitis (Fig. 6.4). In some centres 'tear break-up' time' is another useful measure. A drop of fluorescein is instilled into the eye and the time between the last blink and the appearance of dark non-fluoresceinated areas in the tear film is ascertained. A rapid break-up of the tear film indicates an abnormality of either the mucin or lipid layer.

Complications of untreated sicca syndrome may occur, including secretory conjunctivitis, corneal ulceration, and perforation, which cause uveitis, cataract, and glaucoma.

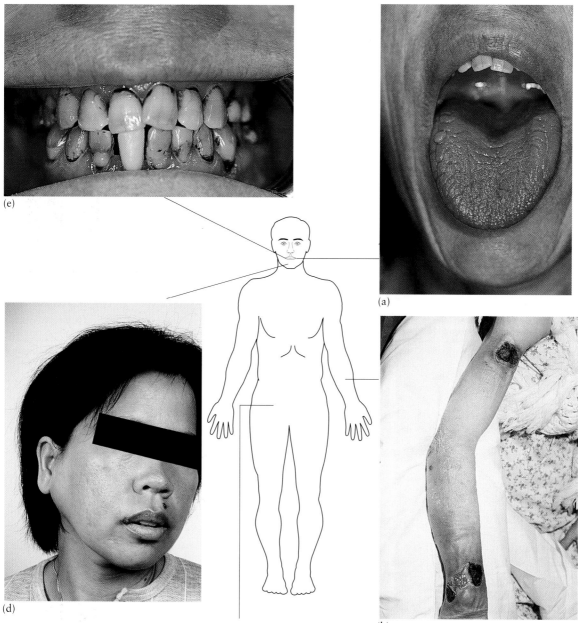

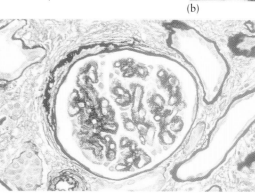

Fig. 6.1. Major clinical features of Sjögren's syndrome. (a) The severe dry tongue of Sjögren's. (b) Lymphoma (unusually of T cell origin) complicating a patient with Sjögren's. (c) Renal involvement is uncommon (in this case membranous glomerulonephritis) but a well-recognized feature of Sjögren's — it is not as severe as in patients with lupus. (d) Dry mouth leads to atrophied gums and recurrent oral infection. (e) Parotid swelling in a patient with Sjögren's.

Table 6.3   Clinical features of keratoconjunctivitis

Symptoms

       Foreign body sensation
       Burning
       Tiredness with/without difficulty in opening the eyes
       Dry feeling often with inadequate response to physical/chemical irritants and emotions
       Redness
       Blurred vision
       Itchiness
       Aches
       Soreness
       Photosensitivity
       Inability to tolerate contact lenses

Signs

       Dilatation of the bulbar conjunctival vessels
       Mild pericorneal injection
       Photophobia
       Irregularity of the corneal image
       Discharge
       Dullness of the conjunctiva and/or cornea

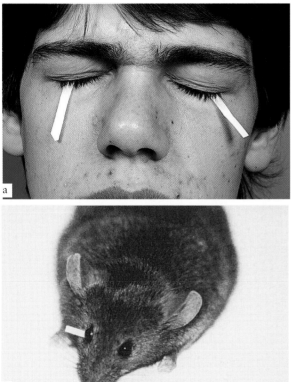

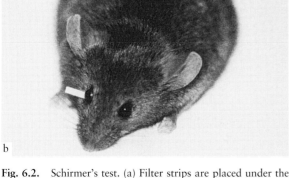

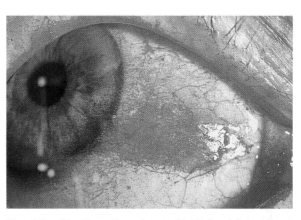

Fig. 6.3. The Rose Bengal stain highlights (pink colour) abnormally dry areas of the conjunctiva.

Fig. 6.2. Schirmer's test. (a) Filter strips are placed under the lower eyelid following gentle eversion. The lids are closed and the strips held in position as shown for 5 minutes. The length to which the strips have been dampened is measured. In healthy individuals the strips will usually be dampened to 15 mm or more. Patients with Sjögren's will often dampen the strips to less than 5 mm. (b) Schirmer's test in the NZB/W mouse.

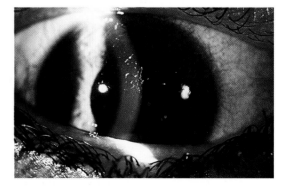

Fig. 6.4. Filamentary keratitis seen on slit lamp examination.

Oral involvement

Nearly all patients with Sjögren's syndrome complain of dryness of the mouth. They may also note lip cracking, difficulty with mastication, and occasional dysphagia. A useful question to ask is whether they have had problems producing sufficient saliva to swallow a dry biscuit or cracker without the help of a glass of water.

On examination the mouth and tongue may look dry with an absence of the salivary pool beneath the tongue. There may also be angular stomatitis, fissuring ulceration of the tongue (Fig. 6.1a), advanced dental caries (see Fig. 6.1d), and secondary candidiasis. It is the dryness of the mouth that predisposes to these complications.

Various tests of varying sensitivity and specificity have been described. Perhaps the simplest test is to ask the patient to produce as much saliva as possible in a measured period of time. However, the naturally occurring fluctuations with age, sex, drug therapy, time of day, etc. make it very hard to establish a normal range for flow rates. Sialography is a radiocontrast method of assessing anatomical changes in the salivary duct system. Unfortunately, some individuals may be allergic to the radio-opaque material. Sialography utilizing water-soluble media is preferred. This method has been shown to correlate quite well with minor salivary gland biopsy changes.

Isotope scanning (scintigraphy) provides a useful functional assessment of the salivary gland for observing the rate, density of the uptake of ^{99m}Tc pertechnate, and the time taken for it to appear in the mouth during a 60-minute period after its intravenous injection. Patients with Sjögren's syndrome have a delayed secretion of saliva using this method. Attempts have been made to analyse the chemical constituents of patients' saliva but, to date, the results have been considered of little value.

Salivary gland enlargement

Salivary gland biopsy remains an integral part of the investigation of Sjögren's syndrome. In this procedure the lower lip is everted and anaesthetized. An incision between 1.5 and 2 cm is made along the labial mucosa and 4–7 nodules of minor salivary gland are obtained and examined histologically. The biopsies (see Fig. 6.5) are scored according to the number of lymphocytes per 4 mm^2 of salivary tissue (> 50 lymphocytes = one focus). Thus, grade 0 = no lymphocytes, grade

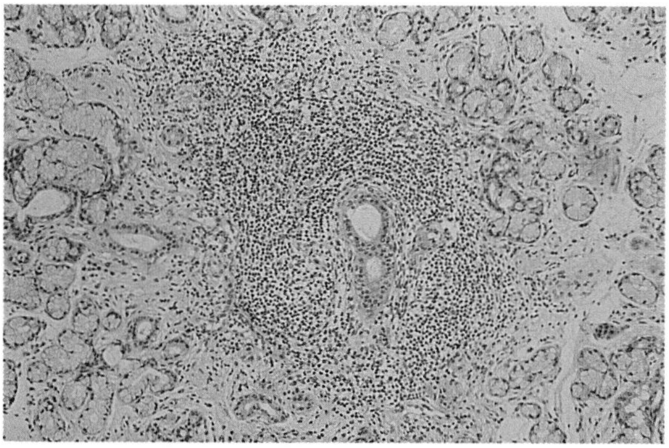

Fig. 6.5. Labial biopsy from a patient with Sjögren's syndrome showing a large focus of inflammatory cells in the central area which has effectively destroyed the normal architecture of the gland (seen on either side). (Courtesy of Dr Meryl Griffiths, × 60.)

1 = slight infiltration, grade 2 = moderate infiltration or less than 1 focus, grade 3 = one focus, grade 4 + = more than one focus.

It seems to be generally agreed that intermittent unilateral swelling appears in up to 25% of patients (see Fig. 6.1e). In contrast, bilateral swelling probably occurs in less than 10% of patients overall. It must be remembered that there are other causes of salivary gland enlargement, including acute infections (infectious mononucleosis, mumps) chronic infections (tuberculosis, leprosy), sarcoidosis, amyloidosis, various tumours, diabetes mellitus, haemachromatosis, and hyperlipidaemia.

Other features of Sjögren's syndrome

A detailed list of the non-ocular and non-oral features that manifest in Sjögren'e syndrome is given in Table 6.4.

Articular

Up to 75% of patients with primary Sjögren's syndrome may complain of arthralgia, although it seems that 10% or fewer have true arthritis. This may be associated with an accompanying myalgia or morning stiffness. It is most unusual in primary Sjögren's patients for X-rays to reveal erosive change. Between 15 and 25% of patients with systemic lupus erythematosus develop Sjögren's syndrome, as do approximately 10–15% of patients with rheumatoid arthritis.

Table 6.4 Systemic manifestations in 66 patients with primary Sjögren's symptoms attending the Autoimmune Rheumatic Disease Clinic at The Middlesex Hospital

Clinical manifestation	n	%	Range in previous studies[*] (%)	Reference
Arthralgia	48	51	64–96	Pavlidis *et al.* (1982) Montecucco *et al.* (1989) Vitali *et al.* (1991) Moutsopoulos *et al.* (1997) Previous studies do not distinguish between arthritis and arthralgia
Arthritis	8	9		
Raynaud's phenomenon	32	34	16–54	Bloch *et al.* (1965) Montecucco *et al.* (1989) Youinou *et al.* (1990) Vitali *et al.* (1991) Moutsopoulos *et al.* (1997)
Fatigue	25	27	69	Vitali *et al.* (1991)
Lymphadenopathy	11	12	14–30	Montecucco *et al.* (1989) Moutsopoulos *et al.* (1997)
Lymphoma	5	5	2–10	Moutsopoulos *et al.* (1997) Pavlidis *et al.* (1982)
Psychiatric disorder	9	10	11–42	Alexander *et al.* (1986) Andonopoulos *et al.* (1989) Montecucco *et al.* (1989)
Peripheral nervous system	7	9	13–41	Pavlidis *et al.* (1982) Andonopoulos *et al.* (1989) Vretham *et al.* (1990) Andonopoulos *et al.* (1990) Moutsopoulos *et al.* (1997)
Central nervous system	6	6	0–25	Alexander *et al.* (1986) Binder *et al.* (1988) Andonopoulos *et al.* (1990) Moutsopoulos *et al.* (1997)
Pulmonary involvement	6	6	10–13	Pavlidis *et al.* (1982) Montecucco *et al.* (1989)
Cutaneous vasculitis	3	3	5–17	Pavlidis *et al.* (1982) Alexander *et al.* (1986) Vitali *et al.* (1991) Moutsopoulos *et al.* (1987)
Overt renal involvement	3	3	2–26	Pokorny *et al.* (1989) Vitali *et al.* (1991) Moutsopoulos *et al.* (1997)
Hypergammaglobulinaemia	8	9		
Pancreatitis	1	2		
Hepatomegaly	0	0	4–25	Pavlidis *et al.* (1982) Moutsopoulos *et al.* (1997)

[*] Shown for comparison.
Each patient met the criteria of Vitali *et al.* (1993).

Dermatological

As indicated above, cutaneous lesions, notably annular erythema affecting mainly the face and trunk, dryness of the skin especially nasal and vaginal dryness, and cheilitis are well recognized. Leucocytoclastic vasculitis and vitiligo are an occasional accompaniment. Marked dryness of the vagina may lead to dyspareunia.

Vascular

Raynaud's phenomenon is present in 35–50% of patients with Sjögren's syndrome. It is frequently present before the onset of the sicca symptoms and may be associated with swelling of the digits. Vasculitis in the form of purpura or urticaria is well recognized. There are said to be two types of inflammatory vascular disease in patients with primary Sjögren's syndrome, namely neutrophilic inflammatory vascular disease and mononuclear inflammatory vascular disease. Both types may cause end-organ damage.

Pulmonary

Significant pulmonary involvement appears to be rather uncommon and is present in approximately 10% of patients only. Symptoms range from a dry cough to dyspnoea from interstitial lung disease. A recent study of high resolution CT scanning of the lungs revealed that in 14 symptomatic patients the main findings were either thickened bronchial walls at the segmental level, or a mild interstitial pattern distributed around the bronchi (Papiris *et al.* 1994). Pulmonary hyperinflation and a link between disturbed lung function tests and elevated β_2-microglobulin levels have also been described (Lahdensuo and Korpela 1995).

Gastrointestinal

Dryness of the oesophagus may lead to dysphagia, which can be troublesome. Atrophic gastritis has also been widely recognized as a complicating factor for the primary and secondary Sjögren's syndrome (Sheikh and Shaw-Stiffel 1995). Sicca syndrome has been described in many patients with primary biliary cirrhosis, as well as some with chronic active hepatitis and cryptogenic cirrhosis. Acute or chronic pancreatitis is rare and significant liver involvement uncommon.

Renal

Renal tubular acidosis is well known to be associated with Sjögren's syndrome. Renal histological examination may demonstrate the infiltration of the tubules and renal parenchyma by lymphocytes and plasma cells. However, this infiltration is secondary to a direct immunological assault, suggested, circumstantially, by the observation in the early stages of renal transplant rejection that patients may develop renal tubular acidosis with lymphocytic infiltration of the tubules. A hypocomplementaemic immune complex-mediated glomerular nephritis has been described. These patients do not have anti-dsDNA antibodies in their serum. Glomerulonephritis has been described in very few patients with Sjögren's syndrome (Fig. 6.1c), invariably in association with high levels of circulating complexes, mixed cryoglobulinaemia, and low levels of complement.

Neuromuscular

Minor sensory abnormalities, including trigeminal neuralgia, mild sensory peripheral neuropathies, or carpal tunnel syndrome, are well-recognized features of patients with Sjögren's syndrome. The studies of Alexander *et al.* (1986) recorded a surprisingly high proportion (up to 25%) of patients with such serious major central nervous system involvement that they were said to be difficult to distinguish from patients with multiple sclerosis. In contrast, studies undertaken in England, Greece, and Scandinavia (see Table 6.4) have shown that while major neurological events can be ascribed to primary Sjögren's syndrome, these events are very rare.

Endocrine

Clinically apparent hypothyroidism is present in 10–15% of patients with Sjögren's syndrome, though subclinical disease is probably more common.

Links to lymphoma

As already mentioned, patients with Sjögren's syndrome have an increased risk of developing lymphomas, which has been estimated to be 44 times that of the general population, although this figure is based on a study undertaken 20 years ago (Kassan *et al.* 1978) and needs to be confirmed using modern diagnostic criteria (Fig. 6.6). Certain clinical parameters, including persistent salivary swelling and monoclonal

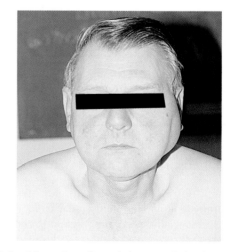

Fig. 6.6. Bilateral swelling of the parotid gland in a patient whose Sjögren's syndrome was complicated by a lymphoma.

immunoglobulins in the urine, may indicate a high risk for individual patients, but their absolute predictive value is uncertain.

In a five-year follow-up study, Tzioufas *et al.* (1996) reported that seven out of 103 consecutively assessed patients developed lymphoma. In six cases a mixed monoclonal cryoglobulin (all IgMκ rheumatoid factors) antedated the appearance of the tumour. They also reported a rather weaker association with two rheumatoid factor cross-reactive idiotypes, 17-109 and G-6.

Most of the lymphomas that develop are low grade B cell lymphomas of the mucosa-associated lymphoid tissue (MALT) type, and most occur within the salivary glands. These lesions are thought to be preceded by a salivary lymphoepithelial lesion. The earliest diagnostic feature of this lesion is a proliferation of centrocyte-like cells around epithelial islands. These cells meet the criteria for a lymphoid neoplasm since they show light and heavy chain monoclonality, but such monoclonality may antedate the development of lymphoma by many years (Diss *et al.* 1993). A study by Jordan *et al.* (1995) suggested that patients with evidence of monoclonality should be regarded as being at high risk of lymphoma development. Such monoclonality was reported to be predictive of disseminated lymphoma in six out of seven cases examined. These authors examined 76 sequential labial salivary glands for immunoglobulin heavy chain monoclonality (by PCR) and found it to be present in 14.5% of cases. Four of these patients subsequently developed evidence of extra-salivary gland lymphomas.

Clearly, however, there is no absolute correlation between the presence of monoclonality and the development of lymphomas and various authors have attempted to link such development with the presence of particular idiotypes and, indeed, evidence of notable cross-reactive idiotypic sharing. As an example, 12 out of 15 monoclonal rheumatoid factors in patients with Sjögren's syndrome reacted with the 17.109 anti-idiotypic antibody (Kipps *et al.* 1989). The authors analysed 17.109 idiotype-positive B cells in the salivary cells of patients with Sjögren's syndrome and found them to be of multiclonal origin in which somatic mutations had accumulated in a non-random fashion, which supports the notion of an antigen-stimulated and T cell-driven process in the expansion of these cells.

Guo *et al.* (1995) have shown that levels of the repairing enzyme for the promutagenic DNA base lesion, O^6-methylguanine, is reduced in patients with Sjögren's syndrome felt to be at risk of developing lymphoma. It has not yet been established whether this is an aetiological factor.

Autoantibodies

An extensive array of both organ- and non-organ-specific autoantibodies may be detected in the serum of patients with both primary and secondary Sjögren's syndrome (see Tables 6.5 and 6.6). Among the organ-specific antibodies, the paucity of salivary duct antibodies in Sjögren's syndrome is notable. Antibodies to gastric parietal cells and thyroid components are found in about one-third of patients with both primary and secondary Sjögren's syndrome. However, antibodies to other organ-specific antigens, including those in the adrenal, ovarian, parathyroid, and pituitary glands, are rare. Among the non-organic-specific antibodies, both rheumatoid factor and anti-nuclear antibodies are frequently found in both primary and secondary Sjögren's syndrome. In primary Sjögren's syndrome the morphological pattern on nuclear immunofluorescence is usually of the speckled variety. This pattern is usually a result of the presence of either or both anti-Ro (SS-A) or anti-La (SS-B) antibodies. While these antibodies are not disease specific, they are more commonly found in patients with Sjögren's syndrome than in any of the other autoimmune rheumatic diseases. Anti-Ro antibodies, in particular, are associated with early

Table 6.5 Non-organ-specific autoantibody profile (%) in primary and secondary Sjögren's syndrome

	1° SS (*n* = 83)	SLE (*n* = 138)	RA (*n* = 50)	SLE + SS (*n* = 27)	RA + SS (*n* = 10)
ANA ⩾ 1:80	58	91	26	100	60
Anti-Ro	42	34	< 5	62	< 5
Anti-La	36	11	< 5	42	< 5
Anti-Sm	2	10	< 5	3	< 5
Anti-RNP	7	16	< 5	23	< 5
Anti-DNA	0	53	< 5	56	< 5

From Kausman *et al.* (1994).

Table 6.6 Organ-specific autoantibody profile (%) in primary and secondary Sjögren's syndrome

	Primary Sjögren's (%)	Secondary Sjögren's (%)
Smooth muscle antibody	30	30
Salivary duct antibody	10–25	50–60
Thyroglobulin-precipitating antibody	15	15
Thyroid microsomal antibody	10–40	10–20
Gastric parietal cells	22–30	25–30

From Kausman *et al.* (1994).

disease onset, recurrent parotid gland enlargement, vasculitis, purpura, hypergammaglobulinaemia, and hypocomplementaemia.

It has been proposed (Manoussakis *et al.* 1986) that the incidence of these antibodies correlates with the intensity of the minor salivary gland infiltration. It has also been shown (Bodeutsch *et al.* 1992) that the total number of immunoglobulin containing plasma cells in labial salivary glands from patents with detectable anti-La autoantibodies is significantly greater than patients with Sjögren's syndrome, whose sera lack these antibodies.

Several attempts have been made to determine the fine specificity of autoantibodies binding to Ro and La, using recombinant antigens and synthetic peptides. The Ro antigen is known to exist in a variety of forms, varying in part with different cell types. The most common variants are known as Ro 60 and Ro 52. Wahren *et al.* (1996) could not distinguish differences in response to Ro 60 kDa, Ro 52 kDa, and La antigens between patients with primary Sjögren's syndrome and

those with SLE and Sjögren's syndrome. However, differences between primary and secondary Sjögren's syndrome were evident in studies by Ricchiuti *et al.* (1994a and b, see also Isenberg 1994). As shown in Table 6.7, the anti-peptide responses were highest in those Sjögren's syndrome patients who also had SLE.

The initiating event in the production of anti-Ro and anti-La antibodies is described elsewhere in this chapter p. 10 (Casciolte-Rosen *et al.* 1994). Apart from possible abnormalities in apoptosis it has also been shown that TNF-α can mediate 52 kDa Ro and La autoantigen surface expression (on human keratinocytes) (Dorner *et al.* 1995).

Prognosis

Kruize *et al.* (1996) studied 112 patients for 10–12 years and concluded that primary Sjögren's syndrome is characterized by a stable and mild course in the majority of cases. The exception being the small number of cases developing lymphoma (see above).

Table 6.7 IgG anti-Ro peptide antibodies in Sjögren's syndrome and other autoimmune diseases (%)

	SLE RA (n = 141)	Primary Sjögren's (n = 89)	SLE + Sjögren's (n = 26)	RA + Sjögren's (n = 31)	RA (n = 31)
Recombinant Ro 52	18	67	46	29	14
Peptides					
2–11	15	15	65	6	7
107–122	6	12	31	3	6
277–292	16	32	54	6	3
365–382	19	19	62	13	11

From Ricchiuti *et al.* (1994*b*).

Immunogenetics

Primary Sjögren's syndrome

An increase of HLA-Dw3(DR3) in patients with primary Sjögren's syndrome was first reported in 1977 (Chusad *et al.* 1977; Hinzova *et al.* 1977). Although this observation was confirmed (Vitali *et al.* 1986; Hietaharjo 1992), an increased frequency of DR3 has not been found among all populations. In a study of Greek patients, DR5 was increased (Papasteriades *et al.* 1988). HLA-DR5 is a serologically defined specificity that was later 'split' into DR11 and DR12. Consistent with findings in the Greek population, an increased frequency of DR11 was found in Israeli Jewish patients, also with no increase of DR3 (Roitberg-Tambur *et al.* 1990).

One possible explanation for differing results, even among Caucasian populations, is that a gene in linkage disequilibrium with DR3 and DR11 is primarily responsible for the observed associations. One such candidate is DR52, encoded for by genes at the DRB3 locus and present on all haplotypes that encode DR3 or DR11 at the DRB1 locus. Wilson *et al.* (1984) addressed this possibility in an analysis of Caucasian patients and controls and found that DR3 was significantly increased among patients, but that the strongest association was with DR52. The relative risk associated with DR3 was 3.3 whereas that associated with DR52 was 7.8. In a study that especially sought male patients with primary Sjögren's syndrome DR52 was significantly increased among both men and women; however, an increase of DR3 was only statistically significant among women (Molina *et al.* 1986).

A model in which the DRB3 locus is the primary susceptibility locus provides a potentially unifying explanation for the results of the above studies. However, it does not provide an explanation for results of other studies. Other studies have found an increase of Dw2(DR2) (Manthorpe *et al.* 1981), and there is no DRB3 locus on DR2-containing haplotypes. In addition, DR52 is also present on haplotypes with DR13 and DR14, which have infrequently been described in association with primary Sjögren's syndrome. Moreover, studies in Japanese patients differ markedly from Caucasian populations. In a study of Japanese patients, no increase of DR52 was found; instead HLA-DR53, encoded by DRB4, was increased among patients (Moriuchi *et al.* 1986), although not significant after correction for multiple comparisons. In this study a class I antigen, B54, was also increased among patients.

No unifying model emerges from serological studies, and investigators have sought better discrimination of HLA antigens by application of DNA-typing techniques. Fei *et al.* (1991) used methods that combined RFLP analysis with DNA probes. These methods provide an intermediate level of discrimination between those of serology and those utilizing complete sequence-specific oligonucleotide probe-typing or sequence-specific primers. HLA-DR3, DR52a, and DQA4 were increased among patients. DR52a is equivalent to the DRB3*0101 allele and the designation 'DQA4' is a grouping that includes the two DQA1 alleles, DQA1*0501 and DQA1*0401. Of note, DQA1*0501 is another candidate primary susceptibility allele because it is in strong linkage disequilibrium with DR3 and also with DR11. (Reitberg-Tambur *et al.* 1993)

DNA-typing techniques with sequence-specific oligonucleotide probe-typing was used in a study that included patients of three ethnic backgrounds reported by Kang *et al.* (1993). Caucasian, Japanese, and Chinese patients were compared with ethnically matched controls. Consistent with serological studies, among Caucasians, DRB1*0301 (encoding DR3) was significantly increased. The extended haplotype associated with primary Sjögren's syndrome among Caucasians was DRB1*0301, DRB3*0101, DQA1*0501, DQB1*0201. Also consistent with serological studies that had previously described an increase of DR53 among Japanese, DRB4*101 (encoding DR53) was increased in Japanese patients. The extended haplotype associated with primary Sjögren's syndrome in Japanese was DRB1*0405, DRB4*0101, DQA1*0301, DQB1*0401. The extended haplotype found among Chinese patients was DRB1*0803, DQA1*0103, DQB1*0601. The results of these studies do not support a primary association with DQA1*0501 since this allele is not found among Japanese or Chinese patients. The results also do not point to an association with a single allele at a class II locus. Inclusion of typing for HLA-DPB1 alleles also failed to demonstrate an allele common to all populations studied. Nevertheless, by examining the amino acid sequences of alleles associated with primary Sjögren's syndrome in each of these populations the authors were able to propose a shared amino acid sequence as a candidate disease-susceptibility sequence. This sequence is encoded by DQB1 alleles *0201, *0401, *0402, and *0601, spans positions 58 through 69 of the first domain of the DQβ1 chain, and encodes as-partic acid at position 67 and isoleucine at position 68.

In another interesting study, DNA-typing techniques were used to determine alleles at DRB1, DQA1, and DQB1 and correlation sought with $\gamma\delta$ T cell receptors in patients with primary Sjögren's syndrome. A significant correlation was found between higher levels of CD45RO$^+$ $\gamma\delta$ cells, lower levels of Vδ1-positive T cells, and the HLA alleles DQA1*0501 and DQB1*0201 (Kerttula *et al.* 1996).

HLA associations of Ro and La antibodies

Autoantibodies to Ro and to La are strongly correlated with particular class II antigens. Many studies suggest that HLA associations with Ro and La antibodies are stronger than those with the diseases in which these antibodies are most frequently found (i.e. Sjögren's syndrome and systemic lupus). Patients with antibodies to Ro and La have an increased frequency of HLA-DR3 (Vitali *et al.* 1986; Hietaharju *et al.* 1992), and in some studies DR3 and DR2 (Wilson *et al.* 1984). Higher levels of *in vitro* production of antibodies to La have been found even among normal individuals who had HLA-DR3 (Venables *et al.* 1988). In contrast to studies in Caucasians, DR3 was not associated with antibodies to Ro among Japanese patients. Instead, an increased frequency of DR52 and DR8 was observed (Miyagawa *et al.* 1992). Again, the question is raised as to whether the primary HLA association might be with genes that are in linkage disequilibrium with HLA-DR either genes that encode DR52 or DQ molecules. There is substantial evidence that the most important HLA association is with HLA-DQ molecules.

A number of studies have reported a striking association of HLA-DQ with antibodies to Ro and La antibodies (Harley *et al.* 1986; Hamilton *et al.* 1988). In 1986, Harley and co-workers reported that heterozygosity for DQ2 and DQ1 was associated with particularly high levels of Ro and La autoantibodies (the former in linkage disequilibrium with DR3 and the latter with DR1) (Harley *et al.* 1986). This association was confirmed in subsequent studies (Arnett *et al.* 1989; Reveille *et al.* 1991). A potential explanation for the synergistic risk observed with a heterozygous combination is that 'hybrid' DQ molecules are created by pairing of a DQα and DQβ encoded in 'trans' (pairing of an α chain encoded by a gene from one parent with a β chain encoded by a gene from the other parent). Results of experiments by Kwok *et al.* (1989), however, argue against this possibility, since these particular DQα and DQβ chains were not found to form stable $\alpha\beta$ heterodimers. Reveille *et al.* (1991) utilized DNA-typing

techniques to examine HLA associations with the anti-Ro response among patients with primary Sjögren's syndrome and systemic lupus. Caucasian andb African-American patients were included in the study. In a careful analysis of amino acid sequences of DQA1 and DQB1 alleles, the authors determined that antibodies to Ro were most frequently found in patients who had DQA1 alleles encoding glutamine at position 34 and DQB1 alleles encoding leucine at position 26. Unfortunately, it is probably not possible to generalize this observation since subsequent studies in Japanese suggest that Ro and La antibodies were associated with DQB1*0401 and DQB1*0601, neither of which encode for leucine at position 26 of the DQβ1 chain (Kang *et al.* 1993). However, the number of primary Sjögren's patients with antibodies to Ro and La is not specifically stated in this report.

The fine specificity of antibodies to Ro proteins, Ro 60 and Ro 52, have also been examined for correlation with HLA antigens. Patients with primary Sjögren's syndrome, and also patients with secondary Sjögren's syndrome associated with SLE, were studied. Both patients with anti-Ro 60 and those with anti-Ro 52 frequently had HLA-DR3; however, whereas antibodies to Ro52 were associated with the extended haplotype A1-B8-DR3, antibodies to Ro 60 were not. The study was not able to address fully a potential role for HLA-DQ antigens because only serological techniques were used; however, the serological specificity DQ1 appeared to be negatively associated with antibodies to Ro 60 (Ricchiuti *et al.* 1994a). See also discussion of the immunogenetics of anti-Ro and anti-La antibodies in patients with systemic lupus and mothers of children with the neonatal lupus syndrome in Chapter 4.

Secondary Sjögren's syndrome

In contrast to the increase of DR3 and DR52 seen among patients with primary Sjögren's syndrome, in a study of Caucasian and some black patients with secondary Sjögren's syndrome (most with SLE or RA) only DR52 was increased (Wilson *et al.* 1984). In a small number of patients with secondary Sjögren's syndrome and rheumatoid arthritis no association with DR3 or DR52 was found and, instead, DR4 was increased (Haralampos *et al.* 1979). Some increase of DR4 was also found in Japanese patients with secondary Sjögren's syndrome and RA in contrast to secondary Sjögren's with other diseases such as SLE, SSC, and overlap (Moriuchi *et al.* 1986). All of the above studies utilized serological techniques. Available data indicate the HLA associations of secondary Sjögren's differ from that of primary Sjögren's, and suggest HLA associations in secondary Sjögren's may be that of the associated disease. Future studies that use DNA-typing techniques and in which larger populations of patients with secondary Sjögren's syndrome are studied categorized according to the specific associated autoimmune disorder will be useful to clarify the latter issue.

Experimental models

A wide variety of attempts have been made to induce the lesions and clinical features of Sjögren's syndrome in animal models over the past 30 years. A review of these induced models is shown in Tables 6.8 and 6.9. They have consisted mainly of the administration of homogenates of salivary glands given together with adjuvants (often Freund's complete adjuvant). In general they have induced a variable degree of sialadenitis, histologically, with a variable degree of clinical effect. These models do not, however, appear to be associated with the typical anti-Ro/La antibody response (though this has been looked for surprising infrequently) and the histological changes are often transient. In the past 20 years there has been much greater focus on the use of inbred strains of mice which spontaneously develop models of secondary Sjögren's syndrome. Thus, the spontaneous development of Sjögren's syndrome in NZB/NZW mice was first described by Kessler (1968). Modified Schirmer's tests (see Fig. 6.2b) and sialochemical studies suggested salivary gland pathology, while histology revealed periductal and perivascular mononuclear cell infiltrates in most animals after four months of age. These infiltrates consisted of small lymphocytes, plasma cells, and

histiocytes, and epimyoepithelial islands were present. The inflammation, which is more marked in females, is most severe in the lachrymal glands.

A periductal mononuclear cell infiltrate in the salivary glands of MRL mice was first reported by Hang (1982). It has since been studied in much more detail (e.g. Jonsson and Holmdahl 1990) and there is general agreement that the salivary gland infiltrate is dominated by CD4[+] T cells, many of which also express MHC class II antigens, suggesting that T cell activation or selective infiltration of activated T cells into the gland has occurred. In the MRL/*lpr* mice, inflammatory lesions are evident in the lachrymal glands by four weeks of age (and at three months of age in the MRL+/+ mice) and these abnormalities persist and indeed increase throughout the life of these animals.

NOD mice, which have more commonly been studied as models of insulin-dependent diabetes, also show the lymphocytic infiltration in the submandibular and lachrymal glands. The sialoadenitis appears at between 8 and 12 weeks in the females and around 14 weeks in the males. It is characterized by small focal infiltrates, located principally around blood vessels. Again, the majority of infiltrating cells are CD4[+] T cells. As reviewed elsewhere (Horsfall *et al.* 1994) there are strong suggestions that the development of insulin-dependent diabetes and sialadenitis in this mouse strain are separate entities.

There have been a number of studies exploring the nature of autoantibody production in the salivary glands from these spontaneous models (reviewed by Horsfall *et al.* 1994). Local reduction of immunoglobulin, in particular IgG, is well recognized in most of these models, but attempts to identify anti-Ro or -La antibodies appear to have been unsuccessful, with the single exception of a report by St Clair *et al.* (1991)

Table 6.8 Experimental models of spontaneously occurring Sjögren's syndrome

Strain	Conjunctivitis	Lachrymal gland inflammation	Salivary gland inflammation	Anti-Ro/La antibodies
NZB	+	+	+	−
NZB/NZW	+	+	+	−
MRL/*lpr*	+	+	+	1 report of anti-La[*]
MRL+	+	+	+	−
NOD	NK	NK	+	−
BDFI[†]	NK	NK	+	−
C57 BL/6[†]	NK	NK	+	−

NK = not known.

[*] St Clair *et al.* (1991).

[†] Sjögren's syndrome in aged non-autoimmune mice (highly age dependent; significant disease occurs only in animals > 12 months).

160

Table 6.9   Induced experimental models of Sjögren's syndrome

Animals injected	Substance	Result	References
Guinea pigs	Submax/CFA	Mild SG inflammation	Chan (1964)
Guinea pigs	SG saline extract + carbonyl iron + *Bordatella pertussis* vaccine	Severe sialadenitis	Whaley and MacSween (1974)
Rats	Submand + CFA + *Bordatella pertussis* vaccine	Sialadenitis severe in nature female donated submand T-cell depletion Decreased sialadenitis	Sharaway and White (1978) White and Casarett (1974) White (1976) Cutler *et al.* (1991)
Mice	SG + CFA	Autoimmune SL/Ni strain developed severe sialadenitis ASDA	Takeda and Ishikawa (1983)
Rats	Submand + CFA	Sialadenitis ASDA	Dean and Hiramoto (1984)
Mice (thymectomized)	Submand + CFA	Thy 1.2+, Lyt 2+ cells infiltrated submand and parotid ASDA	Hayashi (1985)
Rabbits	Lachrymal gland cauterization, removal of nictitan + Harderian glands	Desquamation of corneal epithelium, abnormal Rose Bengal staining. Normal Schirmer test	Gilbard *et al.* (1988)
Mice C3H/He(H-2k) (thymectomized)	Submand + CFA	L3T4+, Lyt 2+ cells infiltrated submand ASDA	Hayashi and Hirakawa (1989)

ASDA, anti-salivary duct antibodies; submax, submaxillary glands; submand, submandibular glands; SG, Salivary gland; CFA, complete Freund's adjuvant.

which described the detection of anti-La antibodies by an ELISA in MRL/*lpr* mice.

Jonsson and Holmdahl (1990), among others, have explored the salivary gland inflammatory lesions for the presence of cytokines, including interferon-γ. Interferon-γ-producing cells were indeed detected in the periphery of large inflammatory infiltrates and were thought to be inducing the expression of MHC class II antigens on epithelial cells. Among the cytokines studied, high levels of IL-6 were found to be spontaneously produced by salivary gland-infiltrating cells, and there was some evidence for IL-3 and interferon-γ in the salivary glands. Studies of local cytokine gene expression have reported the presence of genes for the inflammatory cytokines IL-1β and TNF-α in the salivary glands of MRL/*lpr* mice before the onset of autoimmune sialadenitis (Hamano *et al.* 1993). In addition, IL-6 gene expression was elevated from three months of age when the sialadenitis was apparent. These cytokines were shown, by immunohistochemistry, to be secreted by mononuclear cells within the salivary gland periductal inflammatory lesions. In contrast, the epithelial cells did not stain for a wide variety of cytokines that were studied. These animal data thus contrast with the cytokine data on human patients reported later in this chapter and confirms that one must be cautious about over-interpreting the relevance of these models to the pathogenesis of human disease.

More recently the development of transgenic and 'knock-out' mice has encouraged the development of a new set of animal models for Sjögren's syndrome. Thus Green *et al.* (1989) studied transgenic mice containing the human T lymphotropic virus-1 (HTLV-1) *tax* gene and showed that the animals developed an exocrinopathy involving the salivary and lachrymal glands. During the first few weeks of life, ductal proliferation in the salivary glands was noted to increase considerably, accompanied by lymphocytic infiltration and proliferating epithelial cells. By the time the mice died (aged 6–8 months) there was extensive epithelial island enlargement with lymphocytic infiltration leading to the destruction of acinar architecture. The salivary gland pathology was noted to correlate with the level of *tax* gene expression in ductal epithelial cells. More recently, Mariette *et al.* (1993) have identified the HTLV-1 *tax* gene in the salivary gland epithelium from two out of nine patients with Sjögren's syndrome.

Transforming growth factor-β1 (TGF-β1) knock-out mice develop a notable acute wasting disease approximately 20 days after birth, which, histologically, is characterized by a multi-focal mixed inflammatory cell infiltrate in various glands, including salivary glands, particularly round the ductal epithelium (Shull *et al.* 1992). TGF-β1 is known to downregulate interferon-β-induced expression of MHC class II antigens by both lymphoid and non-lymphoid cells. Thus, its absence could allow the presentation of self-antigens by inappropriate cells, perhaps leading to the autoimmune response.

Other animal models

Haneji *et al.* (1994) developed an animal model of primary Sjögren's syndrome in NFS/*sld* mutant mice thymectomized three days after birth. The T cell receptor Vβ8 gene is preferentially expressed in these inflammatory lesions at the onset of the disease and high concentrations of IgG salivary duct autoantibodies were detected in the sera of these mice. Intriguingly, they did not develop any other autoimmune lesions.

Finally the graft-versus-host (GvH) mouse was first described as a model for autoimmune disease by Gleichmann *et al.* (1976) and was shown by Pals *et al.* (1985) to have lymphocytic infiltrations in the salivary glands reminiscent of the exocrinopathy of Sjögren's syndrome. Some extensions of this model have been studied (reviewed in Horsfall *et al.* 1994), but again there appears to be an absence of anti-Ro or anti-La antibodies, which characterize the human disease serologically.

Aetiopathogenesis

Sjögren's syndrome has long been considered likely to have an important viral aetiological factor because the salivary glands are known to be a site of latency for various viruses. The possible mechanisms by which viruses can induce tolerance bypass include polyclonal activation of B cells, molecular mimicry between viral epitopes and autoantigens, modified self, idiotypic network perturbation, exposure of so-called 'hidden antigens', and direct toxic effects of viruses on target cells (see also Chapter 1). Each of these mechanisms may be applied to Sjögren's syndrome.

Polyclonal activation of B cells by a virus infection is known to occur in Epstein–Barr virus (EBV). Fox *et al.* (1986*b*) originally claimed that EBV was present uniquely in saliva or salivary gland biopsies from patients with primary Sjögren's syndrome, but the many attempts to reproduce this finding have resulted in conflicting results (Venables *et al.* 1994). It thus remains a matter of conjecture as to whether or not EBV is an aetiological agent in Sjögren's syndrome.

The Ro and La autoantigens, a major target of antibodies in patients with Sjögren's syndrome, have been shown to share sequence similarities with some viruses. Kohsaka *et al.* (1990) reported a region of homology (six out of eight consecutive amino acids) between amino acids 88 and 101 in the N terminal region of La containing an immunodominant epitope, and a feline retroviral gag protein. Similarly, Scofield and Harley (1991) showed six regions of homology between the 60 kDa Ro and the nucleocapsid protein of a vesicular stomatitis virus. Thus, these antibodies might be induced by a form of molecular mimicry. However, it is important to remember that these homologies may simply have occurred by chance and be of no aetiological relevance.

Retroviruses have attracted considerable attention as possible aetiological agents in the past five years (see Table 6.10) and Venables *et al.* (1994) have suggested that endogenous retroviruses can cause interferon-γ expression (Fig. 6.7) which stimulates epithelial cells to the express HLA class II antigens and cytoplasmic La. This, in turn, could induce an immune response, resulting in the infiltration of positive CD4 lymphocytes, which can secrete further interferon-γ. This model supports the view first put forward by Talal (1971) that the activated epithelial cell may be the main instigator of autoimmunity in Sjögren's syndrome.

The La autoantigen is involved in the processing of viral RNAs, suggesting that antibodies to La may develop as a result of a combination of La and viral RNA. Some interesting recent work by Zhang and Reichlin (1996), proposing in some cases that anti-La antibodies may act as anti-idiotypic antibodies for anti-

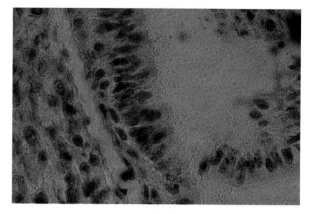

Fig. 6.7. Expression of interferon-γ (red stain) adjacent to the epithelial cells seen in a labial biopsy from a patient with Sjögren's syndrome. (Courtesy of Deborah Rowe, × 100.)

DNA antibodies, suggests a previously unsuspected degree of connection between autoantibody 'families'. However, we still await definitive evidence that perturbation of these idiotypic connections can result in clinical effects. It remains tempting to speculate that organ-specific autoimmune diseases are likely to have organ/tissue-specific autoantigens. Haneji *et al.* (1997) have recently proposed that an actin-binding protein, α fodrin, may be a particular target in Sjögren's syndrome. It is known that the secretion in parotid acinar cells is associated with significant alterations in the cytoskeletal proteins, particularly of α fodrin.

The notion that antigens previously hidden might become exposed and thus potentially autoantigenic has been given a boost by recent studies on apoptosis. Thus Casciola-Rosen *et al.* (1994) have shown that keratinocytes exposed to ultraviolet radiation will induce, during the process of apoptosis, surface blebs that contain nuclear autoantigens including DNA, Ro, and La. This finding suggests a mechanism by which autoantigens 'hidden' inside cells may be exposed to the immune system. The proteolysis of fodrin during apoptosis, a consequence of the enzymatic activity of proteases, could lead to conformational changes that render α fodrin an autoantigen. However, it remains to be explained why, since cells are dying constantly, autoantibody responses to these autoantigens are not a more common feature in healthy individuals and why particular autoantigens seem to be targets in patients with autoimmune diseases, given that approximately 2000 such targets are thought to exist within cells!

The idea that viruses might target and damage particular cells has long been considered a possibility. As

Table 6.10 Links between retroviruses and Sjögren's syndrome

- Infection and persistence in cells of the immune system (e.g. CD4+ T cells, macrophages) in target tissues such as salivary glands.
- Antibodies to the capsid antigen p24 protein of HIV-1 found in the sera of patients with Sjögren's syndrome.
- Endogenous retroviral sequences in minor salivary glands.
- Disease resembling Sjögren's syndrome reported in transgenic mice containing the HTLV-1 *tax* gene.
- Reaction of epithelial cytoplasmic protein from minor salivary glands with monoclonal antibody to p19 gag protein of HTLV-1.

described on page 161 mice transgenic for the human T lymphotrophic virus (HTLV-1) *tax* gene developed a form of proliferative synovitis and it was proposed that this was the direct consequence of the *tax* gene (Green *et al.* 1989), the inflammatory response being due to the upregulation of class II antigens and cytokine production by cells expressing this gene.

Human immunodeficiency virus (HIV) has been linked to salivary gland lymphocyte infiltrates in patients with the acquired immunodeficiency syndrome (AIDS). These patients may have sicca symptoms but in general they do not fulfil the criteria for Sjögren's syndrome. In contrast, an increased prevalence of hepatitis C virus infection has been reported in a group of patients with sicca symptoms who did meet the European criteria (Jorgensen *et al.* 1996). These patients lacked anti-Ro/La antibodies and, if these observations are confirmed, would suggest the existence of a particular subset.

As with responses to EBV, conflicting claims have been made about the presence of antibodies to herpes virus and cytomegalovirus (reviewed in Venables *et al.* 1994) and the role of these viruses as potential aetiological agents thus remains equally uncertain.

Other aetiological factors

The precise reason why it is principally women who suffer from Sjögren's syndrome remains unclear. The possible role of abnormalities in apoptosis in patients with Sjögren's syndrome has been explored in several reports. Rose *et al.* (1995) found no increase in levels of bcl-2 (an oncogene whose expression delays apoptosis) in peripheral blood mononuclear cells from these patients. However, Newkirk *et al.* (1996) have proposed that an Epstein–Barr virus early antigen (BHRF1/p17.1), known to be a viral homologue of bcl-2, could be preventing apoptosis and thus contributing to the accumulation of lymphocyte and/or epithelial cells. In a more detailed study, an unresolved paradox has been reported in which bcl-2 mRNA expression of T cells derived from patients with Sjögren's syndrome was increased, but *in vitro* T cell apoptosis was enhanced (Ogawa *et al.* 1996). Presumably, the balance of other cell death promoters/inhibitors for signals must be crucial.

There has also been a suggestion that changes in IgA glycosylation are detectable in patients with primary Sjögren's syndrome. Thus, Dueymes *et al.* (1995) reported that the proportion of sialylated IgA1 and A2 was augmented, while galactosylated A1 and A2 were reduced compared with controls.

Lymphocyte function

The numbers of peripheral blood lymphocytes and total T and B lymphocytes in patients with Sjögren's syndrome appear to be little different from healthy individuals. There is no general agreement as to whether there are significant differences in the T cell subsets in the peripheral blood lymphocytes of these patients.

In contrast, there is general agreement that most of the infiltrating lymphocytes in the salivary glands of patients with Sjögren's syndrome are T lymphocytes (approximately 80%), the remainder being mainly B lymphocytes and plasma cells, with a few monocytes, macrophages, and NK cells being observed (Speight *et al.* 1990). Among the predominant T cell infiltrate, approximately three times as many carry the CD4 phenotype. The T cells also express mainly the $\alpha\beta$ heterodimer form of the T cell receptor (fewer than 5% bear the $\gamma\delta$ phenotype) (Zumla *et al.* 1991). The T cells also tend to be the of the helper/inducer, memory (CD4/45 Ro$^+$) subtype.

As with virtually all other autoimmune diseases, major attempts have been made to determine whether there is any bias in the repertoire of the T cell receptor usage, which might indicate an infectious aetiology and superantigen-driven disease. There does not seem to be any obvious restriction, although Sumida *et al.* (1992) describe a preferential expression of Vβ2 and Vβ13 receptor transcripts in lesional infiltrates, and other workers have suggested that there may be preferential expression of certain junctional sequences, with an increased frequency of Vβ2/Jβ.2.3 and Vβ13/Jβ.2.1.

Epithelial cells in Sjögren's syndrome biopsies

It has been known for over 10 years that epithelial cells in salivary gland biopsies express HLA-DR (Isenberg *et al.* 1984). Such expression might allow glandular epithelial cells to develop antigen-presenting functions and participate in antigen-driven reactions. Pursuing this idea as, suggested earlier in this chapter, Venables *et al.* (1994) have proposed that the stimulation of the epithelial cells by interferon-γ is responsible for the expression of HLA class II antigens and probably also cytoplasmic La and retroviral antigens.

Cytokines

Table 6.11 provides an overview of cytokine expression seen in the salivary glands of patients with

Table 6.11   Cytokine expression in Sjögren's syndrome

	Mononuclear infiltrate	Acini	Ducts
Interferon-α	Rare	Rare	–
Interferon-β	–/+	–/+	–/+
Interferon-γ	–/+	–/+	+/+
IL-1α	–/+	–/+	–/+
IL-1β	+	+	++
IL-2	–	–	–
IL-4	–	–	–
IL-6	+	–	++
IL-8	–	+	++
TNF-α	+	–	++
TNF-β	–	–	–
TGF	+	+	++
EGF	–	–	++

Adapted from Table I in Fox and Speight (1996).

Sjögren's syndrome. Although different techniques and tissues have been used, the overall message, especially bearing in mind an important study by Cauli *et al.* (1995) which found little difference in such expression with that observed with patients with chronic sialoadenitis, is that the changes seen are unlikely to be found uniquely in Sjögren's syndrome patients. Thus, the cytokine expression that has been reported is probably part of a common inflammatory response that develops whatever the initial damaging event. By analogy, patients with either a brain haemorrhage or ischaemic clot in the right cerebral hemisphere will present with the same type of pyramidal track lesions of the left arm and leg.

Fox *et al.* (1994), using reverse transcription and a semi-quantitative polymerase chain reaction to study cytokine mRNA expression, detected IL-1α, IL-2, IL-10, and interferon-γ in biopsies from patients with Sjögren's syndrome but not in normal salivary tissue. As part of their analysis they showed that the CD4+ T cells were found to contain IL-2, IL-10, and interferon-γ, but not IL-4 or -5. CD8+ T cells expressed TNF-α but not the other cytokines. Salivary gland epithelial cell-enriched fraction also contained mRNA for IL-1α, TNF-α, IL-6, and IL-10. These data confirm that the gland cells as well as the infiltrating lymphocytes produce a number of immunologically active cytokines. Messenger RNAs of the Th1 cytokines (notably IL-2 and interferon-γ) were detected in all the labial salivary glands from 15 patients with Sjögren's syndrome but in none of three controls. The Th2 cytokines (IL-4 and IL-5) were found in about half of the cases, in association with B cell accumulations. IL-6 (especially), IL-10, and TGF-β were also found consist-

ently. The authors (Ohyama *et al.* 1996) proposed that Th1 cytokines together with IL-6, -10 and TGF-β are essential in the induction of Sjögren's syndrome and/or its maintenance, while Th2 cytokines are involved in disease progression, especially local B cell activation. However, on balance, a truly complete study of cytokine expression of the major and minor salivary glands of patients with Sjögren's syndrome remains to be undertaken.

Adhesion molecules

A small number of studies have attempted to investigate these molecules, which mediate cell to cell and cell to matrix interactions. In one study the vascular cell adhesion molecule-1 (VCAM-1) was found on both vascular and ramifying dendritic cells at the centre of large T cell aggregates and in all aggregates in which there was a central clustering of B cells (Fig. 6.8) (Edwards *et al.* 1993). The authors proposed that this may be important in determining the distribution of B rather than T cells in lymphocytic infiltrates in patients with Sjögren's syndrome. Other adhesion molecules, notably ICAM-1 and E-selectin have been found on endothelial cells and ICAM-1 on the epithelium (Aziz *et al.* 1992). This was associated with a strong expression of the β_2-integrins on the infiltrating lymphocytes. However, it is again unlikely that increased expression of adhesion molecules is a specific feature of Sjögren's syndrome or even an initiating factor for its pathogenesis.

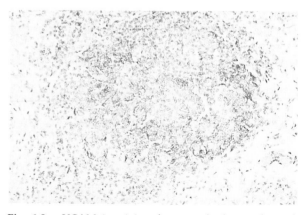

Fig. 6.8.   VCAM-1 staining shown on both vascular and dendritic cells in association with what were found to be T and B cell aggregates.

Summary of the aetiopathogenesis of Sjögren's syndrome

In Fig. 6.9 the factors we have just discussed, which appear to be critical in the development of aetiopathogenesis of Sjögren's syndrome, are drawn together to indicate a hypothetical chain of events that could lead to the clinical expression of Sjögren's syndrome. There are a number of important caveats, however. Although experimental data supports an aetiological role for viruses, confirmatory evidence in patients is lacking. The precise mechanism of the immunogenetic influence on the development of tissue lesions remains obscure, as are the factors that determine those patients more likely to develop the complication of lymphoma (Fox and Speight 1996). Equally uncertain are the reasons why some individuals develop marked extraglandular manifestations and why not all patients with Sjögren's syndrome have the classic anti-Ro/La antibodies. The central role of abnormalities in apoptosis within the salivary gland is also enigmatic.

Treatment

The treatment of Sjögren's syndrome is symptomatic relief of the effects of chronic xerostomia and keratoconjunctivitis sicca by keeping mucosal surfaces moist (Foster *et al.* 1993). Dry eyes should be moistened with artificial tears as often as necessary. A number of preparations are available using one of several different ingredients; hypromellose (hydroxyethylcellulose), which helps to replace the aqueous layer; acetylcysteine, which helps to break down mucus accumulation; and dispersants (polyvinyl chloride, polyethylene glycol, dextran), which spread the aqueous layer. Some patients may become sensitive to the preservatives (benzalkonium chloride, chlorhexidine), stabilizers (disodium edetate), and solubilizer (polysorbate 80). If corneal ulceration develops eye patches and boric acid ointment are required. Drugs that cause a decrease in lachrymation and salivation should be avoided, i.e. diuretics, antihypertensive agents, antidepressants, phenothiazines, decongestants, and heavy smoking. Symptoms may be exacerbated by environments with a low level of humidity, including air-conditioning and dusty, dry, and windy climates. Soft contact lenses can help to protect the cornea but require frequent wetting and great care to avoid infection.

The treatment of xerostomia is difficult. Sugarless, highly flavoured lozenges may be helpful. A variety of saliva substitute solutions are available (van der Reijden *et al.* 1996). Many patients carry water and use sugar-free lemon drops or chewing gum. Sugar must be avoided to prevent rapid dental decay. Regular oral hygiene after meals and dental assessments are strongly advised. Topical oral treatment with fluoride enhances dental mineralization and may slow the damage to the surface of teeth (Daniels and Fox 1992). Bromhexine (48 mg/day) may help sicca symptoms. Vaginal dryness is treated with lubricant jellies (KY jelly or propionic acid gels) and dry skin with

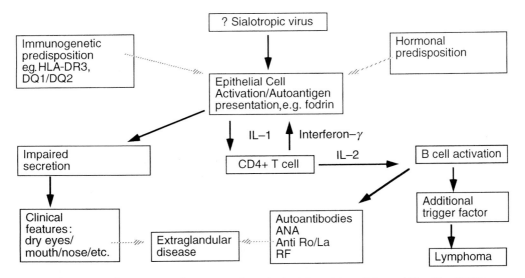

Fig. 6.9. Aetiopathogenesis of Sjögren's syndrome — an hypothesis. Adapted from Price and Venables (1995).

moisturizing creams. Dryness of the nasal passages can be annoying and is usually managed by the use of saline sprays and/or nocturnal humidifiers.

Pilocarpine hydrochloride (5 mg three times daily) can also improve sicca symptoms, through its muscarinic, cholinergic activity (Fox *et al.* 1986a). Flushing and sweating are possible side-effects.

Parotid gland swelling is a feature of Sjögren's syndrome. If the gland becomes tender with permanent enlargement, infection should be ruled out and treatment with tetracycline (500 mg four times per day) instituted.

The joint symptoms of Sjögren's syndrome can be treated effectively with non-steroidal anti-inflammatory drugs or simple analgesics. Hydroxychloroquine (200 mg/day) may be helpful for both the arthralgia and fatigue of Sjögren's syndrome, this also reduces hypergammaglobulinaemia, decreases the titre of IgG antibodies to La/SS-B, and the erythrocyte sedimentation rate, and also increases the haemoglobin (Fox *et al.* 1988), but a controlled trial failed to demonstrate any benefit attributable to hydroxychloroquine (Kruize *et al.* 1993).

Corticosteroids (0.5–1.0 mg/kg/day) and other immunosuppressive drugs are used in patients with severe extraglandular disease, including interstitial pneumonitis, glomerulonephritis, vasculitis, and peripheral neuropathy.

Experimental treatment

Cyclosporin is effective in the MRL/*lpr* mouse in ocular and lacrimal gland inflammation (Jabs *et al.* 1996b). Gunduz and Ozdemir (1994) found that topical 2% cyclosporin in olive oil resulted in a decrease in Rose Bengal staining but that tear production as assessed by the Schirmer tear test was unaffected.

Interferon-α increased saliva production in preliminary studies (Shiozawa *et al.* 1993), but this finding has not yet been confirmed in a placebo-controlled trial.

High dose intravenous immunoglobulin was successful in a single case of refractory vasculitis with primary Sjögren's syndrome (Zeuner *et al.* 1995). Plasma exchange and intravenous immunoglobulin produced partial responses in three patients with Sjögren's syndrome who had severe neuropathy due to vasculitis (Hebbar *et al.* 1995).

Anti-CD4 monoclonal antibodies decrease ocular inflammation in the MRL/*lpr* mouse but not the salivary gland inflammation (Jabs *et al.* 1996a,b).

CD4+ T cells were removed from the lachrymal gland but a diffuse infiltrate of CD8+ T cells developed.

Summary

Sjögren's syndrome is a member of a family of autoimmune rheumatic diseases and is characterized by xerostoma (dry mouth) and xerophthalmia (dry eyes). These two manifestations alone are known as the sicca complex, or primary Sjögren's syndrome, but the disorder is frequently found in association with SLE or rheumatoid arthritis. Serologically, the disease is characterized by antibodies to the extractable nuclear antigens, Ro (SS-A) and La (SS-B), and the function of the parotid and lachrymal glands is compromised by infiltrating lymphocytes as with other diseases of this type. The aetiology of Sjögren's syndrome is unknown but the disease has a genetic and hormonal background. Recently, endongenous retroviruses have been implicated in its pathogenesis. Unlike SLE, most of the patients with this condition are not severely ill, although a tendency to develop lymphomas of B cell origin has been identified. Several strains of autoimmune-prone mice, including MRL/*lpr* and NZB/W, have facilitated studies on experimental therapeutics and immunopathology. The clinical features of dry eyes and dry mouth usually respond in part to symptomatic therapy. Treatment with immunosuppressive agents have yielded disappointing results.

References

Alexander der EL, Malinow K, Lejewski JE *et al.* Primary Sjögren's syndrome with central nervous system disease mimicking multiple sclerosis. *Ann Intern Med* 1986; **104**: 323–30.

Anaya JM, Ogawa N, TN. Sjögren's syndrome in childhood. *J Rheumatol* 1995; **6**: 1152–8.

Andonopoulos AP, Lagos G, Drosos AA *et al.* Neurological involvement in primary Sjögren's syndrome: a preliminary report. *J Autoimmun* 1989; **2**: 485–8.

Andonopoulos AP, Lagos G, Drosos AA *et al.* The spectrum of neurological involvement in primary Sjögren's syndrome. *Br J Rheumatol* 1990; **2**: 21–3.

Arnett FC, Bias WB, Reveille JD. Genetic studies in Sjögren's syndrome and systemic lupus erythematosus. *J Autoimmun* 1989; **2**: 404–13.

Aziz KE, McCluskey PJ, Montanaro A *et al.* Vascular endothelium and lymphocyte adhesion molecules in minor salivary glands of patients with Sjögren's syndrome. *J Clin Lab Immunol* 1992; **37**: 39–49.

Binder A, Snaith ML, Isenberg D. Sjögren's syndrome: a study of its neurological complications. *Br J Rheumatol* 1988; **27**: 275–80.

Bloch KJ, Buchanan WW, Wohl MJ *et al.* Sjögren's syndrome: a clinical, pathological and serological study of 62 cases. *Medicine* 1965; **44**: 187–231.

Bodeutsch D, de Wilde PCM, Kater L. Quantitative immuno-histologic criteria are superior to the lymphocytic focus score criterion for the diagnosis of Sjögren's syndrome. *Arth Rheum* 1992; **35**: 1075–87.

Casciola-Rosen LA, Anhalt G, Rosen A. Autoantigens targeted in systemic lupus erythematosus are clustered in two populations of surface structures on apoptotic keratinocytes. *J Exp Med* 1994; **179**; 1317–30.

Cauli A, Yanni G, Pitzalis C *et al.* Cytokine and adhesion molecule expression in the minor salivary glands of patients with Sjögren's syndrome and chronic sialoadenitis. *Ann Rheum Dis* 1995; **54**: 209–15.

Chan WC. Experimental sialadenitis in guinea pigs. *J Pathol Bacteriol* 1964; **88**: 592–5.

Chused TM, Kassan SS, Opelz G *et al.* Sjögren's syndrome association with HLA-Dw3. *N Eng J Med* 1977; **296**: 895–7.

Cutler LS, Rozenski D, Coolens J *et al.* Experimental auto-allergic sialadenitis in the LEW rat. I. Parameters of disease induction. *Cell Immunol* 1991; **135**: 333–45.

Daniels TE, Fox PC. Salivary and oral components of Sjögren's syndrome. *Rheum Dis Clin North Am* 1992; **18**: 571–89.

Dean DH, Hiramoto RN. Experimental autoallergic sialadenitis in male rats. *J Oral Pathol* 1984; **13**: 63–8.

Diss TC, Wotherspoon AC, Peng HZ *et al.* A single neoplastic clone in sequential biopsy specimens from a patient with primary gastric mucosa associated lymphoid tissue lymphoma and Sjögren's syndrome. *N Eng J Med* 1993; **329**: 172–5.

Dorner T, Hucks M, Mayet WJ *et al.* Enhanced membrane expression of the 52 kDa Ro(SS-A) and La(SS-B) antigens by human keratinocytes induced by TNF alpha. *Ann Rheum Dis* 1995; **54**: 904–9.

Dueymes M, Berdaord B, Pennec YL *et al.* IgA glycosylation abnormalities in the serum of patients with Sjögren's syndrome. *Clin Exp Rheumatol* 1995; **13**: 243–50.

Edwards JCW, Wilkinson LS, Speight P *et al.* Vascular cell adhesion molecule-1 and α4 and β1 integrins in lymphocyte aggregates in Sjögren's syndrome and rheumatoid arthritis. *Ann Rheum Dis* 1993; **52**: 806–11.

Fei HM, Kan H, Scharf S *et al.* Specific HLA-DQA and HLA-DRB1 alleles confer susceptibility to Sjögren's syndrome and autoantibody production. *J Clin Lab Anal* 1991; **5**: 382–91.

Foster HE, Gilroy JJ, Kelly CA *et al.* The treatment of sicca features of Sjögren's syndrome: a clinical review. *Br J Rheumatol* 1993; **33**: 278–82.

Fox PC, Speight PM. Current concepts of autoimmune exocrinopathy: immunologic mechanisms in the salivary pathology of Sjögren's syndrome. *Crit Rev Oral Biol Med* 1996; **7**: 144–58.

Fox P, van der Ven PF, Baum BJ. Pilocarpine for the treatment of xerostomia associated with salivary gland dysfunction. *Oral Surg Oral Med Oral Pathol* 1986a; **61**: 243–6.

Fox RI, Pearson G, Vaughan JH. Detection of Epstein-Barr virus associated antigens and DNA in salivary gland biopsies from patients with Sjögren's syndrome. *J Immunol* 1986b; **137**: 3162–8.

Fox RI, Chan E, Benton Long S *et al.* Treatment of primary Sjögren's syndrome with hydroxychloroquine. *Am J Med* 1988; **85** (Suppl. 4A): 62–7.

Fox RI, Kang H, Aral D *et al.* Cytokine mRNA expression in salivary gland biopsies of Sjögren's syndrome. *J Immunol* 1994; **152**: 5532–9.

Gilbard JP, Rossi SR, Gray KL *et al.* Tear film osmolarity and ocular surface disease in two rabbit models for kerato-conjunctivitis sicca. *Invest Ophthamol Vis Sci* 1988; **29**: 374–8.

Gleichmann E, Gleichmann H, Wilke L. Autoimmunization and lymphoma genesis in parent to F_1 combinations differing at the major histocompatibility complex: model for spontaneous disease caused by altered self antigens? *Transplant Rev* 1976; **31**: 156–224.

Green JB, Hinricks SH, Vogen J *et al.* Exocrinopathy resembling Sjögren's syndrome in HTLV-1 tax transgenic mice. *Nature* 1989; **341**: 72–4.

Gunduz K, Ozdemir O. Topical cyclosporin treatment of keratoconjunctivitis sicca in secondary Sjögren's syndrome. *Acta Ophthalmol* 1994; **72**: 438–42.

Guo K, Major G, Foster N *et al.* Defective repair of O6–methylguanine-DNA in primary Sjögren's syndrome patients predisposed to lymphoma. *Ann Rheum Dis* 1995; **54**: 229–32.

Hamano H, Saito I, Haneji N *et al.* Expressions of cytokine genes during the development of autoimmune sialadenitis in MRL/lpr mice. *Eur J Immunol* 1993; **23**: 2387–91.

Hamilton R, Harley J, Bias W *et al.* Two Ro (SS-A) autoantibody responses in systemic lupus erythematosus. Correlation of HLA-DR/DQ specificities with quantitative expression of Ro (SSA) autoantibody. *Arthritis Rheum* 1988; **31**: 496–505.

Haneji N, Hamano H, Yanagi K *et al.* A new animal model for primary Sjögren's syndrome in NFS/sld mutant mice. *J Immunol* 1994; **153**: 2769–77.

Haneji N, Nakamura T, Takio K *et al.* Identification of α Fodrin as a candidate autoantigen in primary Sjögren's syndrome. *Science* 1997; **276**: 604–7.

Hang L. A spontaneous rheumatoid arthritis-like disease in MRL/l mice. *J Exp Med* 1982; **155**: 1690–701.

Harley JB, Reichlin M, Arnett FC *et al.* Gene interaction at HLA-DQ enhances autoantibody production in primary Sjögren's syndrome. *Science* 1986; **232**: 1145–7.

Hayashi Y. Induction of experimental allergic sialadenitis in mice. *Am J Pathol* 1985; **118**: 476–83.

Hayashi Y, Hirakawa K. Immunopathology of experimental autoallergic sialadenitis in C3H/He mice. *Clin Exp Immunol* 1989; **75**: 471–6.

Hebbar M, Hebbar-Savean K, Hachulla E *et al.* Participation of cryoglobulinaemia in the sensory peripheral neuropathies of primary Sjögren's syndrome. *Ann Med Inte* 1995; **146**: 235–8.

Hietaharju A, Korpela M, Ilonen JJ *et al.* Nervous system disease, immunological features, and HLA phenotype in Sjögren's syndrome. *Ann Rheum Dis* 1992; **51**: 506–9.

Hinzova E, Ivanyi D, Sula K *et al.* HLA-Dw3 in Sjögren's syndrome. *Tissue Antigens* 1977; **9**: 8–10.

Horsfall AC, Skarstein K, Jonsson R. Experimental models of Sjögren's syndrome. In: *Autoimmune Diseases: Focus on Sjögren's Syndrome*, eds Isenberg DA, Horsfall AC. Bios Scientific Publishers, Oxford, 1994: 67–88.

Isenberg DA. Secondary Sjögren's syndrome – the sausage factory revisited. *Clin Exp Rheum* 1994; **12**: 519–21.

Isenberg DA, Rowe D, Tookman A *et al.* An immunohistochemical study of secondary Sjögren's syndrome. *Ann Rheum Dis* 1984; **43**: 470–6.

Jabs DA, Burns WH, Prendergast RA. Paradoxic effect of antiCD4 therapy on lacrimal gland disease in MRL/Mp-lpr/lpr mice. *Invest Ophthalmol Vis Sci* 1996a; **37**: 246–50.

Jabs DA, Lee B, Burek CL *et al.* Cyclosporine therapy suppresses ocular and lacrimal gland disease in MRL/Mp-Lpr/Lpr mice. *Invest Ophthalmol Vis Sci* 1996b; **37**: 377–83.

Jacobsson LTH, Axell TE, Hansen BU *et al.* Dry eyes or mouth – an epidemiological study in Swedish adults, with special reference to primary Sjögren's syndrome. *J Autoimmun* 1989; **2**: 521–7.

Jonsson R, Holmdahl R. Infiltrating mononuclear cells in salivary glands and kidneys in autoimmune MRL/Mp-lpr/lpr mice express IL-2 receptor and produce interferon-γ. *J Oral Pathol* 1990; **19**: 330–4.

Jordan RCK, Diss TC, Lench NJ *et al.* Immunoglobulin gene re-arrangements in lymphoplasmacytic infiltrates of labial salivary glands in Sjögren's syndrome: A possible predictor of lymphoma development. *Oral Surg Oral Med Oral Pathol* 1995; **79**: 723–9.

Jorgensen C, Legouffe MC, Perney P *et al.* Sicca syndrome associated with hepatitis C virus infection. *Arthritis Rheum* 1996; **39**:1166–71.

Kang HI, Fei HM, Saito I *et al.* Comparison of HLA class II genes in Caucasoid Chinese, and Japanese patients with primary Sjögren's syndrome. *J Immunol* 1993; **150**: 3615–23.

Kassan S, Thomas T, Moutsopoulos H *et al.* Increased risk of lymphoma in sicca syndrome. *Ann Intern Med* 1978; **89**: 888–92.

Kausman D, Allen M, Snaith ML *et al.* Autoimmunity and the clinical spectrum of Sjögren's syndrome. In: eds *The Molecular Basis of Autoimmunity: Focus on Sjögren's Syndrome*, Isenberg DA, Horsfall A eds. Bios Publishers, Oxford, 1994; 1–24.

Kerttula TO, Collin P, Polvi A *et al.* Distinct immunologic features of Finnish Sjögren's syndrome patients with HLA alleles DRB1*0301, DQA1*0501, and DQB1*0201. *Arthritis Rheum* 1996; **10**: 1733–9.

Kessler HS. A laboratory model for Sjögren's syndrome. *Am J Pathol* 1968; **52**: 671–8.

Kipps TJ, Tomhave E, Chen PP *et al.* Molecular characterization of a major autoantibody associated cross-reactive idiotype in Sjögren's syndrome and rheumatoid factor associated cross reactive idiotype. *J Immunol* 1989; **142**: 4261–8.

Kohsaka H, Yamamoto K, Fujii H *et al.* Fine epitope mapping of the human SSB/La protein. *J Clin Invest* 1990; **85**: 1566–4.

Kruize AA, Hene RJ, Kallenberg C *et al.* Hydroxychloroquine treatment for primary Sjögren's syndrome: a two year double blind cross over study. *Ann Rheum Dis* 1993; **52**: 360–4.

Kruize AA, Hene RJ, van der Heide A *et al.* Long term follow up of patients with Sjögren's syndrome. *Arthritis Rheum* 1996; **39**: 1166–71.

Kwok W, Thurtle P, Nepom G. A genetically controlled pairing anomaly between HLA-DQα and HLA-DQβ chains. *J Immunol* 1989; **1143**: 3598–601.

Lahdensuo A, Korpela M. Pulmonary findings in patients with Sjögren's syndrome. *Chest* 1995; **108**: 316—9.

Lee LA. Neonatal lupus erythematosus. *J Invest Dermatol* 1993; **100**: 95–135.

Manoussakis MN, Tzioufas AG, Pange PJE *et al.* Serological profiles in subgroups of patients with Sjögren's syndrome. *Scand J Rheum* 1986; **61** (Suppl.): 89–92.

Manthorpe R, Morling N, Platz P *et al.* HLA-D antigen frequencies in Sjögren's syndrome: Differences between the primary and secondary form. *Scand J Rheumatol* 1981; **10**: 124–8.

Mariette X, Agbalika F, Daniel MT *et al.* Detection of human T lymphotropic virus type 1 *tax* gene in salivary gland epithelium from two patients with Sjögren's syndrome. *Arthritis Rheum* 1993; **36**: 1423–8.

Miyagawa S, Dohi K, Shima H *et al.* Absence of HLA-B8 and HLA-DR3 in Japanese patients with Sjögren's syndrome positive for anti-SSA (Ro). *J Rheumatol* 1992; **19**: 1922–44.

Molina R, Provost TT, Arnett FC *et al.* Primary Sjögren's syndrome in men. Clinical, serologic, and immunogenetic features. *Am J Med* 1986; **80**: 23–31.

Montecucco C, Franciotti DM, Coporali R *et al.* Sicca syndrome and anti-Ro antibodies in patients with suspected or definite multiple sclerosis. *Scand J Rheumatol* 1989; **18**: 407–12.

Moriuchi J, Ichikawa Y, Takaya M *et al.* Association between HLA and Sjögren's syndrome in Japanese patients. *Arthritis Rheum* 1986; **29**: 1518–21.

Moutsopoulos HM, Mann DL, Johnson AH *et al.* Genetic differences between primary and secondary sicca syndrome. *N Eng J Med* 1979; **301**: 761–8.

Moutsopoulos HM, Tzioufas AG, Youinou P. Sjögren's syndrome. In: *Oxford Textbook of Rheumatology*, 2nd edn, eds Maddison PJ, Isenberg DA, Woo P, Glass DN. Oxford University Press, Oxford. 1998; 1301–17.

Newkirk MM, Shiroky JB, Johnson N *et al.* Rheumatic disease patients prone to Sjögrens syndrome and/or Lymphoma mount an antibody response to BHRFI, the Epstein Barr viral homologue of bcl-2. *B J Rheumatol* 1996; **35**: 1075–81.

Ogawa N, Dang H, Kong L *et al.* Lymphocyte apoptosis and apoptosis – associated gene expression in Sjögren's syndrome. *Arthritis Rheum* 1996; **39**: 1875–85.

Ohyama Y, Nakamura S, Matsuzaki G *et al.* Cytokine messenger RNA expression in the labial salivary glands of patients with Sjögren's syndrome. *Arthritis Rheum* 1996; **39**: 1376–84.

Pals ST, Radaszkiewicz T, Roozendal L *et al.* Chronic progressive polyarteritis and other symptoms of collagen vascular disease induced by graft-vs-host reaction. *J Immunol* 1985; **134**: 1475–82.

Papasteriades CA, Skopouli FN, Drosos AA *et al.* HLA-alloantigen associations in Greek patients with Sjögren's syndrome. *J Autoimmun* 1988; **1**: 85–90.

Papiris SA, Skopouli FN, Maniati MA *et al.* Brochiolitis in primary Sjögren's syndrome. In: *Sjögren's Syndrome. State of the art*, eds Homma M, Sugai S, Tojo T, Miyakaka N, Akizuki M. Kugher, Amsterdam, 1994; 431–2.

Pavlidis NA, Karsh J, Moutsopoulos HM. The clinical picture of primary Sjögren's syndrome: a retrospective study. *J Rheumatol* 1982; 9: 685–90.

Pokorny G, Sonkondi S, Ivanyi B *et al*. Renal involvement in patients with primary Sjögren's syndrome. *Scand J Rheumatol* 1989; 18: 231–4.

Price EJ, Venables PJW. The etiopathogenesis of Sjögren's syndrome. *Sem Arthritis Rheum* 1995; 25: 117–33.

Reveille JD Macleod MJ, Whittington K *et al*. Specific amino acid residues in the second hypervariable region of HLA-DQB1 chain genes promote the Ro (SS-A)/La (SS-B) autoantibody responses. *J Immunol* 1991; 146: 3871–6.

Ricchiuti V, Isenberg D, Muller S. HLA association of anti-Ro60 and anti-Ro52 antibodies in Sjögren's syndrome. *J Autoimmun* 1994a; 7: 611–21.

Ricchiuti V, Briand JP, Meyer O *et al*. Epitope mapping with synthetic peptides of 52 kDa SSA/Ro protein reveals heterogeneous antibody profiles in human autoimmune sera. *Clin Exp Immunol* 1994b; 95: 397–407.

Roitberg-Tambur A, Brautbar C, Markitzui A *et al*. Immunogenetics of HLA class II genes in primary Sjögren's syndrome in Israeli Jewish patients. *Isr J Med Sci* 1990; 26: 677–81.

Roitberg-Tambur A, Friedmann A, Safirman C *et al*. Molecular analysis of HLA class II genes in primary Sjögrens syndrome. *Human Immunol* 1993; 36: 235–42.

Rose LM, Latchman DS, Isenberg DA. Bcl-2 expression is unaltered in unfractionated peripheral blood mononuclear cells in patients with systemic lupus erythematosus. *Br J Rheumatol* 1995; 34: 316–20.

Scofield RH, Harley JB. Autoantigenicity of Ro/SSA antigen is related to a nucleocapsid protein of vesicular stomatitis virus. *Proc Natl Acad Sci USA* 1991; 88: 3343–7.

Sharaway M, White SC. Morphometric and fine structural study of experimental autoallergic sialadenitis of rat submandibular glands. *Virch Arch (Cell Pathol)* 1978; 28: 255–73.

Sheikh SH, Shaw-Stiffel TA. The gastrointestinal manifestations of Sjögren's syndrome. *Am J Gastroenterol* 1995; 90: 9–14.

Shiozawa S, Morimoto I, Tanaka Y *et al*. A preliminary study on interferon alpha for xerostomia of Sjögren's syndrome. *Br J Rheumatol* 1993; 32: 52–4.

Shull MM, Ormsby I, Kier AB *et al*. Targeted disruption of the mouse transforming growth factor-β1 gene results in multifocal inflammatory disease. *Nature* 1992; 359: 693–9.

Speight PM, Cruchley A, Williams DM. Quantification of plasma cells in labial salivary glands: increased expression of IgM in Sjögren's syndrome. *J Oral Pathol Med* 1990; 19: 126–30.

St Clair EW. Anti-La antibody production by MRL-lpr/lpr mice. Analysis of fine specificity. *J Immunol* 1991; 146: 1885–92.

Sumida T, Yonaha F, Maeda T *et al*. T-cell receptor repertoire of infiltrating T-cells in lips of Sjögren's syndrome patients. *J Clin Invest* 1992; 89: 681–5.

Takeda Y, Ishikawa G. Experimental autoallergic sialadenitis in mice. Histopathological and ultrastructural studies. *Virchows Arch (Pathol Anat)* 1983; 400: 143–54.

Talal N. Sjögren's syndrome, lymphoproliferation and renal tubular acidosis. *Ann Intern Med* 1971; 74: 633–4.

Tzioufas AG, Boumba DS, Skopouli FN *et al*. Mixed monoclonal cryoglobulinaemia and monoclonal rheumatoid factor cross-reactive idiotypes as predictive factors for the development of lymphoma in primary Sjögren's syndrome. *Arthritis Rheum* 1996; 39: 767–72.

van der Reijden W, van der Kwaak H, Vissink A *et al*. Treatment of xerostomia with polymer based saliva substitutes in patients with Sjögren's syndrome. *Arthritis Rheum* 1996; 39: 57–63.

Venables PJW, Rigby S, Memford PA *et al*. Autoimmunity to La (SS-B) in vitro is related to HLA-DR3 in healthy subjects. *Ann Rheum Dis* 1988; 47: 22–7.

Venables PJW, Brookes SM, Price EJ. Viruses in the initiation and perpetuation of autoimmunity of Sjögren's syndrome. In: *Autoimmune Diseases: Focus on Sjögren's Syndrome*, edsIsenberg D , Horsfall A. Bios Scientific Publishers Ltd, Oxford, 1994; 177–88.

Vitali C, Tavoni A, Rizzo G *et al*. HLA antigens in Italian patients with primary Sjögren's syndrome. *Ann Rheum Dis* 1986; 45: 412–16.

Vitali C, Tavoni A, Sciuto M *et al*. Renal involvement in primary Sjögren's syndrome: retrospective-prospective study. *Scand J Rheumatol* 1991; 20: 132–6.

Vitali C, Bombardieri S, Moutsopoulos HM *et al*. Preliminary criteria for the classification of Sjögren's syndrome: results of a prospective concerted action supported by the European Community. *Arthritis Rheum* 1993; 36: 340–7.

Vitali C, Bombardieri S, Moutsopoulos H *et al*. Assessment of the European classification criteria for Sjögren's syndrome in a series of clinically defined cases: results of a prospective multicentre study. *Ann Rheum Dis* 1996; 55: 116–21.

Vretham M, Lindvall B, Holgrem H *et al*. Neuropathy and myopathy in primary Sjögren's syndrome: neurophysiological, neurological and muscle biopsy results. *Acta Neurol Scand* 1990; 82: 126–31.

Wahren M, Solomin L, Pettersson I *et al*. Autoantibody repertoire to Ro/SSA and La/SSB antigens in patients with primary and secondary Sjögren's syndrome. *J Autoimmun* 1996; 9: 537–44.

Whaley K, MacSween RNM. Experimental induction of immune sialadenitis in guinea-pigs using different adjuvants. *Clin Exp Immunol* 1974; 17: 681–4.

White SC. T-cell dependence of experimental autoallergic lesions of rat submandibular glands. *J Dent Res* 1976; 55: B299.

White SC, Casarett GW. Induction of experimental autoallergic sialadenitis. *J Immunol* 1974; 112: 178–85.

Wilson RW, Provost TT, Bias WB *et al*. Sjögren's syndrome. Influence of multiple HLA-D region alloantigens on clinical and serologic expression. *Arthritis Rheum* 1984; 27: 1245–53.

Youinou P, Pennec YL, Katsikis P *et al*. Raynaud's phenomenon in primary Sjögren's syndrome. *Br J Rheumatol* 1990; 29: 205–7.

Zeuner RA, Schroeder JO, Schroder F *et al*. Successful application of high dose intravenous immunoglobulins in Sjögren's syndrome associated arthritis. (letter). *Ann Rheum Dis* 1995; 54: 936.

Zhang W, Reichlin M. Some autoantibodies to Ro/SS-A and La/SS-B are anti-idiotypes to anti-double-stranded DNA. *Arthritis Rheum* 1996; 39: 522–31.

Zumla A, Mathur M, Stewart J *et al*. T cell receptor expression in Sjögren's syndrome. *Ann Rheum Dis* 1991; 50: 691–3.

7 | *Polymyositis*

Introduction

Autoimmune myositis is divided into two major forms, polymyositis and dermatomyositis. Both cause weakness of the proximal muscles but only the latter is associated with a vasculitic skin rash. The general acceptance of diagnostic criteria by Bohan and Peter (1975) has greatly facilitated the assessment of these conditions which are also associated with a variety of disease-specific autoantibodies.

Milestones in the history of myositis

1863   Wagner reported an acute generalized muscular 'affection' with skin involvement — the patient died within six days.

1887–1891   Hepp and Unverricht (from Germany) and Jackson (USA) described cases with more chronic muscle weakness with/without skin involvement. Unverricht used the term dermatomyositis, stressed the proximal muscle involvement, and reported spontaneous recovery in one case.

1899–1903   Oppenheim described ocular and cardiac muscle involvement. Gowers coined the term polymyositis. Steiner described 28 cases from the literature, including childhood onset; 17 had died.

1916   First link between cancer and polymyositis described by Stertz.

1939   Scheurmann estimated that 239 cases had been described in the literature.

1950s/1960s   Corticosteroids introduced for therapy, as reviewed by Pearson (1963).

1958   Walton and Adams attempted the first clinical classification.

1966   Banker and Victor showed that childhood dermatomyositis is probably a distinct entity.

1975   Bohan and Peter described another classification now widely accepted.

1980   First description by Nishikai and Reichlin of an antibody, anti-Jo-1, with disease specificity.

1983   Jo-1 antigen identified by Mathews and Bernstein as tRNA–histidyl synthetase.

The clinical picture

Classification

There are three major forms of myositis:

- polymyositis, a condition limited to involvement of the muscles and which usually responds to immunosuppressive therapy;
- dermatomyositis consisting of cutaneous and muscular manifestations; and
- inclusion body myositis, which is associated with a characteristic histological appearance and poor response to immunosuppressive therapy.

Table 7.1   Comparison of adult-onset forms of myositis

	Polymyositis	Dermatomyositis	Inclusion body myositis
Female:male ratio	$\simeq 2:1$	$\simeq 3.1$	$\simeq 1:3$
Age of onset	40–60	40–60	50–70
Main site of weakness	Proximal muscles, symmetrical	Proximal muscles, symmetrical	Proximal/distal, asymmetrical
Myalgia	$\simeq 50\%$	$\simeq 50\%$	Rare
Dysphagia	10–30%	10–30%	Rare
Overall association with cancer	Yes Odds ratio $\simeq 2$	Yes Odds ratio $\simeq 4$	No
Response to immunosuppressives	Some response usual	Some response usual	Very little
Fibre necrosis	+	+	+
Perifascicular atrophy	–/+	++	–
Ig/C' deposition	+	++	–
Inclusion bodies	–	–	++

A comparison of these three major types is shown in Table 7.1.

Although various classification schemes have been suggested over the years, some controversy remains, notably whether childhood dermatomyositis and dermatomyositis associated with neoplasia represent distinct entities. We advocate the use of the classification scheme outlined in Table 7.2. It should be recognized that when myositis is associated with another autoimmune rheumatic disease the full criteria for this concomitant condition may not be met.

General features

The incidence of polymyositis has been reported as 0.5 cases per 100 000 (Medsger *et al.* 1970) with a prevalence of 8 per 100 000 (DeVere and Bradley 1975). In the former study, from Tennessee, it was noted that black females were much more likely to develop the disease than any other group. This may simply reflect the increased incidence of SLE in the same population. The latter study, from Newcastle, UK, a female/male preponderance of nearly 3:1 was noted especially where there were co-existent features of another 'collagen-vascular disease'. However, in patients with an accompanying neoplasm the incidence was greater in males, by about 2:1. Acute presentations are recognized. These patients usually give a history of a few weeks of intense pain and tenderness in the proximal and trunk muscles. Gross subcutaneous oedema may occur with involvement of the bulbar muscles. Fibre necrosis leading to raised myoglobin levels in the serum and myoglobinuria has been described (Kagan 1971).

Myositis more commonly presents in an insidious fashion with weakness and wasting developing over weeks, months, or even years. Muscle pain and tenderness are found in less than 50% of patients, and pharyngeal weakness in about 20%. The proximal muscles of the lower limbs are usually the first to be affected. This causes difficulty in climbing stairs and rising from a chair. Subsequently, weakness of the upper limb proximal muscles becomes evident, with difficulty in combing the hair or reaching to take down an item from a high shelf.

Clinical assessment of muscle power is a relatively crude way of determining the degree of muscle weakness. Several attempts have been made to devise instruments capable of providing a more objective and reliable method of measuring muscle power. These

Table 7.2   Suggested classification scheme for patients with myositis

Adult-onset idiopathic polymyositis
Adult-onset idiopathic dermatomyositis
Myositis associated with another autoimmune rheumatic disease
Myositis associated with a neoplasm
Childhood-onset dermatomyositis
Inclusion body myositis

include the use of an adapted chair with an ankle strap and a recording device placed over the quadriceps which measures the power generated by the muscle as it extends against the restraining strap (see Fig. 7.1a). A recent and more sophisticated device (Fig. 7.1b,c) allows the testing of several different muscles and is easily transportable (Stoll *et al.* 1995). Certainly, an instrument of this type greatly facilitates assessing the response of the patients' muscle strength to drug therapy.

The tendon reflexes are preserved until late on in the disease (a useful distinguishing feature from muscular dystrophies) and muscle wasting is often surprisingly slight. However, of major significance as far as immediate prognosis is concerned is the fact that the respiratory muscles may be involved in the acutely presenting cases. Serial assessment of lung function may thus be mandatory.

The characteristic skin involvement in patients with dermatomyositis is a lilac discoloration of the eyelids (heliotrope rash) which may extend to involve much of the face (Fig. 7.2) and a patchy oedematous rash over the dorsum of hands and proximal interphalangeal joints, sometimes extending up the forearm. Less frequently the rash may involve the anterior surface of the neck, thorax, shoulders, and neckline. It may be photo-

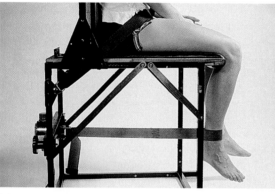

(a)

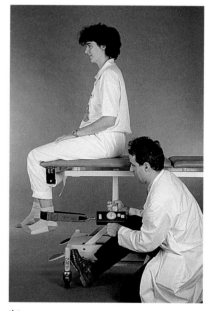

(b)

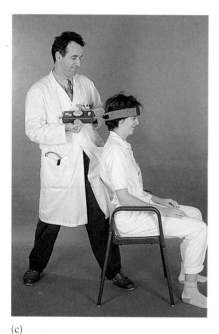

(c)

Fig. 7.1. (a) Testing for muscle strength. The subject is seated on an adapted chair (a muscle power recording device, not shown, placed over the quadriceps) to ascertain the power generated by the muscles as the patient is asked to extend his knee as hard as possible against the restraining strap around the ankle. (Courtesy of Professor D. Newham.) (b) A mobile myometer records quadriceps strength employing a similar principle of forced knee extension against a restraining strap around the ankle, which in this method is attached directly to the recording device. (Courtesy of Dr T. Stoll.) (c) The advantage of this device is that it may be used to record the muscle strength of a variety of muscles, in this case the neck flexors. (Courtesy of Dr T. Stoll.)

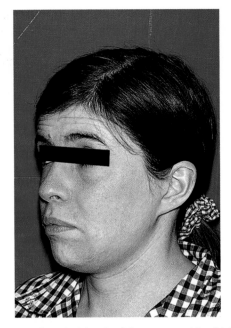

Fig. 7.2. Striking facial rash of dermatomyositis which characteristically spares the area around the lips.

sensitive and is sometimes accompanied by telangiectasia and a fine desquamation (flaking off). In some patients the rash over the hands and forearms appears to consist of discrete papules (papules of Gottron) which are elevated erythematous areas that may subside with treatment but often 'linger on'. There may be hyperaemia round the nails, with some tenderness when the surface of the nail is pressed.

The major features of myositis and some of its complications are shown in Fig. 7.3.

Systemic features

Joint manifestations

Perhaps as many as half of the patients presenting with either idiopathic polymyositis or dermatomyositis suffer from arthralgias (and less frequently true arthritis) affecting the wrists, fingers, shoulders, and knees. This usually settles within a few weeks and does not leave permanent sequelae. Clearly, when the disease co-exists with rheumatoid arthritis or lupus, the joint disease may be far more serious.

Cardiac features

Although clinically overt heart disease is rare, its manifestations include myocarditis, palpitations, pericardial effusions, congestive heart failure, and the consequences of arrhythmias (Love *et al.* 1991; Tami and Bhasin 1993). However, laboratory investigations suggest that the heart muscle may be involved in up to 40% of patients (Taylor *et al.* 1993). Isolated changes on the electrocardiogram are relatively common. More sophisticated investigations, including echocardiography and thallium isotope scanning, confirm that cardiac abnormalities are present in many patients with myositis. Rarely, an endomyocardial biopsy is required to determine whether true myocarditis is present, which may require increasing immuno-suppressive therapy.

Pulmonary manifestations

As with cardiac disease, pulmonary involvement is far more evident on investigation than it is clinically overt. Major respiratory muscle weakness occurs in less than 10% of patients with myositis (Dickey and Myers 1984). Even less frequently, spontaneous pneumo-mediastinum (air in the chest) may occur (Matsuda *et al.* 1993). As indicated later in this chapter, some patients with the anti-Jo-1 antibody have a combination of pulmonary fibrosis and myositis (Love *et al.* 1991).

Radiologically diffuse interstitial fibrosis is recognized and, much more rarely, an inhalation pneumonitis subsequent to inflammation of the pharyngeal and oesophageal muscles can occur. Histologically, Tazelaar *et al.* (1990) reported a variety of lung conditions in patients with myositis, including bronchiolitis obliterans, interstitial pneumonitis, diffuse alveolar damage, and cellular interstitial pneumonia. Of these forms patients with bronchiolitis obliterans had the best outcome (Wells and duBois 1993).

Other systemic manifestations

Involvement of the gastrointestinal tract is observed occasionally but is more common in children (see later in this chapter). Dysphagia is the most common of these symptoms, although abdominal discomfort and malabsorption are recognized rarely. The central and peripheral nervous systems are likewise very rarely involved, though occasionally areflexia has been recorded. Renal disease in the absence of an additional

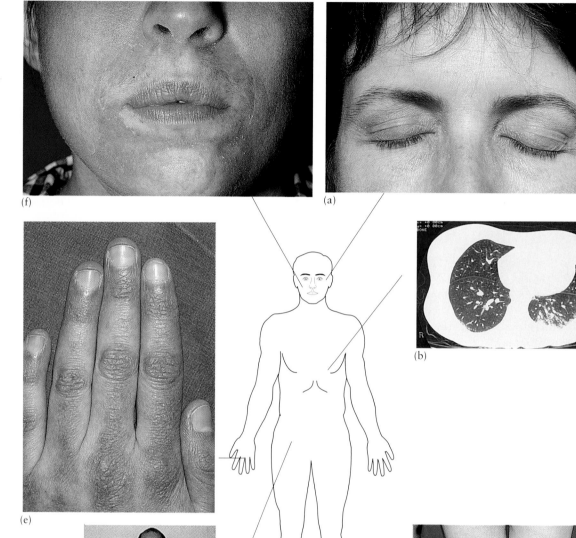

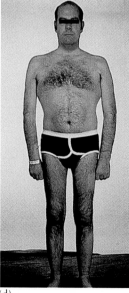

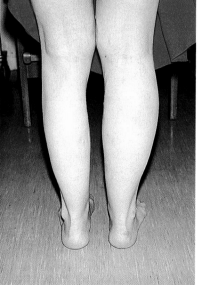

Fig. 7.3. Major clinical features of polymyositis. (a) Heliotrope rash. (b) Fibrosing alveolitis shown on a CT scan complicating a patients with dermatomyositis. (c) Distal, unilateral gastrocnemius muscle wasting (uncommon). (d) Striking proximal weakness of arms and legs. (e) Gottron's papules. (f) Perioral sparing of the facial rash in a patient with dermatomyositis.

autoimmune disease is rare, though a relatively non-specific form of glomerulonephritis is seen occasionally.

Myositis and cancer

Estimates of the frequency of this association have ranged from 15 to 71%, the latter figure is ascribed generally to Shy (1962) who described a 71% rate of cancer in men over 50 with late-onset myopathy. From the data provided, however, it was not clear how many of these patients really had dermatomyositis. Most authors who have reviewed this connection (e.g. Callen 1994) have concluded that dermatomyositis rather than polymyositis represents an increased risk of malignancy and generally that risk is greatest over the age of 50. In a particularly careful study performed in Sweden by Sigurgeirsson *et al.* (1992), 788 patients with dermatomyositis or polymyositis diagnosed from 1963 to 1983 were followed. The relative risk of cancer in the patients with dermatomyositis was 2.4 in males and 3.4 in females, with figures of 1.8 and 1.7 in patients with polymyositis, respectively. In patients with dermatomyositis there was also a higher rate of mortality from cancer. Of particular note was the link between cancer of the ovary with dermatomyositis. It is, however, questionable how intensively a search for a tumour should be carried out on patients with myositis. The problem is further discussed in the section on Treatment.

Dermatomyositis and children

In the UK an incidence of 1.9 per million children under the age of 16 has been reported (Symmons *et al.* 1995). The female:male ratio was 5:1. A similar predominance was found in China (Wang *et al.* 1993) whereas in Japan Hiketa *et al.* (1992) reported a ratio of 3:1 of girls to boys. It is uniformly agreed that dermatomyositis is considerably more common (up to 20 times) than polymyositis in children and that malignancy is, in essence, not a feature of childhood-onset disease.

In children with this condition the skin rashes are often particularly prominent and, unlike adult cases, calcinosis is well recognized and, once it has developed, difficult to treat (Fig. 7.4 and 7.5). However, Callan *et al.* (1994) reported that none of 20 children with dermatomyositis, who had been treated aggressively early in the course of their disease, had developed calcinosis.

Myalgia is a more striking feature in patients with juvenile dermatomyositis, and Gower's sign is well

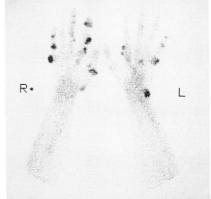

Fig. 7.4. Severe calcinosis shown radiologically in the hands of an adolescent with dermatomyositis.

recognized (the use of the hands on the knees to push up the body in an attempt to stand). Weakness of the neck flexor muscles is a sensitive indicator of muscle impairment.

Gastrointestinal involvement is well recognized in children in whom swallowing, especially of liquids, may be problematic. Oesophageal reflux is another common problem that results in aspiration pneumonia if care is not taken. Vascular involvement may affect any part of the gastrointestinal tract leading to weight loss and mucosal ulceration with potentially life-threatening perforation on occasion. Furthermore, in young children, speech pattern development may be disturbed causing further management problems. As in adults, cardiovascular and respiratory problems are far

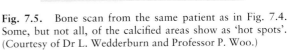

Fig. 7.5. Bone scan from the same patient as in Fig. 7.4. Some, but not all, of the calcified areas show as 'hot spots'. (Courtesy of Dr L. Wedderburn and Professor P. Woo.)

more commonly reported following investigation than are recognized by clinical complaint.

In children, a common persistent finding is thrombosis of dilated vessels of the margin of the upper eyelid. In active disease, retinal changes, including cotton wool spots and/or transient exudates, may be recognized after the occlusion of small blood vessels. Although more than 60% of children with dermatomyositis have anti-nuclear antibodies, hardly any have anti-synthetase antibodies (unlike their adult counterparts, see later). Approximately half of these patients have evidence of endothelial cell damage (Pachman 1995).

Myositis and pregnancy

As myositis is a rare disease it is not surprising that there are few reports of the effects of pregnancy. In the studies of Oddis and Hill (1993) and Ishii *et al.* (1991) it is evident that when a patient with myositis is under reasonable control at the time she becomes pregnant the disease is not more likely to flare during the pregnancy. Corticosteroids are safe to use during pregnancy and azathioprine can be used if necessary. Other immunosuppressive drugs, including methotrexate and cyclophosphamide (see Treatment section) should not be used and should probably be stopped approximately three months before conception. Some patients have been identified whose myositis appears to develop during pregnancy. These patients often have more severe disease, and relatively poor fetal outcome (Ishii *et al.* 1991; Satoh *et al.* 1994).

Laboratory investigations

Serology

The most important enzyme and other muscle factor-associated investigations are shown in Table 7.3. Of these, serum creatine kinase is the most widely available and the most useful. Over 80% of patients with myositis have an elevated CK level at the time of presentation, the levels often rising to between 10 and 50 times the upper limit of normal before the disease is brought under control. The CK level also provides a useful objective assessment of disease activity and is the most widely used serial laboratory measure.

In some patients, unexpectedly, the CK levels are low in the presence of what, clinically, appears to be active disease. Possible causes for this are shown in Table 7.4. Of the various factors mentioned in this table, it is probably true to say that the 'unexplained cause' is the most frequent! An older view that a low CK was a feature of myositis complicating another autoimmune rheumatic disease has been challenged recently. Garton and Isenberg (1997) reviewed their patients with

Table 7.4   Cases of low CK levels in patients with active myositis

Circulating inhibitor
Concurrent autoimmune rheumatic diseases — questionable
Steroid treatment without clinical disease suppression
Advanced disease with significant muscle atrophy
Unexplained (!)

Table 7.3   Enzyme and other muscle-associated factor investigations in patients with suspected myositis

Source	Enzyme/factor	Comment
Serum Enzymes	Creatine kinase (CK)	The most useful, raised in > 80% of patients, good correlation with activity.
	CK–MB isoenzyme	Initially thought to be associated with cardiac involvement but not confirmed.
	Aldolase	May be raised in patients with normal CK.
	Carbonic anhydrase III	Rarely measured but is found exclusively in skeletal muscle.
	Lactate dehydrogenase (LDH)	Often elevated.
	Aspartate trasnsaminase (AST)	Often elevated and reflects disease activity.
Other muscle	Myoglobin	Confined to skeletal and cardiac muscle; associated raised levels are a useful marker of disease factors activity but not widely available.
	Creatine	Its urinary excretion is raised in myositis, but not a good marker of disease activity.
	Measures of muscle mass	Include 24 h urinary creatinine, 3-methyl histidine. Total body potassium — of interest but not in clinical practice.

'primary' myositis and compared them with their lupus patients with myositis. No major differences were evident with respect to the CK levels.

The CK may be raised for reasons other than myositis. These include excessive physical exertion (after running a marathon, the creatine kinase may well be in excess of 50 000 iu/l for several days), other muscle diseases including muscular dystrophy, rhabdomyolysis (a non-immune form of severe degenerative muscle disease), and myocardial infarction. Various endocrine and metabolic disorders (including hyperthyroidism and diabetes) and various drugs (including colchicine, chloroquine, lovistatin, clofibrate, cyclosporin, and vincristine) can cause an elevation in the CK level. Finally, there is good evidence that the normal range for CK varies between ethnic groups. The average CK is thus higher in healthy black men and women (Worrall *et al.* 1990).

Various other enzymes may also be elevated in the presence of myositis (see Table 7.3). Of these the aldolase is perhaps the most useful, since it may be raised in patients with myositis who have a normal CK. Certain enzymes generally regarded as liver function tests, including the aspartate transaminase, are often elevated in patients with myositis.

Among other muscle-associated factors, levels of myoglobin, not normally present in serum or urine, are invariably raised in patients with myositis and can be a useful marker of disease activity. Myoglobin is a haem protein with a single polypeptide chain of molecular weight 17 kDa. Unfortunately, assays for measuring this protein are not widely available. Likewise, although other muscle-related factors, including twenty-four-hour urinary creatinine, 3-methyl histidine excretion, and total body potassium, while of potential value, are little used in clinical practice.

A wide variety of autoantibodies (see Table 7.5) have been identified in patients with myositis (Miller 1993). Anti-nuclear antibodies are present in over 80% of these patients by immunofluorescence. The specific targets of these anti-nuclear antibodies are increasingly well defined. For reasons that remain obscure, a particular target for these antibodies are the synthetase enzymes that link a specific amino acid to its cognate tRNA. Of these anti-synthetase antibodies, anti-Jo-1 (the target is histidyl tRNA–synthetase) is the antibody most frequently identified. The importance of this observation is that, as reported by Marguerie *et al.* (1990) and Love *et al.* (1991), particular clinical features are associated with anti-Jo-1 antibodies (and the other anti-synthetase antibodies). Thus, over 60% of patients with this antibody have a combination of Raynaud's phenomenon, fever, interstitial lung disease, arthralgia, and arthritis, as well as myositis. In addition these patients tend to be HLA-DR3-positive and about 40% have a dermatomyositis rash.

Among other non-specific tests, total immunoglobulins may be raised in about 30% of patients and the erythrocyte sedimentation rate (ESR) in about 40%, but this correlates poorly with disease activity. Complement levels are usually normal in these patients and rheumatoid factor is found in about 15% of them.

Electromyography

Over 85% of patients with active myositis have electromyography (EMG) abnormalities. These abnormalities are principally increased insertional activity, myopathic motor unit action potentials, a myopathic recruitment pattern with increased spontaneous activity but normal nerve conduction, and no fasciculations or myotonic discharges. It is very important to remember that these changes are not specific for myositis, but are helpful in demonstrating the absence of a neuropathy or certain types of myopathy (e.g. myotonic dystrophy).

The myopathic potentials seen in patients with myositis are generally of low amplitude and short duration, with increased polyphasic potential. In certain specialized units, it is possible to undertake single-fibre EMG which is reported to show increased jitter.

Imaging

Technetium-99m (Fig. 7.6) and thallium scans demonstrate increased uptake in muscles affected by active inflammation. While non-specific they can act as a useful guide for determining which muscle to biopsy.

CT scanning has been used to identify inflamed or damaged muscles for over 10 years and may provide a useful guide to the extent of the muscle damage (Fig. 7.7). However, the amount of radiation required for extensive muscle scanning or serial scanning is regarded as a limiting factor. In contrast, magnetic resonance imaging (MRI) has become more popular since no radiation is involved. It is very useful for distinguishing areas of muscle inflammation and fibrous or fatty replacement (Fig. 7.8). T_2-weighted images are optimal for determining those muscles with active inflammation, and have been used to confirm the clinical impression that myositis is often focal even within the same muscle (Fleckenstein and Reimers 1996).

Table 7.5   Autoantibodies and myositis

Antibody	Target	% of all PM/DM	Comment
Anti-Jo-1	Histidyl–tRNA	15–20	Associated with joint/lung/Raynaud's
Anti-PL-7	Threonyl–tRNA	< 3	"
Anti-PL-12	Alanyl–tRNA	< 3	"
Anti-OJ	Isoleucyl–tRNA	< 2	"
Anti-E2	Glycyl–tRNA	< 2	"
Anti-signal recognition Particle	Signal recognition Particle	≃ 4	Found in PM
Anti-kJ	Unidentified translation factor	1	
Anti-Fer	Elongation factor-1a, (translation factor)	1	
Anti-Mi-2	A nuclear protein complex	8	Found in children with DM
Anti-PM-Scl	A nucleolar protein complex	8	
Anti-56 kDa	56 kDa ribonuclear protein	≃ 85%	Found in all subgroups — not yet in clinical usage
Anti-Ro	52/60 kDa RNA protein	< 10	"
Anti-La	48 kDa RNA protein	< 5	Found myositis overlap syndrome
Anti-U1 RNP	U1 sn RNP	≃ 10	"
Anti-U2 RNP	U2 sn RNP	< 2	"
Anti-Ku	DNA-binding protein dimer	< 2	"

Anti-nuclear antibodies (ANA) = ≃ 80% positive by immunofluorescence. PM = polymyositis; DM = dermamyositis
For further details see Arad-Dann et al. 1987; Marguerie et al. 1990; 1992; Oddis et al. 1992; Targoff 1998.

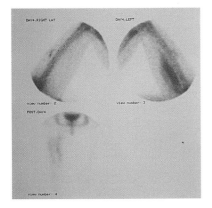

Fig. 7.6. Technetium scan showing increased uptake in muscles affected by active inflammation.

This form of imaging can be used repeatedly to help determine response, or lack of it, to therapy. Its major drawback is its cost.

Biopsy

Even in patients who provide a typical history of myositis with a raised creatine kinase and abnormal EMG or MRI scans, it remains most important to confirm the clinical suspicion by undertaking a muscle biopsy. This should be done because the diagnosis may have to be revised in the light of the biopsy findings. Thus, patients with sporadic forms of muscular dystrophy may be very difficult to distinguish from those with myositis, but the presence of muscle fibre hypertrophy is an essential clue in the diagnosis of dystrophy.

Traditionally, muscle biopsy has been undertaken by the surgical or 'open' technique. A relatively long,

5–10 cm, incision is used, which has the advantage of allowing a relatively large specimen to be obtained, but the disadvantage of creating an unsightly scar with the risks, admittedly minor, of bruising and infection. The alternative technique uses a needle (Fig. 7.9a) or conchotome (Fig. 7.9b) biopsy. This requires a much smaller incision (approximately 1 cm) with fewer side-effects (Edwards *et al.* 1983; Dietrichson *et al.* 1987; Ehrenstein *et al.* 1992). Although individual biopsy specimens are smaller, through the same incision, multiple specimens can be taken at different angles and may thus provide tissue from a larger portion of an individual muscle than is usually obtained by open biopsy. After a few months it is often difficult to determine the site of the incision and this has encouraged patients to permit sequential biopsies. We are aware of one patient who has undergone seven biopsies in the course of her well-documented myositis! (Edwards *et al.* 1979). It is generally regarded as optimal to obtain biopsy material from a muscle that is obviously involved but not atrophied. Technically, it is far more difficult to undertake a needle biopsy from an atrophied muscle and on some patients it is actually impossible to do so. For these patients an open biopsy will be required. In practice, the quadriceps is the muscle most often biopsied, though the more experienced operator can also obtain samples from the calf or deltoid muscles.

The major features of the changes seen on biopsy in patients with myositis are shown in Table 7.6 and Figs 7.10 and 7.11. In essence, a combination of mononuclear cell infiltrates (mainly lymphocytes, but also macrophages, plasma cells, eosinophils, and neutrophils) are present, particularly in the endomysial area round the muscle fibres (in polymyositis) or around the

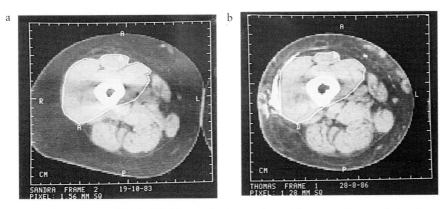

Fig. 7.7.(a) and (b) Serial CT scanning in a patient with progressive muscle wasting.

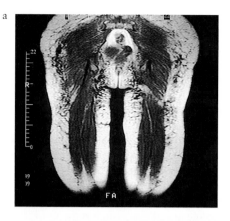

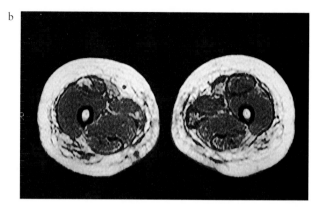

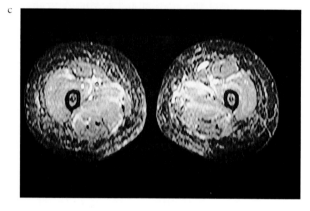

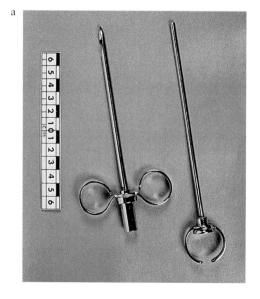

Fig. 7.8. MRI scans from a 42-year-old female with dermatomyositis. The cross-sectional images show (a) coronal, (b) TI, and (c) STIR (short tau invasion recovery sequence, a fat-suppressive technique) views. The STIR image shows increased signal of the muscles in a myofascial distribution, as well as of the skin and subcutaneous tissues. The coronal image shows patchy increased signal of the glutei. The increased signal is due to oedema, presumably caused by inflammation and/or necrosis. The calcinosis is dark on the TI and STIR images. (Courtesy of Dr E. Adams and Dr P. Plotz.)

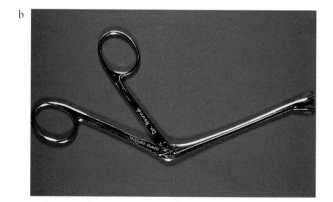

Fig. 7.9. (a) Muscle biopsy needle. (b) Muscle biopsy conchotome.

Table 7.6 Biopsy findings in patients with myositis

Finding	Comment
In polymyositis	
Mononuclear cell infiltrate	Mostly lymphocytes and generally in the endomysial areas
Muscle fibre necrosis	
Muscle fibre phagocytosis	Fibres are invaded by the mononuclear cells
Muscle fibre regeneration	
Internalized nuclei	
In dermatomyositis	
Mononuclear cell infiltrate	Principally around the fascicles and blood vessels
Vasculopathy	Endothelial cell injury (neurosis and capillary thrombosis) with swelling, hyperplasia, vacuolization, and degeneration
In 'end-stage' disease	
Muscle fibre atrophy, fibrosis and fatty replacement	These features may be present to a lesser degree earlier in the disease

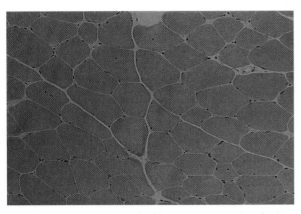

Fig. 7.10. Normal muscle biopsy; cross-sectional view showing roughly hexagonal cells with peripheral nuclei.

fascicles and blood vessels (in dermatomyositis). These features are associated with muscle fibre necrosis, phagocytosis, and often some degree of regeneration. The last of these features is associated with sarcoplasmic basophilia, internalized nuclei, and prominent nucleoli. As the disease progresses, there is increasing evidence of muscle fibre atrophy, fibrosis, and replacement by fat. The main lesion in patients with dermatomyositis is focused on the small blood vessels, with evidence of endothelial cell injury, including necrosis and capillary thrombosis, and subsequently there is a loss of capillaries, resulting in decreased capillary density.

In patients with dermatomyositis, biopsies of lesional skin are often undertaken and these generally show a

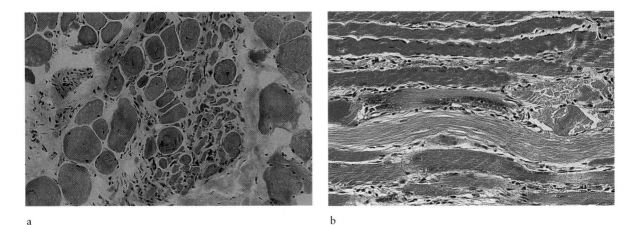

a   b

Fig. 7.11. (a) Cross-sectional muscle biopsy, from a patient with severe myositis showing fibre necrosis, fibre phagocytosis, increase in fibrous tissue and fatty replacement of muscle fibres. (b) Longitudinal view of a biopsy from a patient with myositis showing an attempt at muscle fibre regeneration (central fibre).

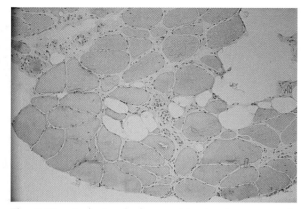

Fig. 7.12. Inclusion body myositis showing a vacuole rimmed by basophilic material.

Patients with inclusion body myositis are characterized histologically by vacuoles rimmed by basophilic material (Fig. 7.12), which have been reported to contain a variety of inclusions, notably amyloid substance, beta amyloid precursor, ubiquitin, Tau protein, apolipoprotein E, and prions (reviewed by Serratrice 1996). However, these changes are not specific for inclusion body myositis. They have, for example, been reported in autosomal recessive familial distal dystrophy. Thus, the diagnosis rests upon the clinical history (an insidious myopathy, involving both proximal and distal muscles, often somewhat asymmetrical prominent quadriceps weakness, loss of knee reflexes within 5 years of onset, and frequent dysphagia) and the histological appearance (Askanas *et al.* 1994; Calabrese and Chou 1994). As well as the vacuoles and inclusions the more typical features of an inflammatory myopathy are also present, especially in the early phase of the disease.

modest mononuclear cell infiltrate at the dermal/epidermal junction in the upper dermis. The basement membrane may be thickened, and oedema and increased mucins seen in the upper dermis. There may be vacuolar change at the basal layer, and the appearance as a whole may be difficult to distinguish from that seen in patients with SLE. However, lupus patients invariably have significant deposition of immunoglobulins and complement at the dermal–epidermal junction of both lesional and non-lesional skin. Such deposition is typically absent in non-lesional tissue biopsies from patients with myositis.

Differential diagnosis

A wide variety of conditions may present with muscle weakness, raised creatine kinase levels, EMG abnormalities, or biopsy changes of inflammation. These are indicated in Table 7.7. In recent times the infectious myopathies resulting from viral infections have attracted a great deal of attention. Viral infection may

Table 7.7 Differential diagnosis of myositis

Infectious	Viruses	HIV, HTLV-1, enteroviruses adenoviruses, hepatitis, herpes
	Bacteria	*Staphylococcus aureus*, Lyme disease
	Parasites	Toxoplasmosis, trichinosis, trypanosomiasis
Granulomatous	Sarcoidosis	
	Crohn's disease	
Eosinophilic myositis		May be relapsing or not, focal or diffuse
Focal myositis		Usually presents as single, painful swelling in the legs
Orbital myositis		
Muscular dystrophies		May be very difficult to distinguish in the early stages, not least because some forms, especially facioscapulohumeral (FSH) dystrophy may have an inflammatory component on biopsy
Mitochondrial myopathy		The appearance of 'ragged red fibres' (subsarcolemmal accumulation of abnormal mitochondria) provides the clue
Metabolic myopathy		Rare, generally genetic defects of glycogen or glucose metabolism
Drug-induced myopathy		Best examples are D-Penicillamine, cimetidine, L-tryptophan, zidovudine, and note steroid-induced myopathy.

cause clinical features and abnormal serology that mimic a variety of autoimmune diseases (reviewed in Morrow *et al.* 1991). Thus, HIV-induced myopathy may closely resemble autoimmune myositis, although a rash typical of dermatomyositis is uncommon. Similarly, human T cell lymphotrophic virus type-1 (HTLV-1) has been identified in particular endemic areas as a cause of myositis. Thus, Morgan *et al.* (1989) found antibodies to HTLV-1 in 13 patients. The clinical symptoms of this disease were similar to idiopathic myositis, clinically, serologically, and histopathologically. In contrast, Smadja *et al.* (1995) emphasized that in seven patients with an inflammatory myopathy and HTLV-1 antibodies, the biopsy findings often showed neurogenic changes and there was a poor response to corticosteroids. This virus should therefore be sought where appropriate. Hepatitis B or C, enteroviruses (including Coxsackie viruses) influenza, and herpesvirus can all cause acute myositic symptoms.

Among bacteria, *Staphylococcus aureus* remains supreme as a cause of pyomyositis (bacterial muscle infection). Lyme disease is a much rarer cause but on occasions the spirochaetes have been identified in muscle tissue (Muller-Felber *et al.* 1993).

There was something of a vogue 10 years ago for linking positive toxoplasma serology to myositis, and such infection may indeed cause a syndrome similar to idiopathic disease. However, it is only rarely that the evidence of acute toxoplasmosis is strong enough to warrant-specific treatment to be utilized. Granulomatous myositis, principally in the form of sarcoidosis, may be troublesome, progressive, and resistant to immunosuppressive treatment. Much less frequently, a granulomatous myopathy is found in patients with Crohn's disease. Eosinophilic myositis may be part of the hypereosinophilic syndrome or may occur separately. Myalgias and tenderness are common and MRI has been found to be useful in identifying areas of active inflammation (Kaufman *et al.* 1993). Focal myositis may present a clinical conundrum since the mass it causes is on occasion confused with a local tumour. Hence, biopsy is invariably required.

As already indicated, muscular dystrophies may confuse the unwary clinician, although the presence of muscle fibre hypertrophy will clinch the diagnosis of the dystrophy. Confusingly, some dystrophies, in particular fascioscapularhumeral dystrophy (FSH), in their early phases have an inflammatory component that can lead to the wrong diagnosis being made. Much less frequently, mitochondrial and metabolic myopathies are confused with myositis. The latter are rare and invariably a result of genetic defects of glycogen and glucose metabolism. Several drugs, including D-penicillamine, cimetidine, and zidovudine, can induce a myopathy. Others, as already indicated, can cause a rise in the CK with myalgia but little weakness (e.g. colchicine, chloroquine, lovastatin, clofibrate, cyclosporin, vincristine, carbimazole, and, rarely, non-steroidal anti-inflammatory drugs). The biopsy appearance of rhabdomyolysis is usually distinctive and should lead to a careful checking of the patient's history for drug abuse, since cocaine, amphetamines, heroin, and barbiturates can all give rise to this picture.

Finally, steroid myopathy remains a practical management problem. Large doses of corticosteroids can induce a type II muscle fibre atrophy (fast twitch) with proximal weakness, though steroids alone are unlikely to induce a rise in the creatine kinase, EMG abnormalities, or muscle biopsy inflammation. However, the picture is often confusing in the patient with active disease treated with large doses of steroids who remains weak. In these instances it is invariably necessary to repeat the biopsy.

Aetiology and pathogenesis

Aetiology

There is strong evidence to support the view that polymyositis and dermatomyositis have an autoimmune pathogenesis. The principal factors include, in common with other autoimmune diseases, an inciting agent and genetic and hormonal factors (Coakley and Isenberg 1996).

Various infections can induce a syndrome that closely resembles myositis in humans or animals (models of myositis are considered later in this chapter, see p. 9). Several attempts have been made to demonstrate that the onset of myositis varies with the season of the year, implicating an infectious trigger (Leff *et al.* 1991; Plotz *et al.* 1995). Viral infections may promote autoimmune reactions by a variety of mechanisms. These include polyclonal activation of lymphocytes, release of subcellular organelles after cellular destruction, and insertion of viral antigens into cellular membranes which promote reactions against self-components. Although culturing viruses from muscle biopsy tissue taken from patients with myositis has rarely been achieved, there are clinical descriptions of acute post-viral polymyositis. Raised post-viral antibody titres have been reported (notably anti-Coxsackie virus) in patients with polymyositis and virally induced mouse models of myositis have been well described (see later, and reviewed in Targoff 1998). In contrast, there is now little doubt that many of the so-called 'viral-like' particles observed in muscle biopsies actually represent simple alterations of the endoplasmic reticulum. Furthermore, the detection of a virus within the skeletal muscle of patients with myositis does not prove it was responsible for the inflammatory muscle disease; it may simply have been an 'opportunistic passenger' in previously damaged muscle.

As indicated above, a variety of drugs are able to induce a form of myositis and could thus act as potential triggers for the autoimmune disease. The mechanism by which such therapy could induce inflammatory muscle disease is not certain. It may occur as a result of direct muscle toxicity, with subsequent antigenic determinants. Alternatively, the drugs might act as haptens. An apt comparison might be with the thrombocytopaenia associated with apronal (Sedormid — a sedative). This drug is thought to combine with platelets, rendering them antigenic, resulting in the formation of antibodies against the drug–platelet complex which then destroys the platelets. Another possible mechanism for drug-induced myositis is an adjuvant or immunostimulatory effect. Drugs, notably penicillamine, might perturb immunological regulation and allow the emergence of clones of lymphocytes that are reactive against muscle fibre and membranes.

The potential causal relationship between neoplasia and myositis is also largely conjectural. Possible links include cross-reacting antigen determinants, shared by muscle membranes and tumours, an immune complex vasculitis, or even the reactivation of latent viruses allowed by the immunosuppressive effects of the tumour.

Immunogenetics

In 1981, Hirsch *et al.* utilized serological methods to determine HLA-DR antigens for 37 patients with myositis, 21 of whom had polymyositis and 16 dermatomyositis. HLA-DR3 was significantly increased among Caucasian patients and DR6 among African-American patients with polymyositis when compared with racially matched local controls. No significant HLA association was found in Caucasian or African-American patients with dermatomyositis.

HLA-DR3 is a common antigen in Caucasian populations. The difference between Caucasians and African-Americans could be a result of differing subtypes of DR3 in Caucasians and African-Americans, or of genes on the extended haplotypes; for example, genes at other loci such as DRB3, DQA1, DQB1, or complement genes. Consistent with the former possibility, the predominant subtype of DR3 in Caucasians is DRB1*0301 (> 90%) and in African-Americans is DRB1*0302 (> 50%) (Tsuji *et al.* 1992). With respect to HLA genes in linkage disequilibrium with DR3, the DQA1 and DQB1 genes that are in linkage disequilibrium with DRB1*0301 and with DRB1*0302 also differ. DQ2, encoded by DQA1*0501 and DQB1*0201, is in linkage disequilibrium with DRB1*0301, and DQ4, encoded by DQA1*0401 and DQB1*0402, is in linkage disequilibrium with DRB1*0302.

Arnett *et al.* (1996) found a strong association of DQA1*0501 among Caucasian patients with polymyositis and an increase of DQA1*0501 and DQA1*0401 among African-Americans. However in Mexican-American and in Japanese patients neither DQA1 allele was increased. In patients with dermatomyositis DQA1*0501 and *0401 were significantly increased in Caucasians only. A study of juvenile-onset dermatomyositis in a Caucasian population also found the strongest association was with DQA1*0501 (Reed *et al.* 1991).

Another explanation that could potentially reconcile observations among different races is if the primary association is with DR52. The DR52 molecule is encoded by the DRB3 locus and is present on haplotypes that have both DR3 and those that have DR6. (DRB3 is also present on haplotypes with DR11 and DR12, and DR52 is also co-expressed with DR8 although not encoded by DRB3.) Studies by Goldstein *et al.* (1990) focused on patients with myositis who had antibodies to histidyl–tRNA synthetase (anti-Jo-1) and reported that 100% of Caucasian and African-American patients had DR52. The frequency of DR52 in controls was also high (67% in Caucasians and 80% in African-Americans), but among Caucasians the difference between patients and controls was nevertheless statistically significant. In the report by Arnett *et al.* (1996) however, in patients with antibodies to Jo1 the strongest association was with DQA1*0501 or 0401. Moreover, these alleles were increased across ethnic groups including Caucasians, blacks, and Mexican-Americans with odds ratios ranging from 9.6 to 5.8.

Love *et al.* (1991) categorized patients according to autoantibody status. Serological techniques were used that define HLA-DR1 to DR10, DR52, DR53, and DQ1 to DQ4. Forty-five patients had autoantibodies to synthetases, seven to signal recognition particles, and eight to Mi-2. In agreement with the prior study of Goldstein *et al.* (1990), patients with antibodies to synthetases, including Caucasians and African-Americans, were found to have a predominance of DR52 (91%). Autoantibodies to synthetase (see Table 7.5) include histidyl–tRNA (anti-Jo-1), threonyl–tRNA (anti-PL-7), alanyl–tRNA (anti-PL-12), isoleucyl–tRNA (anti-OJ), and glycyl– tRNA (anti-EJ). Within this group, patients with antibodies to Jo-1 were more likely to also have DR3 (91%) than those with other anti-synthetase antibodies (18%). Patients with antibodies to signal recognition proteins (anti-SRP) more frequently had DR5 (57%) than those with anti-synthetase antibodies (11%). These studies predated the ability to determine DQA1 alleles and are not inconsistent with a primary role for DQA1.

In contrast to patients with antibodies to synthetase and to those with antibodies to signal recognition particles, patients with antibodies to Mi-2 had an increased frequency of DR7 (75%) and DR53 (100%) (Love *et al.* 1991). In another study of 16 patients with antibodies to Mi-2 and dermatomyositis, Mierau *et al.* (1996) also found a strong association with DR7. The latter study included sequence-specific oligonucleotide probe-typing to determine alleles of DQA1 and DQB1 and found a strong association with DQA1*0201. This is not surprising since DQA1*0201 is in very strong linkage disequilibrium with DR7. The odds ratio for DR7 was 22 and that for DQA1*0201 was 20.2. No association was observed with any DQB1 allele. Although 14 of the 16 patients had DR7, because two patients without DR7 had DR1 or DR2, the authors also suggested the possibility of a shared tryptophan at position 9 of DRβ1 could be important.

In contrast to studies in Caucasian populations, a preliminary report that examined HLA associations in Japanese patients categorized by autoantibodies found an increase of DRB1*0405, DQA1*0302, and DQB1*0401 in patients with antibodies to synthetases, and of DRB1*0802 in patients with antibodies to signal recognition proteins (Hirakata *et al.* 1995). By studying myositis-specific antibodies across four ethnic groups Arnett *et al.* (1996) were able to localize the primary associations to the DQA1 locus. DQA1*0501 and *0401 were increased among patients with anti-

Jol, anti PL-12 and other myositis specific antibodies except in Japanese where DQA1*0102 and *0103 predominated. In predominantly Caucasian populations antibodies to the nucleolar antigen PM-Scl have been found associated with DR3 (Genth *et al.* 1990; Oddis *et al.* 1992; Marguerie *et al.* 1992).

As previously discussed, HLA-DR3 occurs frequently on an extended ancestral haplotype. Because this haplotype frequently includes a null allele at the complement locus C4A, another potential candidate in the analysis of MHC contributions to myositis is the C4A*Q0 (null) allele. However, two studies have examined patients with myositis for the C4A null allele and neither found an association that was independent of linkage disequilibrium with HLA-DR3 (Moulds *et al.* 1990; Reed *et al.* 1991). Occasional reports of myositis with hereditary C2 complement deficiency (Leddy *et al.* 1975) have been described.

Animal models

There are two main categories of animal models of myositis, namely spontaneously occurring disorders and induced models. Hargis *et al.* (1986) have reported the post-mortem findings of an inflammatory myopathy in collies and Shetland sheep dogs. These animals may develop a symmetrical muscle involvement, a characteristically myopathic EMG, histological evidence of myositis, and, on occasion, a form of dermatitis. However, the muscles involved are usually distal rather than proximal and muscle enzymes are not usually elevated in these animals. It has been proposed (Haupt *et al.* 1985) that, in collies, dermatomyositis is inherited as a dominant trait with variable penetrance. Spontaneous polymyositis has also been reported in the South African rodent *Mastomys natalensis* (Snell and Steurart 1975). These animals may develop thymomas and myocarditis but appear to have been little studied as a model of human disease.

Experimentally induced models of myositis were described initially in rats (Pearson 1956) and guinea pigs (Dawkins 1965) after giving repeated injections of homogenized muscle in Freund's complete adjuvant. These models are referred to as experimental allergic myositis (EAM). The main results and implications of work done using EAM models have been to show the following:

(i) It is possible to induce a cell-mediated type of response specifically to muscle antigens in animals. This effect resembles polymyositis histologically.

(ii) Adoptive transfer of lymphocytes, but not serum from sensitized animals, can produce similar symptoms in recipient animals.

(iii) *In vitro* it is possible to demonstrate lymphocyte transformation to muscle antigens and myotoxicity of lymphocytes from the animals sensitized against muscle cells, but not from animals immunized with other tissues.

However, EAM remains an unsatisfactory model for human polymyositis. It does not occur spontaneously and requires frequent 'booster' injections to maintain the pathological appearance. Furthermore, an accompanying adjuvant arthritis may interfere with the assessment of the muscle disease. Most significantly, however, the affected animals do not, in general, appear to be weak.

A syndrome of chronic myositis following Coxsackie group B virus-1 infection (a member of the Picornavirus family) was noted in a susceptible strain of neonatal mice (Ray *et al.* 1979). After the acute muscle infection, these animals developed proximal hind limb myositis with obvious clinical weakness. Subsequently, Strongwater *et al.* (1984) induced myositis in CDI Swiss mice less than two days old, by intraperitoneal injection of a similar strain of B1 Coxsackie virus. The animals developed proximal muscle weakness approximately seven days after the viral challenge, and the symptoms persisted without further injections for 10 weeks. EMG and histological abnormalities were noted throughout this time, although the virus itself was not detected from two weeks after the initial injections. Further studies have shown that the myositis in this model progresses for up to six months. Viral nucleic acid persists for up to four weeks and occasionally for 6–12 months (Tam *et al.* 1994). Production of this form of myositis depends upon the strain of virus and the type of mouse used, and clearly utilizes a form of cell-mediated immunity. The picornaviruses have thus been thought to be promising candidates for a viral trigger in patients with myositis and some (e.g. Yousef *et al.* 1990) but not all (e.g. Leff *et al.* 1992) investigators have detected evidence of these viruses in the muscles of patients with inflammatory myopathy.

Approximately 50% of Macaque monkeys infected with the D-type simian retrovirus, SRV-1, develop a myositis that closely resembles polymyositis as part of AIDS-like disease (Dalakas *et al.* 1987). These monkeys have weakness, raised muscle enzymes, and histological changes showing inflammation necrosis, phagocytosis, and fibrosis.

Pathogenic mechanisms

Studies of peripheral blood cells

Although there has been some dispute, the distribution of T cell subsets in the peripheral blood of patients with myositis has indicated a reduction in the number of CD8+ cells. More contentious have been studies to determine whether lymphocytes in patients with myositis respond to autologous or heterologous muscle. Much of the published data has not been confirmed, few controls have been used, and the results are difficult to interpret. Such cytotoxicity as has been seen in these systems does not appear to be specific for lymphocytes in patients with myositis. Definitive reports of *in vitro* antigen-directed MHC-restricted T cell cytotoxicity from patients with myositis directed against autologous muscle are lacking. However, there does appear to be increased traffic passing from lymphocytes to muscles, and in patients with active myositis a high proportion of peripheral blood T cells carry activation markers (Miller *et al.* 1990).

Muscle biopsy studies: cellular aspects

In a series of papers (Rowe *et al.* 1981, 1983; Isenberg *et al.* 1986) monoclonal antibodies were used to analyse the inflammatory infiltrates in muscle fibre antigen expression in muscle biopsies from patients with myositis. The main findings of this group were shown in Table 7.8 and Figs 7.13–7.15.

Other groups have broadly confirmed and extended these observations. Thus, Arahata and Engel (1986, 1988a, b) and Mantegazza *et al.* (1993) have confirmed that CD4+ T cells predominate in muscle biopsies in patients with active untreated myositis and tend to decrease with treatment. However, on moving from the perivascular to the endomysial region, the proportion of CD8+ cytotoxic T cells increases at the expense of CD4+ T cells and B cells. The biopsies in patients with dermatomyositis show a higher proportion of B cells and a lower proportion of CD8+ T cells than are found in patients with polymyositis. In a study of polymyositis, dermatomyositis, and inclusion body myositis De-Bleecker and Engel (1995) reported a predominance of CD45RO-positive T cells (primed memory cells)

Table 7.8 Analysis of immunohistochemical findings in muscle biopsies from patients with myositis

1. Large number of 'activated' T lymphocytes.

2. Preponderance of T helper/inducer cells within the T lymphocyte population in untreated cases.

3. Diffusion of HLA-DR (class 2)-positive material from the infiltrates into the muscle fibres.

4. Restriction of HLA-ABC (class 1) antigens to damaged muscle fibres and those adjacent to inflammatory infiltrates.

5. Demonstration of α, β, and γ interferons in the same tissue distribution as the class 1 antigens, suggesting that the expression of those antigens has been induced by interferon release.

Based on data from Rowe *et al.* (1981, 1983) and Isenberg *et al.* (1986).

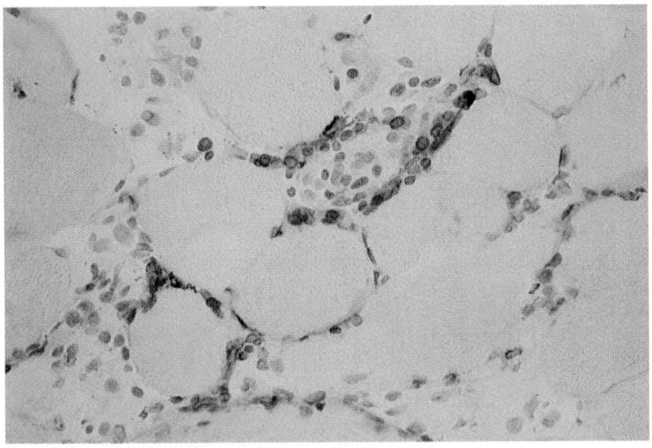

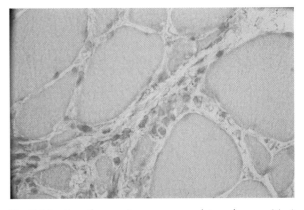

Fig. 7.13. Use of a monoclonal pan T cell marker reveals most of the inflammatory cells in this biopsy from a patient with myositis to be T cells (brown stain = positive). (Courtesy of Dr G. Cambridge.)

Fig. 7.15. Interferon-γ is overexpressed (purple = positive) on the sarcolemma/basement membrane of the muscle fibres and in and around the infiltrating cells — reminiscent of the distribution of the HLA class 1 antigens. (Courtesy of Deborah Rowe and Professor Peter Beverley.)

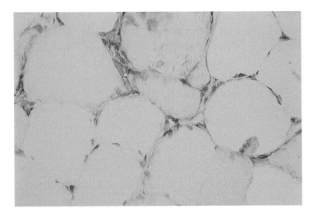

Fig. 7.14. HLA class I antigens are overexpressed (brown stain = positive), mainly on the sarcolemma/basement membrane of myofibres in this patient with myositis.

compared with CD45RA-positive cells (unprimed virgin T cells) in each. While implicating these memory cells in pathogenesis, the results do not distinguish between the possibility that these cells simply have greater transendothelial migratory ability or whether a conversion from virgin to memory cell occurs within the muscle.

Most of the mononuclear cells invading the muscle fibres are CD8+ T cells. Relatively few natural killer cells have been detected and thus they do not seem to be of great importance in the muscle damage that occurs. In recent years, several groups have analysed the T cell repertoire of lymphocytes in affected muscles, since clonality of T cell receptors would suggest an antigen-driven process. It is also important to determine whether the repertoire of these segments inherited by an individual governs the development of myositis. Mantegazza *et al.* (1993) first demonstrated oligoclonality of T cell receptors in muscle-infiltrating

T cells in polymyositis. Using the reverse transcriptase polymerase chain reaction method of analysing muscle biopsies, $V\alpha1$, $V\alpha5$, $V\beta1$, $V\beta15$ gene rearrangements were found in 60–100% of 15 patients, but not in the controls. Ninety per cent of the $V\beta15$ clones had $J\beta2.1$ and a common motif in the CDR3 region, suggesting an antigen-driven process. However, the ethnic group of the patients and controls was not clarified. O'Hanlon et al. (1995) examined nine patients with polymyositis and eight with dermatomyositis, all of whom possessed the anti-Jo-1 antibody. The authors stated that this group was chosen to increase the genetic homogeneity, though it must be pointed out that the patients studied were a mixture of Caucasoids, blacks, and other ethnic groups. Again using a reverse transcriptase polymerase chain reaction method the polyclonal T cell repertoire was found in dermatomyositis but oligoclonality was seen in polymyositis. However, the genes expressed were not in complete accordance with the findings of Mantegazza et al. (1993). $V\alpha1$ and $V\beta6$ were present in 82 and 91% of biopsies, respectively. J gene analysis of four patients with $V\beta6$ showed restricted usage of $J\beta2.1$, $J\beta2.3$, and $J\beta2.7$. Further complexities are suggested by another study of six patients with inclusion body myositis (Fyhr et al. 1996) among whom $V\alpha7$, $V\alpha14$, and $V\beta8$ were clearly overexpressed in muscle tissue. These results suggest an antigen-driven process in polymyositis. The reasons for the differences between the groups are not entirely clear, but non-specific recruitment of T cells to inflammatory lesions, variations in temporal patterns of disease, and technical factors may all play a part.

If the attack on muscle fibres that is thought to occur in polymyositis is due to antigen-directed T cell cytotoxicity it may be anticipated that MHC antigens will be upregulated on the target tissue. MHC antigen expression on muscle fibres is normally low or absent but it is increased in patients with polymyositis and inclusion body myositis. In particular, Emslie-Smith et al. (1989) have shown that all muscle fibres invaded by CD8+ lymphocytes overexpress MHC class 1 antigens.

The upregulation of class I antigens may be induced by interferon-γ and this was shown to be present on the sarcolemma/basement membrane of muscle fibres by Isenberg et al. (1986) (Fig. 7.15). Interferon-γ can also inhibit proliferation and differentiation (an effect that is known to be helped by tumour necrosis factor-α), which could be contributing to the lesions seen in myositis. In a recent study (Lundberg et al. 1995) a similar pattern of cytokine mRNA expression was identified in five patients each with polymyositis, inclusion body myositis, and dermatomyositis. However, the pattern of both predominantly T cell-derived cytokines (Il-2, Il-4, Il-5, interferon-γ) and macrophage-derived cytokines (Il-1, Il-6, and TNF-α) resembled that seen in five patients with Duchenne dystrophy and 'non-weak' controls, albeit the patients with myositis had comparatively increased expression. Thus, involvement of cytokine secretion in the ongoing immune system 'atttack' on muscle fibres is likely to represent a quantitative overall response rather than the development of a novel or unique cytokine.

Humoral aspects

The incidence of disease-specific autoantibodies (as discussed earlier), while not in itself proof of their involvement in the damage that is seen in patients with myositis, does indicate that humoral abnormalities are also present in this disease.

Lisak and Zweiman (1976) have shown raised IgG, IgA, and IgM levels in 9 of 11, 7 of 11, and 4 of 11 polymyositis/dermatomyositis cases, respectively. Furthermore, Kiprov and Miller (1984) have described three cases of a monoclonal IgGκ gammopathy in association with myositis. Humoral abnormalities are likely to be more important in dermatomyositis, where a vasculopathy involving small vessels and capillaries is an important mechanism of damage. Emslie-Smith and Engel (1990), while finding no structural change by routine examination in patients with early-onset dermatomyositis, found definite microvascular abnormalities by electron microscopy. Such damage is likely to be mediated by complement. Kissel et al. (1991) found the deposition of the complement membrane attack complex in the walls of the muscle microvasculature, confirming that local activation of complement had occurred. These observations were most pronounced in patients with juvenile-onset dermatomyositis and in some cases of adult dermatomyositis, but not in adult-onset polymyositis. Precisely how the complement is activated, however, remains uncertain. Deposition of immunoglobulin muscle blood vessels is not seen in healthy muscle tissue, but is found in muscle disease of many different types (Isenberg 1983) and its relationship to the MAC deposition is unknown. Immunoglobulin deposition has been described in the muscle blood vessel walls, the muscle fibres themselves, and on the sarcolemma and basement membrane of the fibres.

Antigenic stimuli and tissue targeting

The missing piece in the immunological puzzle that is myositis remains the reason why skeletal muscle is the principal target, at least in patients with poly- as opposed to dermato-myositis. Despite many efforts this puzzle has not been solved. Some insight, however, has been gained into the possible role of histidyl–tRNA synthetase as an autoantigen in at least a proportion of patients with myositis (reviewed by Plotz 1994). He reviewed the evidence that this enzyme, or a mimic of it, is a key autoantigen. Plotz and colleagues (Raben *et al.* 1994) have demonstrated that the first 60 amino acids that constitute histidyl–tRNA synthetase contain a motif that is shared among other aminoacyl–tRNA synthetases. This motif is essential for the enzymatic activity and contains the major autoantigenic epitope. Other possible mechanisms include the notion that following infection by a particular virus, the viral RNA and histidyl–tRNA could form a complex that is perceived as foreign, the result being an autoimmune response leading to an anti-Jo-1 antibody. Alternatively, antibodies might be generated by the host, against an infecting virus, with molecular mimicry responsible for the formation of the anti-Jo-1 antibodies.

None of these ideas really explains how or why the B cells are exposed to intact histidyl–tRNA synthetase, or the role of T cells in the drive to produce these antibodies and in stimulus to B cell production of disease-specific antibodies.

Treatment of myositis in adults

Treatment of polymyositis should be initiated speedily once the diagnosis has been confirmed. Delay in starting treatment is associated with a worse outcome (Oddis and Medsger 1989). In certain cases, particularly those with severe weakness, dysphagia, respiratory distress, cardiac, or systemic involvement, treatment should be begun before final confirmation of the diagnosis.

Corticosteroids

Corticosteroids started at high doses (prednisolone 60–80 mg/day) are the mainstay of treatment, although there are no good controlled trials. At least 90% of patients respond at least partially to prednisolone (Henriksson and Sandstedt 1982). High dose steroids

should be continued until the serum creatinine kinase is normal (or nearly normal) and there is improvement in muscle strength. This usually takes 1–2 months. At that time the dose of prednisolone can be reduced to approximately 15–25% of the existing dose until a stable maintenance dose is obtained. Such a treatment schedule is associated with a better response (Oddis and Medsger 1988) that can be assessed using clinical symptoms, muscle strength (measured either clinically or by formal isometric strength testing, see Fig. 7.2), and serum creatine kinase.

Alternate day prednisolone may reduce side-effects while maintaining efficacy (Uchino *et al.* 1985). High dose intravenous methylprednisolone may achieve a rapid effect in severely ill patients (Yanagisawa *et al.* 1983).

Oral corticosteroids at high doses are associated with numerous side-effects (see Chapter 3). Consideration should be given to prophylaxis against osteoporosis with calcium and vitamin D, hormone replacement therapy, or a bisphosphonate. Patients on high doses should be closely monitored for side-effects such as hypertension, diabetes, and infection.

Steroid myopathy is also a potential complication and should be considered in patients in whom the CK falls but weakness persists. Other possibilities in this situation include malignancy, other types of muscle disease, including metabolic myopathy, or inclusion body myopathy. In about 25% of patients corticosteroids are ineffective (weakness and CK elevation persist) and additional immunosuppression should be considered using azathioprine, methotrexate, cyclosporin, cyclophosphamide, or a combination thereof. These drugs are frequently utilized to help reduce the corticosteroid requirement.

Other immunosuppressive drugs

Azathioprine is used by many clinicians as the immunosuppressive of first choice, although methotrexate is gaining popularity. In a prospective double-blind-controlled trial of azathioprine and prednisolone versus prednisolone alone there was no significant difference in muscle strength, biopsy appearance, or CK (Bunch *et al.* 1980), open follow-up of 28 of these patients for three years suggested that the combination was better (Bunch 1981). In a retrospective study Ramirez (1990) reported that azathioprine and prednisolone produced satisfactory results in most patients and permitted use of lower doses of steroids.

Methotrexate (low dose maximum 20 mg/week) is increasingly used as an adjunct to prednisolone. Retrospective analysis suggests a better and more rapid response rate (Joffe *et al.* 1993). A recent randomized crossover study of 30 patients with refractory myositis showed that a combination of oral methotrexate and azathioprine was more successful than intravenous methotrexate (Villalba *et al.* 1998). Intramuscular methotrexate should be avoided because of its tendency to elevate the serum CK.

Cyclosporin has been used in few patients with myositis with some clinical benefit (Dawson *et al.* 1997), but there are no randomized trials to support its use.

Intermittent, intravenous pulse cyclophosphamide was felt to be ineffective in a group of 11 patients with steroid-resistant disease. Only one patient improved and there was significant toxicity (infection) (Cronin *et al.* 1989). However, Bombardieri *et al.* (1989) successfully treated 10 patients with intravenous cyclophosphamide. As with other drugs, there are no controlled trials to support the use of cyclophosphamide.

Other therapeutic strategies

As with other autoimmune diseases, plasmapheresis has been tried. This technique seems to be more effective in the acute phase (Herson *et al.* 1989). In resistant cases leucopheresis and plasma exchange are no more effective than sham apheresis (Miller *et al.* 1992). Intravenous immunoglobulin (IVIg) produces clinical improvement in patients with refractory disease (Cherin *et al.* 1991). A more recent study from the same group suggested that IVIg as first-line therapy showed little benefit (Cherin *et al.* 1994) and that it should not be considered to be a therapy of first choice. However, Dalakas *et al.* showed that IVIg was significantly better than placebo is a double blind, cross over study in adults with dermatomyositis.

Treatment of extra muscular manifestations

The rash of dermatomyositis may respond to immuno-suppression with corticosteroids or other immuno-suppressive agents. If the rash persists, or there is a photosensitive component, hydroxychloroquine may be useful. In the latter case high factor sun block should also be used. Calcinosis is particularly difficult to treat. Adequate treatment of inflammatory disease helps prevent calcinosis but has no effect on established disease.

Rehabilitation

During active inflammation active exercise is not advisable. However, passive motion exercises are important to prevent joint contractures. As the patient improves, active exercises may be slowly introduced.

Treatment of childhood disease

As with adult disease there are few controlled trials to guide therapy. Oral prednisolone is the established primary therapy for childhood-onset disease and has improved the outcome. In patients with steroid-resistant disease or unacceptable steroid toxicity, immunosuppression with azathioprine, methotrexate, cyclosporin, or IVIg should be considered.

Summary

Polymyositis/dermatomyositis are organ-specific members of the autoimmune rheumatic disease family. Patients with myositis are commonly female and often carry the HLA-B8/HLA-DR3 antigens. The disease mainly affects the proximal skeletal muscles but it is now appreciated that more extensive involvement, notable cardiac, often occurs. Myositis carries a guarded prognosis and the usual immunosuppressive regimes used for treatment offer limited improvement in its morbidity and mortality. The immunopathology of polymyositis is poorly understood, although as with other diseases of this type it is likely that both humoral and cell-mediated mechanisms play a role. The disease is distinguished by antibodies to the Jo-1 antigen which has been identified as tRNA–histidyl transferase. The tissue tropism of the disease is still a mystery and investigations into the origins of polymyositis are hampered by the lack of a good animal model.

References

Arad-Dann H, Isenberg DA, Shoenfeld Y *et al.* Autoantibodies against a specific nuclear RNA protein in the sera of patients with autoimmune rheumatic diseases associated with myositis. *J Immunol* 1987; **138**: 2467–8.

Arahata K, Engel AG. Monoclonal antibody analysis of mononuclear cells in myopathies III: immunoelectron microscopy aspects of cell-mediated muscle fibre injury. *Ann Neurol* 1986; **19**: 112–15.

Arahata K, Engel AG. Monoclonal antibody analysis of mono-nuclear cells in myopathies V: identification and quantitation of T8+ cytotoxic and T8+ suppressor cells. *Ann Neurol* 1988a; **23**: 493–9.

Arahata K, Engel AG. Monoclonal antibody analysis of mononuclear cells in myopathies IV: cell mediated cytotoxicity and muscle fibre necrosis. *Ann Neurol* 1988b; **23**: 168–73.

Arnett FC, Targoff IN, Mimori T *et al.* Interrelationship of major histocompatability complex class II alleles and autoantibodies in four ethnic groups with various forms of myositis. *Arthritis Rheum* 1996; **39**: 1507–18.

Askanas V, Engel WK, Mirabella M. Idiopathic inflammatory myopathies inclusion myositis, polymyositis and dermatomyositis. *Curr Opin Neurol* 1994; **7**: 448–56.

Bohan A, Peter JB. Polymyositis and dermatomyositis. *N Engl J Med* 1975; **292**: 344–7.

Bombardieri S, Hughes GRV, Neri R *et al.* Cyclophosphamide in severe polymyositis. *Lancet* 1989; **i**: 1138–9.

Bunch TW, Worthington JW, Combs JJ *et al.* Azathioprine with prednisolone for polymyositis. A controlled trial. *Ann Intern Med* 1980; **92**: 365–9.

Bunch TW. Prednisolone and azathioprine for polymyositis; long term follow up. *Arthritis Rheum* 1981; **24**: 45–8.

Calabrese LH, Chou SM. Inclusion body myositis. *Rheum Dis Clin North Am* 1994; **20**: 955–72.

Callen JP. Myositis and malignancy. *Curr Opin Rheumatol* 1994; **6**: 590–4.

Callen AM, Pachman LM, Hayford JR *et al.* Intermittent high-dose intravenous methylprednisolone (IV pulse) therapy prevents calcirosis and shortens disease course in juvenile dermatomyositis (JDMS). *Arthritis Rheum* 1994; **37**: 810.

Cherin P, Herson S, Wechsler B *et al.* Efficacy of intravenous gammaglobulin therapy in chronic refractory polymyositis and dermatomyositis: an open study with 20 adult patients. *Am J Med* 1991; **91**: 162–8.

Cherin P, Piette JC, Wechsler B *et al.* Intravenous gammaglobulin as first line therapy in polymyositis and dermatomyositis: an open study in 11 adult patients. *J Rheumatol* 1994; **21**: 1092–7.

Coakley G, Isenberg DA. Inflammatory muscle disease: theoretical aspects. *Rheum Eur* 1996; **25**: 60–3.

Cronin ME, Miller FW, Hicks JE *et al.* The failure of intravenous cyclophosphamide therapy in refractory idiopathic inflammatory myopathy. *J Rheumatol* 1989; **16**: 1225–8.

Dalakas M, Gravell M, London WT *et al.* Morphological changes of an inflammatory myopathy in Rhesus monkeys with simian acquired immunodeficiency syndromes. *Proc Soc Exp Biol Med* 1987; **185**: 368–76.

Dalakas MC, Illa I, Dambrosia JM *et al.* A controlled trial of high dose intravenous immune globulin infusions as treatment for dermatomyositis. *N Eng J Med* 1993; **329**: 1993–2000.

Dawkins RL. Experimental myositis associated with hypersensitivity to muscle. *J Path Bact* 1965; **90**: 619–25.

Dawkins RL, Garlepp MJ, McDonald BL. Immunopathology of muscle. In: *Skeletal Muscle Pathology*, eds Martaglia FL, Walton J. Churchill Livingstone, Edinburgh, 1982; 761–82.

Dawson JK, Abernethy VE, Lynch MP. Effective treatment of anti-Jo-1 antibody positive polymyositis with cyclosporin. *Br J Rheumatol* 1997; **36**: 144–5.

De-Bleeker JL, Engel AG. Immunocytochemical study of CD45 T cell isoforms in inflammatory myopathies. *Am J Pathol* 1995; **146**: 1178–87.

DeVere R, Bradley MG. Polymyositis: its presentation, morbidity and mortality. *Brain* 1975; **98**: 637–66.

Dickey BF, Myer, AR. Pulmonary disease in polymyositis/ dermatomyositis. *Sem Arthritis Rheum* 1974; **14**: 60–76.

Dietrichson P, Coakley J, Smith PEM *et al.* Conchotome and needle percutaneous biopsy of skeletal muscle. *J Neurol Neurosurg Psych* 1987; **50**: 1761–71.

Edwards RHT, Wiles CM, Round JM *et al.* Muscle breakdown and repair in polymyositis: a case study. *Muscle Nerve* 1979; **2**: 223–8.

Edwards RHT, Round JM, Jones DA. Needle biopsy of skeletal muscle: a review of 10 years experience. *Muscle Nerve* 1983; **6**: 676–83.

Emslie-Smith AM, Engel AG. Microvascular changes in early and advanced dermatomyositis: a quantitative study. *Ann Neurol* 1990; **27**: 343–56.

Emslie-Smith AM, Arahata K, Engel AG. Major histocompatibility complex class I antigen expression, immunolocalization of interferon subtypes and T cell-mediated cytotoxicity in myopathies. *Hum Pathol* 1989; **20**: 224–31.

Fleckenstein JL, Reimers CD. Inflammatory myopathies: radiologic evaluation. *Radiol Clin North Am* 1996; **34**: 427–39.

Fyhr JM, Moslemi AR, Tarkowski A *et al.* Limited T-cell receptor V gene usage in inclusion body myositis. *Scand J Immunol* 1996; **47**: 109–16.

Garton M, Isenberg DA. Clinical features of lupus myositis versus idiopathic myositis. A review of 30 cases. *Br J Rheumatol* 1997; **36**: 1267–74.

Genth E, Mierau R, Genetzky P *et al.* Immunogenetic associations of scleroderma-related antinuclear antibodies. *Arthritis Rheum* 1990; **33**: 657–65.

Goldstein R, Duvic M, Targoff IN *et al.* HLA-D region genes associated with autoantibody responses to histidyl-transfer RNA synthetase (Jo-1) and other translation-related factors in myositis (review). *Arthritis Rheum* 1990; **33**: 1240–8,

Hargis KH, Prieur D, Haupt KH *et al.* Post mortem findings in four litters of dogs with familial canine dermatomyositis. *Am J Pathol* 1986; **123**: 480–96.

Haupt KH, Prieur D, Moore MP *et al.* Familial canine dermatomyositis: clinical, electrodiagnostic and genetic studies. *Am J Vet Res* 1985; **46**: 1861–9.

Henriksson KG, Sandstedt P. Polymyositis — treatment and prognosis. A study in 107 patients. *Acta Neurol Scand* 1982; **65**: 280–300.

Herson S, Lok C, Ronjeau JC. Plasma exchange in dermatomyositis and polymyositis. Retrospective study of 38 cases of plasma exchange. *Ann Med Interne (Paris)* 1989; **140**: 453–5.

Hiketa T, Matsumoto Y, Ohashi M *et al.* Juvenile dermatomyositis: a statistical study of 114 patients with dermatomyositis. *J Dermatol* 1992; **19**: 470–6.

Hirakata M, Suwa A, Nakamura K. Myositis-specific antibodies are associated with HLA class II alleles in Japanese patients. *Arthritis Rheum* 1995; **38** (Suppl.): S2321 (abstract).

Hirsch TJ, Enlow RW, Bias WB *et al.* HLA-D related (DR) antigens in various kinds of myositis. *Hum Immunol* 1981; **3**: 181–6.

Isenberg DA. Immunoglobulin deposition in skeletal muscle in primary muscle disease. *Q J Med* 1983; **52**: 297–310.

Isenberg DA, Rowe D, Shearer M *et al.* Localisation of interferons and IL-2 in polymyositis and muscular dystrophy. *Clin Exp Immunol* 1986; **63**: 450–8.

Ishii N, Ono H, Kawaguchi T, Nakajima H. Dermatomyositis and pregnancy: case report and review of the literature. *Dermatologica* 1991; **183**: 146–9.

Joffe MM, Love LA, Leff RL *et al.* Drug therapy of the idiopathic inflammatory myopathies: predictors of response to prednisolone, azathioprine, methotrexate and comparison of their efficacy. *Am J Med* 1993; **94**: 379–87.

Kagen LJ. Myoglobulinaemia and myoglobinuria in patients with myositis. *Arthritis Rheum* 1971; **14**: 457–64.

Kager LJ. Approach to the patient with myopathy. *Bull Rheum Dis* 1987; **33**: 1–8.

Kaufman LD, Kephart GM, Seidman RJ *et al.* The spectrum of eosinophilic myositis. Clinical and immunopathogenic studies of three patients and review of the literature. *Arthritis Rheum* 1993; **36**: 1014–24.

Kiprov DD, Miller RG. Polymyositis associated with monoclonal gammopathy. *Lancet* 1984; **ii**: 1183–7.

Kissell JT, Hatterman RK, Rammohan KW *et al.* The relationship of complement-mediated microvasculopathy to the histologic features and clinical duration of disease in dermatomyositis. *Arch Neurol* 1991; **48**: 26–30.

Leddy JP, Griggs RC, Klemperer MR *et al.* Hereditary complement (C2) deficiency with dermatomyositis. *Am J Med* 1975; **58**: 83–91.

Leff RL, Burgess SH, Miller FW *et al.* Distinct seasonal patterns in the onset of adult idiopathic inflammatory myopathy in patients with anti Jo-1 and antisignal recognition particle autoantibodies. *Arthritis Rheum* 1991; **34**: 1391–6.

Leff RL, Love LA, Miller FW *et al.* Viruses in idiopathic inflammatory myopathy absence of candidate viral genomes in muscle. *Lancet* 1992: **339**: 1192–5.

Lisak RP, Zweiman B. Serum immunoglobulin levels in myasthenia gravis, polymyositis and dermatomyositis. *J Neurol Neurosurg Psychiatr* 1976; **39**: 34–7.

Love LA, Laff RL, Fraser DD *et al.* A new approach to the classification of idiopathic inflammatory myopathy: myositis specific autoantibodies define useful homogeneous patient groups. *Medicine* 1991; **70**: 360–74.

Lundberg J, Brengman JM, Engel AG. Analysis of cytokine expression in muscle in inflammatory myopathies. Duchenne dystrophy and non-weak controls. *J Neuroimmunol* 1995; **63**: 9–16.

Mantegazza T, Andreata F, Bernasconi P *et al.* Analysis of T cell receptor repertoire of muscle-infiltrating T lymphocytes in polymyositis. Restricted V alpha/beta rearrangements may indicate antigen driven selection. *J Clin Invest* 1993; **91**: 2880–6.

Marguerie C, Bunn C, Beynon HLC *et al.* Polymyositis, pulmonary fibrosis and autoantibodies to aminoacyl-tRNA synthetase. *Q J Med* 1990; **77**: 1019–38.

Marguerie C, Bunn CC, Copier J *et al.* The clinical and immunogenetic features of patients with autoantibodies to the nucleolar antigen PM-Scl. *Medicine* 1992; **71**: 327–36.

Matsuda Y, Tomii M, Kashiwazaki S. Fatal pneumomediastinum in dermatomyositis without creatine kinase elevation. *Intn Med* 1993; **32**: 643–7.

Medsger TA Jr, Dawson WN Jr, Masi JT. The epidemiology of polymyositis. *Am J Med* 1970; **48**: 715–23.

Mierau R, Dick T, Bartz-Bazzanella P *et al.* Strong association of dermatomyositis-specific Mi-2 autoantibodies with a tryptophan at position 9 of the HLA-DRβ chain. *Arthritis Rheum* 1996; **39**: 868–76.

Miller FW. Myositis-specific autoantibodies. *JAMA* 1993; **270**: 1846–9 (review).

Miller FW, Love LA, Barbieri SA *et al.* Lymphocyte activation markers in idiopathic myositis: changes with disease activity and differences among clinical and autoantibody subgroups. *Clin Exp Immunol* 1990; **81**: 373–9.

Miller FW, Leitman SF, Cronin ME *et al.* Controlled trial of plasma exchange and leucopheresis in polymyositis and dermatomyositis. *N Eng J Med* 1992; **326**: 1380–4.

Morgan St.O.C, Mora C, Rodgers-Johnson P, Char G. HTLV-1 and polymyositis in Jamaica. *Lancet* 1989; **ii**: 1184–2.

Morrow WJW, Isenberg DA, Sobol RF *et al.* AIDS virus infection and autoimmunity: a perspective of the clinical, immunological and molecular origins of the autoallergic pathologies associated with HIV disease. *Clin Immunol Immunopathol* 1991; **58**: 163–80.

Moulds JM, Rolih C, Goldstein R *et al.* C4 null genes in American Whites and Blacks with myositis. *J Rheumatol* 1990; **17**: 331–4.

Muller-Feiber W, Reimers CD, de Koning J *et al.* Myositis in Lyme borreliosis: an immunohistochemical study of seven patients. *J Neurol Sci* 1993; **118**: 207–12.

Oddis CV, Hill P. Pregnancy outcome in women with inflammatory myopathy. *Arthritis Rheum* 1993; **36**: S 255.

Oddis CV, Medsger TA Jr. Relationship between serum creatinine level and corticosteroid therapy in polymyositisdermatomyositis. *J Rheumatol* 1988; **15**: 807–11.

Oddis CV, Medsger TA Jr. Current management of polymyositis and dermatomyositis. *Drugs* 1989; **37**: 382–90.

Oddis CV, Okana Y, Rudert W *et al.* Serum autoantibody to the nucleolar antigen PM-Scl *Arthritis Rheum* 1992; **35**: 1211–7.

O'Hanlon TP, Messersmith WA, Dalakas MC *et al.* Gammadelta T cells receptor gene expression by muscle-infiltrating lymphocytes in the idiopathic inflammatory myopathies. *Clin Exp Immunol* 1995; **100**: 519–28.

Pachman LM. An update on juvenile dermatomyositis. *Curr Opin Rheumatol* 1995; **7**: 437–41.

Pearson CM. Development of arthritis, periarthritis and periostitis in rats given adjuvants. *Proc Soc Exp Biol Med* 1956; **91**: 95–101.

Pearson CM. Patterns of polymyositis and their responses to treatment. *Ann Intern Med* 1963: **59**: 827–38.

Plotz PH. Reverse immunology: the lessons from myositis. *Clin Immunol Immunopathol* 1994; **72**: 204–7.

Plotz PH, Rider LG, Targoff IN *et al.* Myositis: immunologic contributions to understanding cause, pathogenesis and therapy. *Ann Intern Med* 1995; **122**: 715–24.

Raben N, Nichols R, Dohlman J *et al.* A motif in human histidyl-tRNA synthetase which is shared among several amino-tRNA synthetases is a coiled-coil that is essential for enzymatic activity and contains the major autoantigenic epitope. *J Biol Chem* 1994; **269**: 24277–83.

Ramirez G, Asherson RA, Khamashta MA *et al.* Adult onset polymyositis-dermatomyositis: description of 25 patients with emphasis on treatment. *Sem Arth Rheum* 1990; **20**: 114–20.

Ray CG, Minnich LL, Johnson PC. Selective polymyositis induced by Coxsackie b1 in mice. *J Infect Dis* 1979; **140**: 239–43.

Reed AM, Pachman L, Ober C. Molecular genetic studies of major histocompatibility complex genes in children with juvenile dermatomyositis: increased risk associated with HLA-DQA1*0501. *Hum Immunol* 1991; **32**: 235–40.

Rowe DJ, Isenberg DA, McDougall J *et al*. Characterisation of polymyositis infiltrates using monoclonal antibodies to human leucocyte antigens. *Clin Exp Immunol* 1981; **45**: 290–8.

Rowe DJ, Isenberg DA, Beverley PCL. Monoclonal antibodies to leucocyte antigens in polymyositis and muscular dystrophy. *Clin Exp Immunol* 1983; **54**: 327–36.

Satoh M, Ajmani AK, Hirakata M *et al*. Onset of polymyositis with autoantibodies to threonyl-tRNA synthetase during pregnancy. *J Rheumatol* 1994; **21**: 1564–6.

Serratrice G. La myosite à inclusions. *Presse Med* 1996; **25**: 985–8.

Shy GM. The late onset myopathy: a clinico-pathological study of 131 patients. *World Neurol* 1962; **3**: 149–60.

Sigurgeirsson B, Lindelof B, Edhag O *et al*. Risk of cancer in patients with dermatomyositis or polymyositis: a population-based study. *N Eng J Med* 1992; **326**: 363–7.

Smadja D, Ballance R, Cabre P *et al*. Clinical characteristics of HTLV-1 associated dermatopolymyositis. Seven cases from Martinique. *Acta Neurol Scand* 1995; **92**: 3206–12.

Snell KC, Stewart HL. Spontaneous disease in a closed colony of Praomys (mastomys) natalensis. *Bull World Health Org* 1975; **52**: 645–50.

Stoll T, Bruhlmann P, Stucki G *et al*. Muscle strength assessment in polymyositis and dermatomyositis evaluation of the reliability and clinical use of a new, quantitative easily applicable method. *J Rheumatol* 1995; **20**: 473–7.

Strongwater SL, Dorovin-Zis K, Bell RD *et al*. A murine model of polymyositis induced by Coxsackie B1 (Tuscan strain). *Arthritis Rheum* 1984; **27**: 433–42.

Symmons DPM, Sills JA, Davis SM. The incidence of juvenile dermatomyositis: results from a nation-wide study. *Br J Rheumatol* 1995; **43**: 732–5.

Tam PE, Schmidt AM, Ytterberg SR *et al*. Duration of viral persistence and its relationship to inflammation in the chronic phase of coxsackie virus B1-induced murine polymyositis. *J Lab Clin Med* 1994; **123**: 346–56.

Tami LF, Bhasin S. Polymorphism of the cardiac manifestations in dermatomyositis. *Clin Cardiol* 1993; **16**: 260–4.

Targoff IN. Polymyositis and dermatomyositis in adults. In: eds *Oxford Textbook of Rheumatology*, 2nd edn, Maddison PJ, Isenberg DA, Woo P, Glass DN. Oxford University Press, Oxford, 1997; **8**: 1249–87.

Taylor AJ, Wortham DC, Burge JR *et al*. The heart in polymyositis: a prospective evaluation of 26 patients. *Clin Cardiol* 1993; **16**: 802–8.

Tazelaar HD, Viggiano RW, Pickersgill J *et al*. Interstitial lung disease in polymyositis and dermatomyositis. *Am Rev Respir Dis* 1990; **141**: 727–33.

Tsuji K, Aizawa M, Sasazuki T (eds). *HLA 1991. Proceedings of the Eleventh International Histocompatibility Work-shop and Conference*, held in Yokohama, Japan, 6–13 November, 1991. Oxford University Press, New York, 1992.

Uchino M, ArakiS, Yoshino O *et al*. High single dose alternate day corticosteroid regimens in treatment of polymyositis. *J Neurol* 1985; **232**: 175–8.

Villalba L, Hicks JE, Adams EM *et al*. Treatment of refractory myositis: a randomized crossover study of two new cytotoxic regimens. *Arthritis Rheum* 1998; **41**: 392–9.

Wang YJ, Lii YP, Lan JI *et al*. Juvenile and adult dermatomyositis among Chinese: a comparative study. *Chinese Medical Journal (Taipei)* 1993; **52**: 285–92.

Wells AV, duBois RM, Bronchiolitis in association with connective tissue disorders. *Clin Chest Med* 1993; **14**: 655–60.

Worrall JG, Phongsathorn V, Hooper RJL *et al*. Racial variation in serum creatine kinase unrelated to lean body mass. *Br J Rheumatol* 1990; **29**: 371–3.

Yanagisawa T, Sueski M, Nawata Y *et al*. Methylprednisolone pulse therapy iondermatomyositis. *Dermatologia* 1983; **167**: 47–51.

Yousef GE, Isenberg DA, Mowbray JF. Detection of enterovirus specific RNA sequences in muscle biopsy specimens from patients with adult onset myositis. *Ann Rheum Dis* 1990; **49**: 310–5.

8 | *Scleroderma*

Introduction

Scleroderma encompasses a spectrum of disorders that range from localized forms such as morphoea with limited cutaneous involvement, which may involve the internal organs after long periods, to diffuse cutaneous disease invariably accompanied by early internal organ involvement.

Milestones in the history of scleroderma

1753   Curzio from Naples provided what was probably the first good description of an authentic case.

1836   Giovanni Fantonetti used the term 'skleroderma' in describing a woman with an uncertain dermatosis.

1842–1846   Chowne and Startin, from London, described more typical cases.

1847   Forget first described joint involvement in scleroderma.

1862   Maurice Raynaud (Paris) described the phenomenon that bears his name.

1883   Auspitz in Vienna first described death owing to renal failure.

1876   Westphal noted skeletal muscle involvement in scleroderma.

1878   Weber first described calcinosis.

1899   Hutchison (London) linked Raynaud's phenomenon and systemic sclerosis.

1903   Ehrmann (Vienna) suggested that dysphagia is due to scleroderma involving the oesophagus.

1910   Thibierge and Weissenbach (Paris) established the link between calcinosis and scleroderma.

1914   Bramwell linked silica exposure to scleroderma development — the first environmental association.

1943   Soma Weiss detailed cardiac involvement in scleroderma.

1964   Winterbauer first suggested the existence of a CREST subset (calcinosis, Raynaud's, oesaphagitis, sclerodactyly, and telangiectasia).

1970s   Identification of the disease-specific, anti-nucleolar, anti-Scl-70, and anti-centromere antibodies.

1980s   Scl-70 antigen shown to be topoisomerase I.
         Use of ACE-inhibitor to control high blood pressure in patients with renal involvement.

Clinical features

The skin changes of scleroderma are characterized by induration, abnormalities of the capillaries, arterioles and small blood vessels, and fibrosis. There is excessive

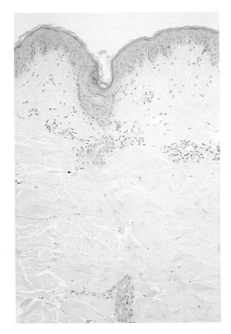

Fig. 8.1. Excessive collagen deposition in the skin is the hallmark of scleroderma.

Table 8.1 Prevalence (%) of Raynaud's phenomenon in autoimmune rheumatic diseases

Rheumatoid arthritis	< 5
Systemic lupus erythematosus	20–30
Sjögren's syndrome	20–50
Myositis	20–40
Scleroderma	> 95

deposition of collagen in the skin and internal organs (Fig. 8.1). In the small arteries, endothelial cell proliferation and mucoid deposition and the appearance of fine collagen fibres in the intima are found. The arterioles may develop intimal sclerosis, fibrinoid change, and necrosis. Blood vessels, including skin capillaries, atrophy and their numbers may be severely depleted. These changes may be observed using nail-fold capillaroscopy, newer techniques for which are now being described (Kabasakal *et al.* 1996).

The diagnosis of scleroderma should be doubted in the absence of Raynaud's phenomenon. This condition, described by the French clinician Maurice Raynaud in 1862, is characterized by episodic, clearly demarcated, two or three phase colour change of the fingers, and sometimes the toes (less commonly the nose, tongue, or ears) in response to the cold or, less often, to emotion (Fig. 8.2). The initial colour change is to white (because of ischaemia), then often to blue (owing to stasis), and finally to red (reactive hyperaemia). Raynaud's phenomenon occurs in up to 5% of an otherwise healthy population. Over 90% of patients with Raynaud's phenomenon are female. At the time of presentation they are often aged under 25. Up to 5% of patients presenting with the condition eventually develop an autoimmune rheumatic disease. The prevalence of Raynaud's phenomenon in these diseases is shown in Table 8.1.

Epidemiology

Scleroderma is more common among women, with a female predominance of 4:1 overall and in the child-bearing years of up to 15:1. It has a peak onset between 30 and 50 years of age and it is estimated to occur in 2–12 individuals per million per year (Medsger and Masi 1971). A more recent estimate of the incidence of morphoea (localized scleroderma) stated a figure of 27 per 1 000 000 population (Peterson *et al.* 1997). The prevalence in this study at 80 years of age was about 2 in 1000. In contrast, the incidence of hospital-diagnosed scleroderma among residents of Pittsburgh and Allegheny County, USA (1963–1982), has been reported as 13.9 per million. Black women had the highest incidence (21.2 per million) and overall the disease was rare in men under 35 and in children (Steen *et al.* 1997). Scleroderma is found in virtually all climates and racial groups (Laing *et al.* 1997).

Clinical subsets

The major subsets of scleroderma are known as 'limited cutaneous' and 'diffuse cutaneous'. The major

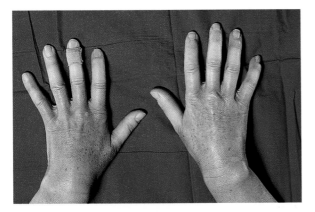

Fig. 8.2. Raynaud's phenomenon seen in a patient with scleroderma.

Table 8.2   Major subsets of scleroderma

Limited cutaneous scleroderma

 Raynaud's phenomenon for years (sometimes decades) before the start of the skin involvement.

 Skin involvement is limited to the hands, face, feet, and forearms.

 Many patients develop pulmonary hypertension (after 10 years or more) which may be accompanied by interstitial lung disease, trigeminal neuralgia, skin calcifications, telangiectasia.

 Anti-centromere antibodies (in 70–80%).

 Dilated nailfold capillary loops usually without capillary drop-out.

Diffuse cutaneous scleroderma

 Skin changes (puffy or hidebound) within one year of the onset of Raynaud's phenomenon.

 Skin involvement of trunk and extremities.

 Tendon friction rubs.

 Early and significant incidence of interstitial lung disease, renal failure, diffuse gastrointestinal disease, and myocardial involvement.

 Anti-topoisomerase (Scl-70) antibodies in 30% of patients.

 Dilated nailfold capillary loops and capillary drop-out.

---

features of these conditions are shown in Table 8.2 and Fig. 8.3.

Limited cutaneous scleroderma

Patients with limited cutaneous scleroderma [which is akin to the previously used acronym CREST — calcinosis, Raynaud's, (o)esophagitis, sclerodactyly, telangiectasia — subgrouping] (see Fig. 8.3) have invariably developed Raynaud's phenomenon (which is often relatively mild) many years before the skin disease is evident. They are susceptible to the development of pulmonary hypertension which may be lethal, though this is usually 10 years or more after the skin changes appear. These patients often have relatively stable, non-progressive disease, albeit associated with calcium deposits in the skin, painful digital scars and ulcers, dilated blood vessels (telangiectasia), and oesophageal dysmotility and reflux. There are few, if any, constitutional symptoms and skin fibrosis is often restricted to sclerodactyly and microstomia with little progression. Although the swelling of the ends of the fingers may be of relatively little concern, unsightly puckering, wrinkling, and tightening of the skin around the mouth are more troublesome.

In those patients in whom internal organ disease does develop, as indicated above, pulmonary hypertension can be prominent and associated with pulmonary interstitial disease. There may also be significant involvement of the gastrointestinal tract. The anti-centromere antibody is present in up to 80% of patients with the limited cutaneous variant of the disease.

Diffuse cutaneous scleroderma

This more serious condition usually develops within weeks or months of the onset of Raynaud's phenomenon, which may be severe. It is associated with marked oedematous change in the fingers, hands, and face. The skin may also be itchy. During the first few years of this variant the patients often complain of fatigue and weight loss. Internal organ involvement (see Table 8.3) is particularly common in the lung and gastrointestinal tract. Less often renal, articular, and muscle involvement is present. These patients require regular reassessment of end-organ involvement.

The thickening of the skin, which invariably appears first in the fingers or toes, spreads rapidly up the limbs and/or on to the trunk, usually within a matter of months. A number of different scoring systems have been proposed to assess skin thickness in patients with scleroderma (Silman *et al.* 1995). Involvement of the face leads to a pinched, taut expression round the mouth as the normal skin folds disappear. It may become increasingly difficult to open the mouth to eat solid food. Hyperpigmentation and hypopigmentation may occur, the latter being more obvious in non-white patients. Rapid progression of skin disease may be accompanied by renal failure (presenting as hypertensive renal crisis) as well as pulmonary interstitial and early cardiac disease.

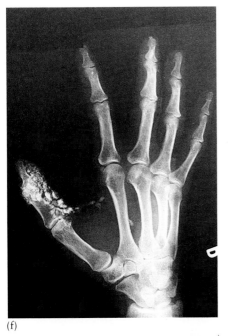

(f)

Fig. 8.3. Major clinical features of scleroderma. (a) 'Tight-lipped' appearance and telangiectasia of a patient with scleroderma affecting the face. (b) Flat, 'featureless' bowel with loss of the normal haustral pattern, which signifies scleroderma affecting the large bowel. (c) Gangrene affecting the fingers in a patient with scleroderma. (d) Gangrene affecting the toes. (e) Morphoea affecting the thigh. (f) Calcinosis seen on X-ray in a patient with long-standing scleroderma.

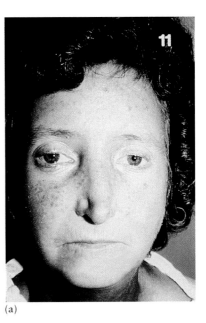

(a)

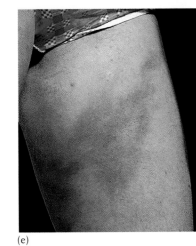

(e)

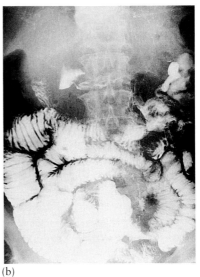

(b)

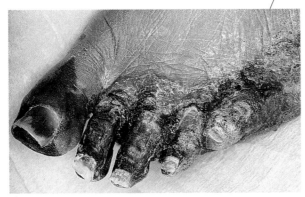

(d)

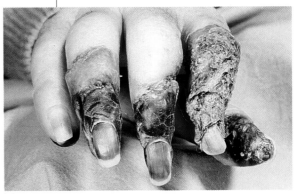

(c)

Table 8.3 Internal organ involvement in scleroderma

Organ	Clinical feature
Gastrointestinal tract	
Oesophagus	Hypomobility and incompetence of the lower oesophageal sphincter leading to: dysphagia, hiatus hernia, stricture.
Duodenum	Duodenal/jejunal hypomobility leading to malabsorption.
Colon	Hypomobility, wide-mouth sacculations leading to constipation.
Lungs	Cough and dyspnoea on exertion.
	Pleurisy and pleural effusion.
	Pulmonary hypertension + cor pulmonale.
	Diffuse interstitial lung disease + bronchitis.
Heart	Pericarditis/pericardial effusion
	Secondary effect from lung involvement, notably right heart failure.
Muscle	Myositis.
Joints	Symmetrical, non-erosive (usually), seronegative polyarthropathy.
Kidney	Increasing thickness of blood vessel walls leading to proteinuria, hypertension, and if severe to acute–chronic renal failure.
Nervous system	Peripheral neuropathy.
	Trigeminal neuralgia.

Approximately five years after the onset of this type of scleroderma, the constitutional symptoms of fatigue and weight loss begin to subside. The so-called 'atrophic' phase which follows may last for many years, with the musculoskeletal problems leading to deformity and wasting. The internal organ disease often progresses, although the risk of new organs being affected is reduced. Auto-antibodies to Scl-70 (topoisomerase-I) are characteristically present in about 30% of this subgroup (see later).

Internal organ involvement

The gastrointestinal tract is frequently affected in scleroderma (both diffuse and so-called limited). The lower end of the oesophagus is a particularly common site for involvement, with the fibrosis leading to hypomotility, and acid reflux from the stomach causing ulceration, hiatus hernia, and stricture.

Although less common, small bowel disease can be troublesome. When it does occur, patients often complain of frequent loose motions, which are associated with malabsorption that in turn leads to significant weight loss and cachexia. Poorly functioning small bowel encourages bacterial overgrowth which may be linked to the malabsorption and is very difficult to manage.

Loss of tone and hypomobility of the large bowel (Fig. 8.3b), rectum, and sigmoid colon, can lead to either constipation or anal incontinence. Management is difficult and on occasion surgical removal of non-functioning large bowel has been attempted, with unpredictable results.

Cardiopulmonary disease

Pulmonary disease is probably second only to oesophageal involvement in the frequency of internal organ manifestations of scleroderma. With the significant improvement in the management of end-stage renal disease, pulmonary involvement is now associated with the greatest risk of mortality in patients with diffuse disease. Altmann *et al.* (1990) reported a median survival of 78 months in those with diffuse skin disease and pulmonary involvement, but lacking cardiac or renal disease. Fibrosing alveolitis and pulmonary vascular disease are the most common clinical manifestations. The interstitial lung disease presents clinically with a combination of breathlessness and a dry cough. The occurrence of interstitial lung disease is poorly correlated with the type of skin involvement (Kane *et al.* 1996). Pleuritic pain and haemoptysis are much less common; indeed, the presence of the latter should encourage a search for an alternative diagnosis, including neoplasm. The most common clinical sign on examination is bilateral basal crepitations.

On X-ray, patients with lung involvement may show evidence of reticulonodular shadowing, especially at the lung bases (Fig. 8.4), but pulmonary function tests are a far more sensitive way of detecting early lung involvement. The diffusing capacity (DL_{co}) is the most sensitive early change reflecting early decreased lung

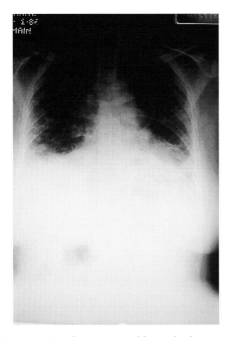

Fig. 8.4. Lung involvement notably at the bases seen on X-ray.

compliance and ventilatory volumes. Subsequently, total lung capacity, vital capacity, and forced vital capacity may also fall, and occasionally patients may demonstrate an obstructive pattern of disease.

Fine cut, high resolution, computerized tomographic (CT) scanning of the lung is now widely available and frequently used to determine whether pulmonary disease is present. An early finding of interstitial lung disease is the peripheral presence of high attenuation in the lower lobes. Another early feature is the presence of reticulonodular appearances, which later change to larger cystic air spaces. These scans may also confirm the presence of pleural involvement or mediastinal lymphadenopathy. Harrison *et al.* (1989) showed that over 40% of patients with scleroderma who had been reported to have a normal chest X-ray had detectable abnormalities on CT scan.

Other investigations widely used in patients who have lung disease include bronchoalveolar lavage (BAL) and lung biopsy. BAL is used to demonstrate the presence of active inflammation of the lower respiratory tract with the presence of abnormal numbers of granulocytes, notably neutrophils and eosinophils. Active alveolitis, as identified by BAL, is associated with progressive pulmonary disease (Behr *et al.* 1996). Histological abnormalities include fibrosis of the interstitium, alveolar septae, and bronchial walls, accompanied by congestion of capillaries with oedema. Small blood vessels frequently show concentric intimal proliferation, perivascular fibrosis causing lumen narrowing, and a proliferation of vessels. A severe vasculopathy is very likely to lead to pulmonary hypertension in due course.

Cardiac involvement in scleroderma is not clinically as apparent as lung disease. However, a variety of symptoms, including dyspnoea, arrhythmias, orthopnoea, oedema, palpitations, and chest pains may be ascribed to the disease, although hard on occasion to distinguish from renal or lung involvement. In a detailed prospective study of 63 patients using Doppler echocardiography, thallium-201 perfusion scintigraphy, and radionucleotide venticulography it was concluded that although the frequency of cardiovascular symptoms was low in scleroderma (limited form) a significant rate of abnormalities is detectable by non-invasive techniques (Candell-Riera *et al.* 1996). Post-mortem examinations have reported myocardial fibrosis in up to 70% of patients, compared with 37% in the control group (Follansbee *et al.* 1990). True myocardial fibrosis, according to Weiss *et al.* (1943), who first described it, occurs in random patchy areas and is associated with a so-called contraction band necrosis. It has been proposed that this scarring may be the consequence of Raynaud's phenomenon affecting the small myocardial vessels, thus causing repeated ischaemic changes with reperfusion.

Pericardial effusion is a well-recognized cardiac complication and on occasions the effusions may be substantial. However, the cause of greatest concern is the development of pulmonary hypertension which, paradoxically, is more frequently seen in patients with the so-called limited cutaneous involvement. It is usually secondary to interstitial lung disease, associated clinically with shortness of breath, an increased pulmonary second heart sound, and a marked decrease in diffusing capacity for carbon monoxide (to less than half of that seen in healthy individuals). As might be anticipated, the pulmonary arteries show intimal and medial hyperplasia. The condition carries a very poor prognosis.

Musculoskeletal system

Perhaps one-fifth of patients with scleroderma have a form of myopathy with rather mild weakness and wasting of muscles, a marginal rise in the creatine phosphokinase, and histological features that, while lacking significant inflammatory change, do show some focal replacement of myofibres with collagen and an increase in perimysial and epimysial fibrosis. Much less frequently, a true myositis is present. A useful indication is the presence of antibodies to the PM-Scl antigen (see Chapter 7, Table 7.5). The myopathy requires no specific treatment, but true myositis occurring in the context of scleroderma should be treated no differently from the primary disease (see Chapter 7).

A relatively mild, non-erosive, symmetrical arthritis is noted in a minority of patients with scleroderma. Fibrosis in the tendons, ligaments, joint capsule, and, rarely, in the synovium itself, are the cause of the stiff and painful hands that may be seen in these patients. Tendon friction rubs can be heard and felt. Recently, a subset of patients who fulfil the criteria for RA and scleroderma has been identified (Misra *et al.* 1995). These patients tend to show limited skin involvement but are positive for both rheumatoid factor and anti-centromere antibodies.

Renal disease

Significant renal involvement in scleroderma invariably presents within five years of the onset of the disease. It has long been recognized (Kovalchik *et al.* 1978) that epithelial and endothelial renal lesions are demonstrable before either fibrosis occurs or there is clinical evidence of renal disease.

Proteinuria, hypertension, and impaired glomerular filtration rate are markers of renal involvement, though the prevalence of 50% suggested by autopsy cases is considerably more than the 10–20% of patients suspected of having significant renal involvement during life.

A well-recognized pattern of renal involvement is the development of acute or subacute renal hypertensive crisis. Traub *et al.* (1984) have suggested a set of criteria to diagnose a scleroderma renal crisis (shown in Table 8.4). Renal histology confirms the intimal thickening of the small and medium sized arteries with lumenal occlusion, fibrinoid necrosis, and periadventitial fibrosis (Fig. 8.5).

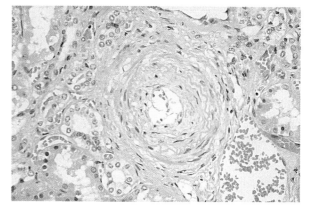

Fig. 8.5. Intimal thickening of a medium size renal artery leading to lumenal occlusion; with periadventitial fibrosis.

In common with the other features of scleroderma, it has proved difficult to prevent the development of the pathological changes seen in the kidney, but the great advances in the management of the consequences of renal damage, notably new and more effective anti-hypertensive drugs, improved dialysis facilities, and renal transplantation, have meant a greatly improved outlook for patients with renal involvement.

Nervous system

Involvement of the nervous system is relatively uncommon in scleroderma, but a potential set of clinical features includes trigeminal neuralgia, carpal tunnel syndrome, peripheral neuropathy (involving both the sensory and motor nerves), autonomic neuropathy, and very rarely a subacute combined degeneration of the cord. The last of these features is usually secondary to small bowel involvement.

Other subsets

A small group of patients have the typical organ involvement of scleroderma on occasions with an

Table 8.4   Criteria to diagnose scleroderma renal crisis

- Abrupt onset of arterial hypertension > 160/90 mmHg
- Hypertensive retinopathy of grade III severity
- Rapid deterioration of renal function and elevated plasma renin activity

Other features include

- Microangiopathic haemolytic blood film
- Hypertensive encephalopathy leading to convulsions

accompanying Raynaud's phenomenon and typical autoantibodies, but without any skin changes. This group is known rather confusingly as scleroderma *sine* scleroderma!

Morphoea is a form of localized scleroderma occurring at any age and virtually any site. It seems to spare skin with apocrine glands such as the vulva and breast nipples. It may begin as small discrete areas of erythematous or violaceous skin (guttate morphoea). Subsequently, larger areas may become involved (morphoea *en plaque*). However, it can present with large plaques of affected skin. The lesions may evolve to become thickened, sclerotic, and waxy coloured. Central depigmentation and peripheral hyperpigmentation (or vice versa) can develop and persist. Some patches may heal spontaneously but others undergo a considerable dissemination involving the trunk and extremities (generalized morphoea).

Scleroderma in childhood

Scleroderma is found rarely in childhood (DeNardo *et al.* 1994). It shows no racial predilection and has a male:female ratio of approximately 1:3 (Singsen 1986). No significant familial incidence has been reported. As in adult cases, disease expression is heterogeneous but localized forms are common in children (Vancheeswaran *et al.* 1996) among whom a significant association with trauma was also noted. Localized scleroderma in children exists in three major forms: morphea, linear scleroderma, and 'en coup de sabre'. 'En coup de sabre' is a variant of linear scleroderma on the face or scalp, which may cause a most unpleasant form of hemiatrophy of the head, potentially extending to the trunk and extremities (David *et al.* 1991). Morphoea varies from a few circumscribed plaque-like lesions to a far more generalized form. Linear scleroderma is usually uni-

lateral, crossing joint lines and leading to contractures. The inflammation and fibrosis impair development and growth, leading to inequality in limb length and fixed deformities in the hand and foot. In addition, vascular deformities of the brain have been observed in this form.

Diffuse cutaneous systemic sclerosis is essentially the same as the adult disease, frequently presenting with Raynaud's phenomenon, arthritis or arthralgia, and internal organ involvement. Among the relatively few children with systemic sclerosis, gastrointestinal involvement has a tendency to be more widespread than in adults and pulmonary disease is almost inevitable. Renal involvement occurs in approximately half of these childhood cases, often presenting with severe hypertension. In contrast with adult diseases, normal levels of vascular activation, T cell activation, and collagen synthesis have been recorded in children with scleroderma who also, in general, lack anti-centromere antibodies (Vancheeswaran *et al.* 1996).

Conditions resembling scleroderma

Many chemicals and drugs can induce a disorder resembling idiopathic scleroderma (see Table 8.5). A particularly tragic example is that of the contaminated rape-seed oil, sold as cooking oil in part of Madrid in the early 1980s. In an epidemic affecting approximately 20 000 people, a denaturing contaminant, aniline, was implicated as the causative agent. The ensuing illness occurred in two phases. The first acute phase consisted of fever, rash, gastrointestinal upset, neurological features, and acute interstitial pneumonia. Those who survived this phase were later found to develop indurated, thickened skin, Raynaud's phenomenon, dysphagia, pulmonary hypertension, alopecia, dryness of mouth, arthritis, and flexion contractures

Table 8.5 Chemicals and drugs that have been linked to scleroderma

Agent	Examples
Chemicals	
Plastics	e.g. polyvinyl chloride, epoxy resins
Solvents	e.g. trichloroethylene, perchloroethylene, trichloroethene, benzene, toluene, zylene
Drugs	Bleomycin
	L-5-Hydroxytryptophan
	Pentazocine
	Certain appetite suppressants, e.g. mazindol, fenfluramine
	Carbidopa
Others	Silica
	'Contaminated' rape-seed oil

(Spurzem and Lockley 1984). It is thought that over 800 people succumbed to the condition.

Although Bramwell (1914) was the first to link scleroderma to an environmental factor (silica exposure in stone masons), vinyl chloride (VC) disease and bleomycin-induced scleroderma are perhaps the best known examples of this type. Both are associated with increased synthesis of collagen by dermal fibroblasts, as occurs in idiopathic disease. Similar vascular and nailfold capillary changes have also been found in VC disease. The presence of raised serum immunoglobulin levels and immunoglobulin complement and fibrinogen deposits in the blood vessel walls of patients with this condition underlines its similarity with the naturally occurring scleroderma. Unlike the idiopathic disease, however, patients with VC disease lack the classical anti-centromere and anti-Scl-70 antibodies. Nevertheless, it has been suggested that VC exposure, especially in genetically predisposed individuals, can induce an immune complex disease. This leads to vascular occlusion, ischaemia, and fibrosis.

Eosinophilic fasciitis is a condition whose dermatological features resemble systemic sclerosis. The inflammation and induration of the skin and subcutaneous tissues are found mostly on the hands, forearms, feet, and legs. Eosinophilia and hypergammaglobulinaemia are usually found in the blood, and large numbers of lymphocytes, plasma cells, eosinophils, and histiocytes are present in the affected tissues. Raynaud's phenomenon and involvement of the internal organs are notably absent. Evidence has been presented that IgG mast cell-dependent eosinophil cytotoxicity may be an important immunopathological mechanism in this disease. Unlike systemic sclerosis a low dose of corticosteroids will often provide satisfactory treatment.

The eosinophilia–myalgia syndrome (EMS) is thought to be caused by L-tryptophan which was available 'over the counter' as a treatment for insomnia and depression (Silver 1991). Several thousand people are thought to have suffered from this condition. Its initial symptoms were those of arthralgia, shortness of breath, and severe myalgia. Erythematous macules appeared on the trunk and limbs with significant swelling of the skin. The laboratory features include a significant peripheral eosinophilia and, curiously, a raised serum aldolase in the presence of a relatively normal creatine kinase. Peripheral neuropathy and neurocognitive dysfunction are relatively common. A link has been established with contamination by 1,1-ethylidene, with bis (L-tryptophan) detected by high performance liquid chromatography in batches of contaminated L-tryptophan. Steroids may provide some relief of these symptoms but the condition may well become chronic. There has been a heated debate in the past decade as to whether silicone breast implants are likely to induce autoimmune conditions, including scleroderma. As larger, better controlled studies have been published the claimed association had won increasingly less support. Thus, in a study of 837 women with scleroderma compared with 2507 race-matched controls, no significant association between such implants and scleroderma was found (Hochberg *et al.* 1996). An even larger study of 7442 women with implants for cosmetic reasons or for reconstruction after surgery for breast cancer also concluded that there was no evidence to link breast implants and scleroderma (and/or other autoimmune rheumatic diseases (Nyrén *et al.* 1998)).

Survivors of human allogeneic bone marrow transplantation are prone to a condition called chronic graft-versus-host disease (GVH) which resembles both systemic sclerosis and Sjögren's syndrome. The patients may develop thickened skin with contractures, ulceration, gastrointestinal involvement, and, less commonly, pulmonary disease and myositis. Very rarely, renal glomerular disease with irregular thickened laminae, intimal thickening of arcuate and interlobular arteries, mesangial sclerosis, and hypercellularity (all features described in the kidneys of patients with scleroderma) have been found in GVH disease Immunological investigations of GVH disease have frequently demonstrated hypergammaglobulinaemia and autoantibodies. Decreased suppressor T cell activity is evident and IgM and complement have been found along the dermal/epidermal junction of the affected skin. In a study of autoantibodies associated with this condition, Bell *et al.* (1996) reported that four patients with GVH that they studied had antibodies to Scl-70 and two had antibodies against PM-Scl, which are generally regarded as characteristic of idiopathic scleroderma (see later). The development of scleroderma after bone marrow transplantation is seen with increasing frequency, the greater the degree of mismatch between donor and recipient.

Immunopathology of scleroderma

Autoantibodies associated with Raynaud's phenomenon and scleroderma

Patients presenting with Raynaud's phenomenon who are found to have anti-nuclear antibodies should be

Table 8.6 Autoantibodies in scleroderma

Antibody	Antigen/molecular characteristics	IF pattern	Clinical association
Anti-Scl-70	Topoisomerase-I (100 kDa enzyme in the nucleolus)	Nuclear (diffuse, fine, speckled)	Present in ≃ 30% of diffuse cutaneous scleroderma
Anti-centromere	Conserved protein in kinetochore of metaphase chromosomes (17, 18, 140 kDa)	Centromere	Present in up to 80% of limited cutaneous scleroderma
Anti-nucleolar	RNA polymerase I, II, or III (complex set of proteins 12.5–210 kDa)	Nucleolar	Present in up to 25% of diffuse cutaneous scleroderma
	Fibrillarin (34 kDa protein component of U3 RNP)		Marker for severe disease
Anti-PM-Scl	Complex of 11 proteins (20–110 kDa)	Nucleolar	Usually associated with scleroderma/myositis overlap
Anti-mitochondrial M2	70 kDa protein (dihydrolipoamide acetyltransferase)	Cytoplasmic (rod-like)	Present in up to 95% of patients with primary biliary cirrhosis; in up to 25% of those with limited cutaneous scleroderma

IF = immunofluorescence

followed up carefully as these are the patients most likely to develop an autoimmune disease. Kallenberg *et al.* (1988) in a prospective study confirmed this observation and suggested that the evolution to an autoimmune rheumatic disease was usually towards scleroderma. In addition, the presence of an anti-centromere antibody had a predictive value for the development of limited systemic sclerosis (sensitivity 60%, specificity 98%) and anti-Scl-70 for diffuse systemic sclerosis (sensitivity 38%, specificity 100%). In addition, from our own observations patients with anti-nucleolar antibodies are also those most likely to go on and develop scleroderma.

A variety of autoantibodies have now been associated with scleroderma (see Table 8.6). Anti-Scl-70 antibodies are actually binding a 100 kDa DNA topoisomerase-I protein. This is an enzyme involved in uncoiling DNA prior to replication. It is localized to the nucleolus [as are other enzymes that are targeted by antibodies in patients with scleroderma, notably RNA polymerase I, II, and III (fibrillarin and others)]. Anti-centromere antibodies appear to react with a conserved protein localized at the kinetochore structure of the metaphase chromosomes. The presence of anti-centromere antibodies is strongly associated with an absence of interstitial lung disease (Kane *et al.* 1996). Anticentromere antibodies and anti Scl-70 are useful in diagnosing and classifying scleroderma variants and in

predicting the natural course of the disease (Steer *et al.* 1988). In contrast, anti-U3 RNP antibodies have been linked to severe pulmonary hypertension in patients with diffuse scleroderma (Black and Denton 1998). The details and clinical associations of the most common autoantibodies reported in patients with scleroderma are indicated in Table 8.6. Among others that have been described, Sato *et al.* (1995) have proposed that there may be a link between anti-histone antibodies and severe pulmonary fibrosis in patients with diffuse scleroderma. Approximately 30% of patients with scleroderma have antibodies to epitopes on native and/or heat-denatured collagens, types I, II, IV, and V (Riente *et al.* 1995).

Routine laboratory tests

The erythrocyte sedimentation rate (ESR) is slightly raised in up to two-thirds of patients. Some have a mild normochromic, normocytic anaemia. Erythrocytes from patients with systemic sclerosis show slightly increased rigidity and adherence and this may play a role in the mechanism of vascular abnormalities and disease. Rarely, a haemolytic anaemia has been described.

Where renal disease becomes evident, the plasma creatinine and urea rise, while the creatinine clearance falls. Liver function tests usually remain normal.

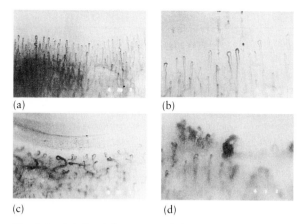

Fig. 8.6. (a) Top left (× 21) and (b) top right (× 35) show normal distribution of capillary blood vessels in the nail bed. In contrast, (c) bottom left (× 26) and (d) bottom right, patients with scleroderma show fewer capillaries which are larger, dilated, and of irregular form and give rise to telangiectasia. Photographs courtesy of Francis Lefford.

Capillary microscopy is also more widely available and provides a simple way of determining whether the capillary blood vessels in the nail beds are abnormal, as is invariably the case in patients with scleroderma (Fig. 8.6).

Histological changes

Skin biopsies from patients with systemic sclerosis show a marked increase in the collagen fibres found mostly in the normal dermis, type I and type III collagen, associated with hyalinization and obliteration of the small blood vessels (see Fig. 8.1). There is also loss of the normal dermal appendages and thinning of the epidermis. In the skin of patients with systemic sclerosis, the upper dermis appears to be composed of normal 'mature' collagen. The lower dermis and subcutaneous tissues are replaced by more immature forms. Electron microscopic examination of the skin confirms the presence of many narrow-calibre collagen fibres. There are also double-stranded beaded filaments identical to those found in embryonic, although not in normal adult, skin.

Mononuclear cell infiltrates are found in the dermis of about 50% of untreated cases. They consist mostly of activated T lymphocytes with an increased ratio of CD4:CD8 cells (2:1 approximately) owing to a decrease in the CD8[+] T cells (Roumm *et al.* 1984).

The calcification, either intra- or subcutaneous, seen in some patients with systemic sclerosis, is due to the deposition of calcium hydroxyapatite. The cause is

uncertain, though a local abnormality in the affected tissues rather than a generalized problem of calcium metabolism is likely.

The range of vascular features found in patients with systemic sclerosis, including Raynaud's phenomenon, digital pitting, ulceration, and gangrene is reflected by many pathological changes. These predominate in the small arteries and arterioles. There is a marked proliferation of endothelial cells leading to intimal thickening. Endothelial cells normally provide a lining function for all blood vessels. In addition, glycosaminoglycan deposition is found, together with fibrinogen or fibrin. The blood vessels may be surrounded by fibrous tissues and/or the type of mononuclear cell infiltrates described above. The lumen of the blood vessel may become occluded and replaced by fibrosis. The blood vessels then atrophy and their numbers may be severely depleted (see Fig. 8.6). Those that remain may dilate and become visible in the skin as telangiectases.

Histological abnormalities within the internal organs are broadly similar to those found in the skin. Up to 90% of patients with systemic sclerosis may show microscopic renal changes, although the number with the clinical features of kidney disease is less than half. Cortical scarring may be observed. The most marked vascular changes in the cortex are usually found in the interlobular arteries in the efferent arterials. The changes include fibromucoid intimal thickening, which results in narrowing of the lumen, focal thinning of the lumen, and occasionally adventitial fibrosis (see Fig. 8.5). Thrombotic inclusions of small arteries and arterioles may also be found. Glomerular involvement is usually focal with various abnormalities, including endothelial cell proliferation and thickening of the basement membrane. The kidney tubules, epithelial degeneration and regeneration, and necrotizing vascular lesions have been described. Interstitial fibrosis is found with a frequency that reflects the duration of the disease.

Within the lungs of patients with systemic sclerosis, interstitial fibrosis is the most commonly found histological abnormality. Usually the lesions consist of an increased number of fibroblasts, capillary congestion, and an increased elastic content of the alveolar walls. Subsequently, increasing collagen deposition causes an increased separation of capillaries from the alveoli. The intima of the arterioles becomes thickened and occlusion of both pulmonary and bronchiolar vessels can occur. Arteriolar thickening is often associated with pulmonary hypertension.

The whole of the gastrointestinal tract is prone to varying degrees of replacement of the submucosa, muscularis, and serosal layers by densely hyalinized fibrous connective tissue. At the lower end of the oesophagus there is a particular tendency for smooth muscle to atrophy and to be replaced by fibrous tissue. In the early stages of the disease, as in other organs, a mononuclear cell infiltrate is found. As indicated earlier in this chapter, chest X-ray, fine cut, high resolution CT scanning, bronchiolar lavage, and lung biopsy are used routinely to assess the extent of the disease.

Within the myocardium, random, focal fibrosis is found in about half of the patients. Interestingly, despite the relatively high incidence of conduction defects described clinically, the conducting tissue is not usually found to have histological abnormalities. The conduction disturbances may thus be the consequence of damage to functioning myocardium. The small coronary blood vessels are usually not affected by the process of systemic sclerosis.

Variable inflammatory and fibrotic changes in the synovial tissue are present in most patients. Lymphocytes and plasma cells may form small aggregates or be scattered diffusely throughout the synovium. These inflammatory changes have been linked to the presence of rheumatoid factor in the serum. This is found both in the serum and synovial fluid in about one-third of patients with systemic sclerosis, usually in low titre. In the absence of rheumatoid factor, moderate or dense fibrosis with little mononuclear cell infiltration is found. As elsewhere, small blood vessel changes consisting of thickened walls and lumenal obliteration may occur. In addition, a notable deposition of fibrin within the synovium has been described. It seems likely that active collagen production occurs in the synovium.

In the terminal phalanges, subcutaneous calcification may occur. Less frequently, an unexplained osteoporosis or even complete resorption occurs. Rarely, this loss of bone substance may extend proximally.

Within the skeletal muscle the most frequently recorded abnormalities are the interstitial and perivascular fibrosis, interstitial and perivascular inflammatory infiltrates, myofibre atrophy, necrosis, and degeneration. Generally, however, the inflammatory changes are much less marked than the polymyositis, although, as discussed in Chapter 9, the two conditions may overlap.

Outcome

The diversity of clinical features in patients with scleroderma has made it difficult to provide accurate mor-

bidity and mortality figures for these patients overall. As indicated from the foregoing sections, morbidity may be significant, particularly from the patients with diffuse disease. Abu-Shakra and Lee (1995) compared the mortality rate in patients with scleroderma with that of the general population. They applied standardized mortality ratios for 230 patients with scleroderma, followed prospectively using sex-specific mortality rates in Ontario for a 14-year period, from 1976. They showed that the mortality rate is increased compared with that of the general population, particularly in the subset with diffuse disease. Although the disease itself, especially where the kidneys and lungs are involved, may be directly responsible for death, other possible causes include side-effects of the drugs sometimes used to treat it. There has also been a suggestion of an increased risk of cancer among patients with systemic sclerosis (Rosenthal *et al.* 1995). These authors analysed patients in Sweden with a discharge diagnosis of systemic sclerosis or localized scleroderma from a database distinguishing hospital discharges for the years 1965–1993. In all, 917 patients with systemic sclerosis, and 102 with localized scleroderma were identified. Using a form of record linkage analysis with the Swedish National Cancer Registry, the authors showed a standardized incidence ratio (the ratio of observed to expected incidence) for the patients with diffuse systemic sclerosis of 1.5, with specific cancer risks for lung cancer, non-melanoma skin cancers, and primary liver disease. In contrast, cancer risks in the similarly ascertained patients with localized scleroderma were no different from those in the general population.

Immunogenetics

HLA associations with scleroderma and scleroderma-related autoantibodies

Many studies of HLA antigens in patients with scleroderma, particularly early studies, have used the classification of diffuse or limited disease. More recently analyses of HLA antigen associations with scleroderma have examined patient subsets categorized by autoantibody status. With few exceptions anti-Scl-70 or anti-centromere antibodies (ACA) are found only in patients who have diffuse or limited disease, respectively. Thus, analyses of HLA antigens in patients categorized by autoantibodies can be related to those that utilize clinically defined disease subsets.

However, as antibodies to Scl-70 are present in only 30% of patients with diffuse disease and ACA in at most 80% of patients with limited disease, results from studies utilizing clinical and autoantibody categorizations can be considered only in part as overlapping.

Limited scleroderma, antibodies to centromere, and Pm-Scl

A number of studies have found an increase of DR1 (Whiteside *et al.* 1983; Black *et al.* 1984) and others an increase of HLA-DR11 (DR5) (Black *et al.* 1984; Dunckley *et al.* 1989; Maddison *et al.* 1993) in patients with limited scleroderma. When patients were categorized according to the presence or absence of ACA, Steen and *et al.* (1984) found a significant increase of DR1. However, other studies have variably found no association particularly after correcting for multiple comparisons (Morel *et al.* 1995; Genth *et al.* 1990). Differing results could potentially be reconciled based on either differences in racial/ethnic compositions of populations studied or if genes in linkage disequilibrium with DR are primarily responsible for the ACA response. Using DNA typing techniques, Reveille and colleagues studied a large number of patients with ACA (Reveille *et al.* 1992a) and found an association of ACA with DQB1*0301. In another large study Morel *et al.* (1995a) found that DQB1*0501 was increased among patients with ACA. In both studies DQB1*0201 was protective. DQB1*0301 is in linkage disequilibrium with DR11, DQB1*0501 with DR1, and DQB1*0201 with DR7.

Based on a comparison of the amino acid sequences of DQB1*0301 and DQB1*0501, Reveille *et al.* (1992a) proposed that the absence of a leucine at position 26, might underlie susceptibility to ACA production. However, in a Japanese study, the majority of patients lacked this allele and a composite analysis for association with a non-leucine residue at position 26 was negative (Kuwana *et al.* 1995a). Limited information is available for HLA-DP. In one study an increase of DPB1*1301 was not significant when corrected for multiple comparisons (Reveille *et al.* 1992b), and in another study no DPB1 association was observed (Stephens *et al.* 1993).

Considered together, studies to date have not generated a model in which a common sequence of DQβ1 can be attributed to the ACA response. Of interest, in the study by Kuwana *et al.* (1995a) higher titres of ACA were found to correlate with some alleleic variants of DR1, DR4, and DR13 (DRB1*0101, *0405, *1302)

and it remains possible that DR and DQ genes are interactive in their contributions to ACA.

Antibodies to Pm-Scl which are most often found in patients with limited scleroderma with overlap are associated with DR3 (Genth *et al.* 1990).

Diffuse scleroderma and anti-Scl-70 antibodies

The most consistently described HLA-DR associations with diffuse scleroderma have been with DR11 (DR5) and DR2. Occasional studies describe an increase of DR3 (Langeritz *et al.* 1992; Maddison *et al.* 1993). Earlier reports of an association with DR5 were probably due to DR11; these studies predated the availability of reagents that 'split' DR5 into DR11 and DR12. An increase of DR11 (DR5) has been described in numerous Caucasian populations (Gladman *et al.* 1981; Dunckley *et al.* 1989; Langevitz *et al.* 1992). In Asian populations the predominant association has been with DR2 (Panicheewa *et al.* 1991; Satoh *et al.* 1994; Takeuchi *et al.* 1994), and in one study that determined specific DRB1 alleles, the association was found to be due to the DR2 allele DRB1*1502 (Takeuchi *et al.* 1994). The latter study also found an increase of DRB1*0802 among DRB1*1502 negative patients. DRB1*0802 differs from DRB1*0803 [which is twice as common among healthy Japanese controls], in having a charged amino acid, aspartic acid, at position 57 (versus a serine), and at position 67, phenylalanine (versus an isoleucine).

Similar to reports for diffuse scleroderma, studies that have examined patients categorized by the presence of antibodies to topoisomerase I, have found associations with DR11 and DR2. An increase of DR11 has been reported in a number of studies (Genth *et al.* 1990; Reveille *et al.* 1992c; Morel *et al.* 1994). Two of the studies included the determination of specific DRB1 alleles. In one of the studies the association with DR11 was found to be mostly owing to an increase of the DRB1*1104 allele. However, the other study did not find a preferential association with any particular DR11 allele. An increase of DR2 has been reported in Japanese patients with anti-Scl-70 (Satoh *et al.* 1994; Takeuchi *et al.* 1994), and attributed to the DR2 allele DRB1*1502.

Studies that have determined DQB1 alleles and analysed patients with antibodies to Scl-70 have found associations in Caucasians and blacks with DQB1*0301 (Reveille *et al.* 1992c; Morel *et al.* 1994) and in Japanese with DQB1*0601 (Kuwana *et al.*

1993). These observations are consistent with those observed for DRB1 since in Caucasian populations DQB1*0301 is in linkage disequilibrium with DR11 and in Japanese, DQB1*0601 is in linkage disequilibrium with DR2, DRB1*1502. Reveille *et al.* have proposed that the primary association of anti-Scl-70 antibodies is with DQB1 with an amino acid sequence encoded by both DQB1*0301 and DQB1*0601, 'TRAELDT', from positions 71 to 77 and tyrosine at position 30. Support for this hypothesis has been generated by studies in US populations (Morel *et al.* 1994) and in Japanese (Kuwana *et al.* 1993). However, this sequence is also found on some other DQβ1 chains (see Table 8.7), and in the Japanese study the strongest association was with tyrosine at position 26. An association of DRB1*1302 and DQB1*0604 has recently been described in patients with scleroderma who have antibodies to fibrillarin (Arnett *et al.* 1996).

A proposed model for HLA associations with diffuse scleroderma and antibodies to topoisomerose

The most consistent observations are the association of DRB1*11 and *02 and DQB1*0301, and *0601 with diffuse scleroderma and with anti-Scl-70 antibodies. Sequence identity is present on the DQβ1 chain encoded by DQB1*0301 and DQB*0601 from amino acid positions 71 to77, and also at positions 30 and 26. DRB1*11 and *02 do not share sequence homology. However, importantly, there is sequence homology of DRβ1 and DRβ5 molecules. Thus the amino acid sequence 'FLEDR' (Table 8.7) is encoded by some alleles of DR11, and also by some alleles of DR51 that are in linkage disequilibrium with DR2 (as well as the DR2 allele DRB1*1601). (Linkage disequilibrium patterns among class II genes is discussed in further detail in Chapter 1 (see Fig. 1.8).) Moreover, this same sequence is encoded by some DR8 allelic variants, including DRB1*0802, which has been found in Japanese. Thus, it seems most likely that a common sequence of DRβ1 and DRβ5, as well as a common sequence of DQβ1, contributes to disease susceptibility and autoantibody production. Consistent with a role for both, *in vitro* T cell proliferative response to topoisomerose 1 was blocked by both anti-DR and anti-DQ monoclonal antibodies (Kuwana *et al.* 1995*b*).

Finally, it is also useful to consider genes that may afford protection from disease. In this regard it is striking that no study in any population has described risk of diffuse scleroderma or antibodies to topoisomerase-I with any haplotypes in the DRB4* family (DR53 associated). These considerations suggest that a model such as that which has been proposed for HLA associations with rheumatoid arthritis (Zanelli *et al.* 1995) may be applicable to scleroderma, i.e. one in which both DQ and DR genes are contributory and in which both susceptibility and protective effects are considered.

Other genes in the major histocompatibility region may also contribute to susceptibility to scleroderma. Briggs *et al.* (1993) have reported a significant increased risk of scleroderma associated with the C4A null phenotype (C4AQ0), as have another group (Maddison *et al.* 1993).

Animal models

While no good animal model of the vascular component of systemic sclerosis exists, some models purporting to show similar collagen abnormalities have been reported. Perhaps the best described is the tight-skin mouse (TSK) (Fig. 8.7). This naturally occurring mutant strain was isolated by Helen Bunker in 1968 at the Jackson Research Laboratories. A comparison of the histopathological, physical, and biochemical properties from the skin of a TSK mouse and skin from patients with systemic sclerosis is shown in Table 8.8. Although the animal does have inelastic skin because of an increase in connective tissue in the dermis and epidermis, other features do not tally as well with the human disease. For example, the ultrastructural changes of disruption of the fibrous architecture and active fibroblasts are found mainly in the upper dermis of the TSK model but in the lower dermis of humans. In addition, the TSK model does not show the mononuclear cell infiltrate often seen in the earlier stages of systemic sclerosis, and the dermal appendages are much better preserved in the mouse. Nevertheless, the similarity in the biochemical abnormalities is striking. Specifically, the TSK mice, like their human counterparts, have increased dermal glycosaminoglycans and hydroxyproline and an increased synthesis of immature collagen (Osborn *et al.* 1983; Jimenez *et al.* 1984).

Unfortunately, the TSK model lacks internal organ disease. Its lesions appear within one week of birth. Thus, although it does provide a useful model for studying abnormalities in collagen synthesis, as

Table 8.7 Shared amino acid sequences of DQβ1 and DRβ1 and DRβ5 associated with antibodies to topoisomerase I and diffuse scleroderma

DQB1 alleles ◆

				Amino acid number					
	26	30	71	72	73	74	75	76	77
0501, 0502, 0503	G	H	A	R	A	S	V	D	R
0601, 0301	*Y*	*Y*	*T*	*–*	*–*	*E*	*L*	*–*	*T*
0602, 0605, 0302, 0303	L	Y	T	–	–	E	L	–	T
0603, 0604	I	–	T	–	–	E	L	–	T
0201	I	S	K	–	–	A	–	–	–
0401, 0402	–	Y	D	–	–	–	–	–	T

DRB1 alleles ◆

			Amino acid number		
	67	68	69	70	71
0101, 0102, 0403–8, 1402	L	L	E	Q	R
1101, 1104, 0801, 0802, 0804, 1202, 1601	*F*	*–*	*–*	*D*	*–*
1103	F	–	–	D	E
1403, 1602	I	–	–	D	–
0103, 0402, 1102, 1301, 1302	I	–	–	D	E
0701, 0803, 1201, 1203	I	–	–	D	–
1001, 1401, 1404–5	F	–	–	D	–
0901	F	–	–	R	–
1501–3	I	–	–	–	A
0301, 0302, 0401	–	–	–	–	K

DRB5 alleles ~

	67	68	69	70	71
0101, 0102 ^	*F*	*–*	*–*	*D*	*–*
*0201, 0202, 0203 #	I	–	–	–	A

DRB3 alleles ◆ ~

	67	68	69	70	71
DRB3 alleles ◆ ~	–	–	–	R	K
DRB4 alleles ◆ ~	–	–	–	R	–

◆ Some uncommon alleles are not listed. The DRB1 'FLEDR' sequence is also encoded by some other rare alleles of DRB1*16, *11, *08, *04, *13, and *14.
~ DRB5, DRB3, and DRB4 are present only on some haplotypes and encode for molecules that are co-expressed on the cell surface, DR51, DR52, and DR53 respectively (see Chapter 1).
^ DRB5 often encodes a DR51 molecule with this sequence when the DRB1*02 allele is either DRB1*1501 or *1502.
# DRB5 often encodes a DR51 molecule with this sequence when the DRB1*02 allele is either DRB1*1601 or *1602.

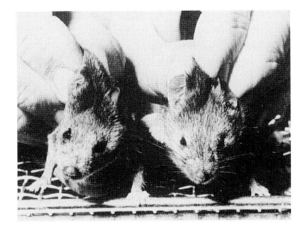

Fig. 8.7. The tight-skin mouse (TSK) described as a model for scleroderma [from Green *et al.* (1976)]. Photograph courtesy of Dr Margaret Green.

a model of systemic sclerosis it clearly lacks many attributes.

Another model, described several years prior to the TSK mouse, is homologous disease of the rat (Stasny *et al.* 1963) which develops after the injection of large numbers of lymphoid cells from an unrelated strain of donor animals. The initial manifestation of disease is erythema and oedema of the skin, followed by the development of a dermatitis and a variety of other systemic features. Thereafter, marked atrophy of the epidermis, increased collagen content of the dermis and

Table 8.8 Comparison of the TSK mouse and human systemic sclerosis

	TSK mouse	Systemic sclerosis skin
Histopathology		
Collagen, upper dermis	++	+
Collagen, lower dermis	+	++
Immature fibrils	?	++
Physical properties		
Thickness	+	+
Wet weight	+	+
Dry weight	+	−
Biochemical properties		
Hydroxyproline content	+	+
Soluble collagen	+	+
Glycosaminoglycans	+	+
Biosynthetic studies		
Protein	+	+
Collagen	+	+

Adapted from Fig. 1 of Russell (1983).

the disappearance of skin appendages become evident in some animals, and these features resemble scleroderma. These mice frequently develop a positive ANA and antibodies to topoisomerase-I (reviewed by Bona *et al.* 1994). These authors have also explored the effects of injecting bone marrow cells from TSK mice into healthy strain C57Bl/6 mice. Intriguingly, it was shown that the injected mice developed histopathological changes reminiscent of systemic sclerosis and an increase in the titre of anti-topoisomerase-I and RNA polymerase I antibodies.

A disease in white leghorn chickens has been described which also shows some similarities with systemic sclerosis (Gershwin *et al.* 1981). A mononuclear cell infiltration and fibrosis develops in the skin and internal organs. However, the disease is more acute than its human counterpart, the inflammatory response is more intense, a marked muscle hypertrophy is found, and a true glomerulonephritis (rare in systemic sclerosis) frequently develops.

Pathogenesis of scleroderma

Any attempt to explain the pathogenesis of scleroderma must take into account the vascular abnormalities, the immunological perturbations, and the disordered collagen synthesis. It seems likely that the primary vascular event found in the small blood vessels, is the proliferation of the endothelial cells in the intimal layer. Fleischmajer and Perlish (1980) have shown, using electron microscopy, that the earliest detectable changes in the capillaries of patients with scleroderma are large gaps between endothelial cells. These cells permit the passage of plasma fluids into the extracellular matrix. This might explain the oedematous changes found in the early skin lesions. Subsequently, the endothelial cells themselves become swollen and are known to produce a wide variety of molecules, including growth factors and cytokines, extracellular matrix and adhesion proteins, anticoagulation factors, and vasoactive proteins. The endothelium is known to regulate many aspects of vascular stability, including the control of vascular tone, permeability, thrombotic potential, and leucocyte trafficking (Kahaleh and Mattuci-Cerinic 1995).

Among the evidence for endothelial cell dysfunction in scleroderma are changes in circulating levels of endothelial cell products, including von Willebrand factor, endothelium-1, plasminogen activator, and angiotensin-converting enzyme; the presence of autoantibodies that bind to endothelial cells; increased capillary permeability demonstrated using tracer molecules; increased endothelial cell surface expression *in vivo*; and elevated circulating levels of the adhesion molecules, intracellular adhesion molecule 1 (ICAM-1) and vascular cell adhesion molecule-1 (VCAM-1) and E-selectin. The mechanism of vasospasm in scleroderma is likely to involve interactions between extracellular matrix products such as nitric oxide, endothelium-1 and prostacyclins, platelet release products, e.g. serotonin, β-thromboglobulin, and neuropeptides, e.g. calcitonin gene-related peptide and vasoactive intestinal polypeptide.

The question of what induces the changes in the endothelial cells is clearly crucial to the pathology observed in the blood vessels. The endothelial cell damage may occur in response to ischaemia, and there is evidence of both immune and non-autoimmune ytotoxicity. The sequence of pathological events seems to be as follows: after the endothelial damage there is subendothelial oedema, followed by platelet aggregation and lymphocyte migration of both CD4[+] and CD8[+] T cells. Following activation (and damage) of the vascular endothelium, adhesion molecules such as E-selectin, VCAM-1, and ICAM-1 are upregulated in response to cytokines and other factors. These adhesion molecules bind to specific ligands on T and B lymphocytes and a variety of other cells, including platelets, neutrophils, monocytes and even natural killer cells. The consequence is to facilitate their adhesion to vascular endothelium and their subsequent migration through 'leaky vessels' into the extracellular matrix.

Collagen abnormalities

Probably the greatest amount of research into the pathogenesis of scleroderma has gone into studies of collagen structure and its metabolism. This is because the thickening and rigidity of the skin, which are the hallmarks of the disease are a result of the increased amount of collagen found in the subcutaneous tissue in deep layers. This increase appears to be a consequence of an accelerated rate of fibroblast collagen synthesis. Techniques for culturing fibroblasts have been studied extensively. Skin grafts from patients with scleroderma have often been shown to synthesize increased quantities of fibronectin, proteoglycan, core proteins, and several of the collagen types, notably type I and type III.

The amounts of nRNA for matrix components have been shown to be increased, and have been localized,

mainly to areas surrounding dermal blood vessels. Not all fibroblasts are activated to produce more collagen but rather a particular group of high quality producers appears to be responsible. The transcriptional rate of genes encoding pro-α2 (I) collagen is increased in fibroblasts from patients with scleroderma, suggesting a change in regular transcription factors in these cells. The mechanisms for this dysregulation is unknown.

Integrating the pathogenic factors

Both circumstantial and direct evidence support the notion that abnormal immune function is an integral part of the pathogenesis of scleroderma. Clinically the disease has been described in association with Sjögren's syndrome, SLE, dermatomyositis, Hashimoto's thyroiditis, and biliary cirrhosis. The invariable presence of autoantibodies, including anti-centromere and anti-Scl-70 antibodies, that show marked disease specificity, supports the notion that scleroderma has a humoral-mediated component. As indicated above, cellular infiltrates composed of lymphocytes, plasma cells, and macrophages are commonly found, especially as a perivascular cuff in the early stages of skin and internal organ involvement. In the skin lesions the majority of cells are T lymphocytes (Roumm *et al.* 1984). This inflammatory response may be accompanied by complement-fixing serological factors and the deposition of immune complexes on the small blood vessel walls. There is some evidence supporting a cell-mediated immune dysfunction in scleroderma. For example, tissue samples extracted from the skin and other organs of patients with systemic sclerosis were shown to be capable of inducing lymphokines from leucocyte preparations of these patients, but not from control subjects (Kondo *et al.* 1976). Furthermore, the marked similarity in chronic skin lesions of graft-versus-host disease and systemic sclerosis also suggests that new mechanisms must be involved in its pathogenesis. In Fig. 8.8 an attempt has been made to show how some of these immunopathological observations might be linked. As is evident, the development of both the fibrous and the vascular lesions is complex and likely to involve various concurrent events.

Treatment

Scleroderma is a difficult disease to treat, but therapies are available to alleviate some symptoms, prevent end-

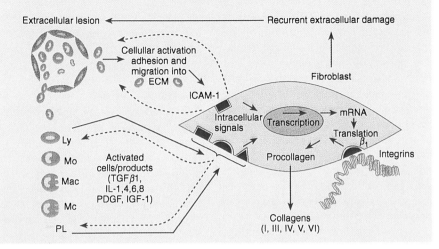

Fig. 8.8. Scleroderma — the overall likely aetiopathogenic links. (Reproduced from Fig 1, Chapter 5.8 Oxford Textbook of Rheumatology, Oxford University Press 1988).

organ damage, and improve quality of life. Choice of treatment depends on disease subset and stage of disease and should treat the vascular, immune, and fibrotic components of the disease. For many treatments there are little or no data from good controlled trials to support their use.

Raynaud's phenomenon

Raynaud's phenomenon is almost universal in patients with scleroderma and patients are at risk of developing digital ulcers. Patients should be advised to avoid cold, temperature change, stress, and to stop smoking. Electrically heated gloves can be helpful. Oral vasodilator therapy with calcium channel blockers such as nifedipine or amlodipine are effective but sometimes poorly tolerated, with headaches and light-headedness. The response to individual calcium channel blockers may be idiosyncratic and it may be necessary to try several different agents. Iloprost is a potent intravenous vasodilator which gives long-lasting relief after daily infusion for 3–5 days (Rademaker *et al.* 1989). Iloprost reduces the frequency and severity of Raynaud's phenomenon and helps to heal active digital ulcers.

Ketanserin is a specific serotonin antagonist. It has been used in an uncontrolled study for the treatment of Raynaud's phenomenon and ischaemia in patients with scleroderma and it improved cutaneous blood flow (Klimiuk *et al.* 1989). Ketanserin does not improve structural vascular disease. Dipyramidole and aspirin reduce circulating β-thrombomodulin and platelet aggregates but were not effective in a controlled trial.

Calcitonin gene-related peptide (CGRP) is a potent endogenous vasodilator that may be involved in the regulation of the peripheral circulation and its response to cold. CGRP improves digital blood flow, digital temperature, and helps to heal digital ulcers in patients with Raynaud's phenomenon (Bunker *et al.* 1993).

Sympathetic blocks may be helpful during severe attacks of Raynaud's phenomenon, including stellate ganglion block and lumbar sympathetic block. Digital sympathectomy is also a promising technique but its place still has to be evaluated.

Scleroderma treatment

Numerous therapies have been attempted for generalized scleroderma, although none have achieved marked success. Some of these regimens are discussed below.

Drugs

D-Penicillamine and colchicine have been used for many years to treat scleroderma. Although both drugs have been given to patients for many years there really is no convincing evidence that either is able to stop the fibrotic process.

A number of immunosuppressive agents have been tried in scleroderma. Chlorambucil and 5-flurouracil were ineffective in placebo-controlled trials. The role of cyclophosphamide is still uncertain, either as a single agent or in combination with corticosteroids or plasmapheresis. The antimetabolites 6-thioguanine and azathioprine are reported to be useful but in uncontrolled studies. Low dose weekly methotrexate appears to be more effective than placebo in patients with active systemic sclerosis (van den Hoogen *et al.* 1996).

Cyclosporin has been used with encouraging improvements in skin thickening but there have been reports of hypertension and renal crisis (Denton *et al.* 1994). Low doses (5mg/kg/day) are used but confirmation of benefit is needed.

Long-term steroids have no place in the management of scleroderma and they may be toxic (Steen *et al.* 1994), being implicated in normotensive renal crisis. The use of corticosteroids is restricted to patients with myositis, arthritis, tenosynovitis, serositis, or the early oedematous phase of skin disease.

Immunomodulatory therapy

Several different immunomodulatory strategies have been attempted in scleroderma. Interferon-α and -γ are both being used in experimental studies. Recombinant interferon-γ is a potent inhibitor of collagen production by both normal and scleroderma fibroblasts *in vitro*. Interferon-α, although less potent as an inhibitor of collagen synthesis, does not activate HLA class II surface antigens which may be advantageous in an HLA-linked disease. Recombinant interferon-γ has been used in open studies with improvement or stabilization of skin thickening and no deterioration in visceral disease (reviewed in Varga 1997). These agents should only be used in early disease.

Studies of rabbit anti-thymocyte globulin are being conducted but are not encouraging (Matteson *et al.* 1996).

Photophoresis using extracorporeal photoactivated 8-methoxypsoralen inhibits T cells and is still under investigation.

Autologous haemopoietic stem cell transplantation has recently been reported, to produce both clinical (improvement in skin) and serological improvement in a single case, (Tyndall *et al.* 1997).

Treatment of organ involvement

Renal disease

The prognosis for scleroderma renal crisis has improved with the use of angiotensin-converting enzyme inhibitors (ACE). Blood pressure and intra-vascular volume must be carefully controlled. ACE inhibitors may be prophylactic in high risk patients.

Bowel

Scleroderma causes oesophageal dysmotility with decreased oesophageal sphincter pressure and reflux oesophagitis with dysphagia and dyspepsia. A proton pump inhibitor (e.g. omeprazole) is highly effective (Sjögren 1994). H_2 antagonists also provide good relief. Oesophageal spasm may respond to cisapride. Midgut and anorectal complications are difficult to treat. Bacterial overgrowth may be diagnosed by the hydrogen breath test and can be treated with cyclical antibiotics (ciprofloxacin, doxycycline, and metronidazole) (Kaye *et al.* 1995). Somatostatin analogues are helpful for diarrhoea.

Pulmonary disease

Interstitial lung disease is a major cause of mortality. The optimum therapy is unknown. Cyclophosphamide and prednisolone improve the vital capacity but not the diffusion capacity (Silver *et al.* 1993). Vasodilator therapy has a short-term effect. Intravenous iloprost lowers mean pulmonary artery pressures but the long-term efficacy is not known (Delamata *et al.* 1994).

Cardiac complications

Pericarditis and pericardial effusion can be treated with NSAIDs and corticosteroids. Arrythmias are treated in the conventional manner. Calcium channel blockers may improve myocardial perfusion (Duboc *et al.* 1991).

Calcinosis

Calcinosis is common in scleroderma and there is no satisfactory therapy. Recent reports have suggested that calcium antagonists may be helpful (Dolan *et al.* 1995).

Summary

Scleroderma or systemic sclerosis is an unpleasant, often progressive, disease characterized by induration and thickening of the skin. Raynaud's phenomenon is invariably present, usually in a severe form. Of all the diseases discussed so far, scleroderma has the least definitive link with autoimmunity. However, notable immunological defects have been observed. These patients have anti-nuclear antibodies and disease-specific autoantibodies, notably anti Scl-70 anti-nuclear and anti-centromere antibodies. At the cellular level abnormalities in lymphocyte production have been linked with disordered collagen synthesis. Histologically, a wide range of changes in the small blood vessels walls is found with an accelerated rate of fibroblast and collagen synthesis and an inflammatory infiltrate. The prognosis of scleroderma depends upon the degree of internal organ involvement. Renal complications and lung disease carry the worst prognosis.

The aetiology of scleroderma remains to be elucidated and, unlike other autoimmune rheumatic diseases, there is no easily identifiable target for autoimmune attack. However, some recent findings suggest that scleroderma might be a graft-versus-host-type disorder in which the host immune system is reacting to the presence of residual maternal lymphocytes. The tight-skin mouse serves as a partial model for experimental studies into scleroderma.

References

Abu-Shakra M, Lee P. Mortality in systemic sclerosis: a comparison with the general population. *J Rheumatol* 1995; **27**: 2100–2.

Altmann RD, Medsger TA Jr, Bloch DA *et al*. Predictors of survival in systemic sclerosis (scleroderma). *Arthritis Rheum* 1990; **34**: 403–13.

Arnett F, Reveille J, Goldstein R *et al*.. Autoantibodies to fibrillarin in systemic sclerosis (scleroderma). *Arthritis Rheum* 1996; **39**: 1151–60.

Behr J, Vogelmeier C, Beinert J *et al*. Bronchoalveolar lavage for evaluation and management of scleroderma disease of the lung. *Am J Resp Crit Care Med* 1996; **154**: 400–6.

Bell SA, Faust H, Mittermuller J *et al*. Specificity of anti-nuclear antibodies in scleroderma like chronic graft versus host disease: clinical correlation and histocompatibility locus antigen association. *Br J Dermatol* 1996; **134**: 848–54.

Black CM, Welsh KI, Maddison PJ *et al*. HLA antigens, autoantibodies and clinical subsets in scleroderma. *Br J Rheumatol* 1984; **23**: 267–71.

Black CM, Denton CP. Scleroderma and related disorders in adults and children. In: *Oxford Textbook of Rheumatology*. Maddison PJ, Isenberg DA, Liss P, Glass DN eds. 2nd edn. Oxford University Press, Oxford, 1998; 1217–47.

Bona C, Shiabata S, Daian C *et al*. Role of immunocompetent cells in skin sclerosis and autoimmunity in tight skin mice. In: *Autoimmunity: Experimental Aspects*, ed. Zouali M, NATO ASI Series. Springer Verlag, Berlin, 1994; 229–44.

Bramwell B. Diffuse scleroderma: its frequency, its occurrence in stone-masons: its treatment by fibrolysin–elevations of temperature due to fibrolysin injections. *Edin Med J* 1914; **12**: 387–401.

Briggs D, Stephens C, Vaughan R *et al*. A molecular and serologic analysis of the major histocompatibility complex and complement component C4 in systemic sclerosis. *Arthritis Rheum* 1993; **36**: 943–54.

Bunker CB, Reavley C, O'Shaughnessy DJ *et al*. Calcitonin gene related peptide in the treatment of severe vascular insufficiency in Raynaud's phenomenon. *Lancet* 1993; **342**: 80–3.

Candell-Riera J, Armadans-Gil L, Simeon CP *et al*. Comprehensive non-invasive assessment of cardiac involvement in limited systemic sclerosis. *Arthritis Rheum* 1996; **39**: 1138–45.

David J, Wilson J, Woo P. Scleroderma 'en coup de sabre'. *Ann Rheum Dis* 1991; **50**: 260–2.

Delamata J, Gomezsanchez MA, Aranzana M *et al*. Long term iloprost infusion therapy for severe pulmonary hypertension in patients with connective tissue diseases. *Arthritis Rheum* 1994; **37**: 1528–33.

DeNardo BA, Tucker LB, Miller LC *et al*. Demography of a regional pediatric rheumatology patient population. *J Rheumatol* 1994; **21**: 1553–61.

Denton CP, Sweney P, Abdulla A *et al*. Acute renal failure occurring in scleroderma treated with cyclosporin A. A report of 3 cases. *Br J Rheumatol* 1994; **33**: 90–2.

Dolan AL, Kissimou D, Gibson T *et al*. Diltiazem induces remission of calcinosis in scleroderma. *Br J Rheumatol* 1995; **34**: 576–8.

Duboc D, Kaham A, Maziere B *et al*. The effect of nifedipine on myocardial perfusion and metabolism in systemic sclerosis. *Arthritis Rheum* 1991; **34**: 198–203.

Dunckley H, Jazwinska EC, Gateby PA *et al*. DNA-DR typing shows HLA-DRw11 RFLPs are increased in frequency in both progressive systemic sclerosis and CREST variants of scleroderma. *Tissue Antigens* 1989; **33**: 418–20.

Fleischmajer R, Perlish JS. Capillary alterations in scleroderma. *J Am Acad Dermatol* 1980; **2**: 161–70.

Follansbee WP, Miller TR, Curtiss EI *et al*. A controlled clinicopathologic study of myocardial fibrosis in systemic sclerosis (scleroderma). *J Rheumatol* 1990; **17**: 656–62.

Genth E, Mierau R, Genetzky P *et al*. Immunogenetic associations of scleroderma-related antinuclear antibodies. *Arthritis Rheum* 1990; **33**: 657–65.

Gershwin MF, Abplanalp H, Castles JJ *et al*. Characterization of a spontaneous disease of white leghorn chickens resembling progressive systemic sclerosis (scleroderma). *J Exp Med* 1981; **1534**: 1640–59

Gladman DD, Keystone EC, Baron M *et al*. Increased frequency of HLA-DR5 in scleroderma. *Arthritis Rheum* 1981; **24**: 854–856.

Green, MC, Sweet HO, Bunker LP. Tight-skin mouse, a new mutation of the mouse causing excessive growth of connective tissue and skeleton. *Am J Pathol* 1976; **82**: 493–512.

Harrison NK, Glanville AR, Strickland B *et al*. Pulmonary involvement in systemic sclerosis: the detection of early changes by thin section CT scan, bronchoalveolar lavage and 99mTc-DTPA clearance. *Respir Med* 1989; **83**: 403–14.

Hochberg MC, Perlmutter DL, Medsger TA Jr *et al*. Lack of association between augmentation mammoplasty and systemic sclerosis. *Arthritis Rheum* 1996; **39**: 1125–31.

Jimenez SA, Sigal SH. A 15 year prospective study of treatment of rapidly progressive systemic sclerosis with D-penicillamine. *J Rheumatol* 1991; **18**: 1496–503.

Jimenez SA, Millan D, Bashey RI. Scleroderma-like alterations in collagen metabolism occurring in the TSK (tight skin mouse). *Arthritis Rheum* 1984; **27**: 180–5.

Kabasakal Y, Elvins DM, Ring EF *et al*. Quantitative nailfold capillaroscopy findings in a population with connective tissue disease and in normal healthy controls. *Ann Rheum Dis* 1996; **55**: 507–12.

Kahaleh MB, Mattuci-Cerinic M. Raynaud's phenomenon and scleroderma: dysregulated neuroendothelial control of vascular tone. *Arthritis Rheum* 1995; **38**: 1–4.

Kallenberg CGM, Wonda AA, Hoet MH *et al*. Development of connective tissue disease in patients presenting with Raynaud's phenomenon: a six-year follow-up with emphasis on the predictive value of antinuclear antibodies as detected by immunoblotting. *Ann Rheum Dis* 1988; **47**: 634–41.

Kane GC, Varga J, Conant EF *et al*. Lung involvement in systemic sclerosis: relation to classification based on extent of skin involvement or autoantibody status. *Respir Med* 1996; **90**: 223–30.

Kaye SA, Lim SG, Taylor M *et al*. Small bowel bacterial overgrowth in systemic sclerosis. Detection using direct and indirect methods, and treatment outcome. *Br J Rheumatol* 1995; **34**: 265–9.

Klimiuk PS, Kay EA, Mitchell WS *et al*. Ketanserin: An effective treatment regimen for digital ischaemia in systemic sclerosis. *Scand J Rheumatol* 1989; **18**: 107–11.

Kondo H, Robin BS, Rodnan GP. Cutaneous antigen-stimulating lymphokine production by lymphocytes of patients with progressive systemic sclerosis (scleroderma). *J Clin Invest* 1976; **50**: 1388–94.

Kovalchik MT, Guggenheim GJ, Robertson JS *et al*. The kidney in progressive systemic sclerosis: a prospective study. *Ann Int Med* 1978; **89**: 881–7.

Kuwana M, Kaburaki J, Okano Y *et al*. The HLA-DR and DQ genes control the autoimmune response to DNA topoisomerase I in systemic sclerosis (scleroderma). *J Clin Invest* 1993; **92**: 1296–301.

Kuwana M, Okano Y, Kaburaki J *et al*. HLA class II genes associated with anticentromere antibody in Japanese patients with systemic sclerosis (scleroderma). *Ann Rheum Dis* 1995a; **54**: 983–7.

Kuwana M, Medsger TA, Jr, Wright TM. T cell proliferative response induced by DNA topoisomerase 1 in patients with systemic sclerosis and healthy donors. *J Clin Invest* 1995b; **96**: 586–96.

Laing TJ, Gillespie BW, Toth MB *et al*. Racial differences in scleroderma among women in Michigan. *Arthritis Rheum* 1977; **40**: 734–42.

Langevitz P, Buskila D, Gladman DD *et al*. HLA alleles in systemic sclerosis: association with pulmonary hypertension and outcome. *Br J Rheumatol* 1992; **31**: 609–13.

Maddison PJ, Stephens C, Briggs D *et al*. United Kingdom Systemic Sclerosis Study Group. Connective tissue disease and autoantibodies in the kindreds of 63 patients with systemic sclerosis. *Medicine* 1993; **72**: 103–12.

Matteson EL, Shbeeb MI, McCarthy TG *et al*. Pilot study of antithymocyte globulin in systemic sclerosis. *Arthritis Rheum* 1996; **39**: 1132–7.

Medsger RA, Masi A. Epidemiology of systemic sclerosis (scleroderma). *Ann Int Med* 1971; **74**: 714–21.

Misra R, Darton K, Jewkes RF *et al*. Arthritis in scleroderma. *Br J Rheumatol* 1995; **39**: 831–7.

Morel PA, Chang HJ, Wilson JW *et al*. HLA and ethnic associations among systemic sclerosis patients with anticentromere antibodies. *Hum Immunol* 1995; **42**: 35–42.

Morel PA, Chang HJ, Wilson JW *et al*. Severe systemic sclerosis with anti-topoisomerase I antibodies is associated with an HLA-DRw11 allele. *Hum Immunol* 1994; **40**: 101–10.

Nyrén O, Yin L, Josefsson S *et al*. Risk of connective tissue disease and related disorders among women with breast: a nation-wide retrospective cohort study in Sweden. *Brit J Med* 1998; **316**: 417–21.

Osborn TG, Bauerr NE, Ross SC *et al*. The tight skin mouse: physical and biochemical properties of the skin. *J Rheumatol* 1983; **10**: 793–6.

Panicheewa S, Chitrabamrung S, Verasertniyom O *et al*. Diffuse systemic sclerosis and related disease in Thailand. *Clin Rheumatol* 1991; **10**: 124–9.

Peterson LS, Nelson AM, Su WPD *et al*. The epidemiology of morphoea (localised scleroderma) in Olmsted County 1960–1993. *J Rheumatol* 1997; **24**: 73–80.

Polisson RP, Gilkeson GS, Pyun EH *et al*. A multicenter trial of recombinant human interferon gamma in patients with systemic sclerosis: effects on cutaneous fibrosis and interleukin 2 receptor levels. *J Rheumatol* 1996; **23**: 654–8.

Rademaker M, Cooke ED, Almond NE *et al*. Comparison of intravenous infusions of iloprost and oral nifedipine in treatment of Raynaud's phenomenom in patients with systemic sclerosis. *Br Med J* 1989; **298**: 561–8.

Reveille JD, Owerbach D, Goldstein R *et al*. Association of polar amino acids at position 26 of the HLA-DQB1 first domain with the anticentromere autoantibody response in systemic sclerosis (scleroderma). *J Clin Invest* 1992a; **89**: 1208–13.

Reveille JD, Brady J, MacLeod-St.Clair M *et al*. HLA-DPB1 alleles and autoantibody subsets in systemic lupus erythematosus, Sjogren's syndrome and progressive systemic sclerosis: a question of disease relevance. *Tissue Antigens* 1992b; **40**: 45–8.

Reveille JD, Durban E, MacLeod-St.Clair M *et al*. Association of amino acid sequences in the HLA-DQB1 first domain with the antitopoisomerase I autoantibody response in scleroderma (progressive systemic sclerosis). *J Clin Invest* 1992c; **90**: 973–80.

Riente L, Marchini B, Dolcher MP *et al*. Anti-collagen antibodies in systemic sclerosis and in primary Raynaud's phenomenon. *Clin Exp Immunol* 1995; **102**: 354–9.

Rook AH, Freundlich B, Jegasothy BV *et al*. Treatment of systemic sclerosis with extracorporeal photochemotherapy. Results of a multicentre trial. *Arch Dermatol* 1992; **128**: 337–46.

Rosenthal AK, McLaughlin JK, Gridley G *et al*. Incidence of cancer among patients with systemic sclerosis. *Cancer* 1995; **76**: 90–4.

Roumm AD, Whiteside TL, Medsger TA Jr *et al*. Lymphocytes in the skin of patients with progressive systemic sclerosis. *Arthritis Rheum* 1984; **27**: 645–53.

Russell ML. The tight-skin mouse: is it a model for scleroderma? *J Rheumatol* 1983; **10**: 679–81.

Sato S, Ihn H, Kikuchi K *et al.* Antihistone antibodies in systemic sclerosis. Association with pulmonary fibrosis. *Arthritis Rheum* 1995; **38**: 1024–5.

Satoh M, Akizuki M, Kuwana M *et al.* Genetic and immunological differences between Japanese patients with diffuse scleroderma and limited scleroderma. *J Rheumatolatol* 1994; **21**: 111–14.

Silman A, Harrison M, Brennan P. Is it possible to reduce observer variability in skin score assessment of scleroderma? The ad hoc international group on the assessment of disease outcome in scleroderma. *J Rheumatol* 1995; 22: 1217–19.

Silver RM. Unravelling the eosinophilia-myalgia syndrome. *Arch Dermatol* 1991: **127**: 1214–16.

Silver RM, Warrick JH, Kinsella MB *et al.* Cyclophosphamide and low dose prednisolone therapy in patients with systemic sclerosis (scleroderma) with interstitial lung disease. *J Rheumatol* 1993; **20**: 838–44.

Singsen BH. Scleroderma in childhood. *Ped Clin N Am* 1986; **33**: 1119–39.

Sjögren RW. Gastrointestinal motility disorders in scleroderma. *Arthritis Rheum* 1994; **37**: 1265–82.

Spurzem JR, Lockley JE. Toxic oil syndrome. *Arch Intern Med* 1984; **144**: 249–50.

Stasny P, Stembridge VA, Ziff M. Homologous disease in the adult rat, a model for the autoimmune disease. I. General features and cutaneous lesions. *J Exp Med* 1963; **118**: 635–48.

Steen VD, Ziegler GL, Rodnan GP *et al.* Clinical and laboratory associations of anticentromere antibody in patients with progressive systemic sclerosis. *Arthritis Rheum* 1984; **27**:125–31.

Steen VD, Powell DL, Medsger TA. Clinical correlations and prognosis based on serum autoantibodies in patients with systemic sclerosis. *Arthritis Rheum* 1988; **31**: 196–203.

Steen VD, Constantin JP, Shapiro AP *et al.* Outcome of renal crisis in systemic sclerosis relation to angiotensin converting enzyme (ACE) inhibitors. *Ann Intern Med* 1993; **113**: 352–7.

Steen VD, Conte C, Mesger TA. Case controlled study of corticosteroid use prior to scleroderma renal crisis (abstract). *Arthritis Rheum* 1994; **37** (Suppl.): S360.

Steen VD, Oddis CV, Conte DG *et al.* Incidence of systemic sclerosis in Allegheny County, Pennsylvania. *Arthritis Rheum* 1997; **40**: 441–5.

Stephens CO, Briggs DC, Vaughan RW *et al.* The HLA-DP locus in systemic sclerosis — no primary association. *Tissue Antigens* 1993; **42**: 144–5.

Takeuchi F, Nakano K, Yamada H *et al.* Association of HLA-DR with progressive systemic sclerosis in Japanese. *J Rheumatol* 1994; **21**: 857–63.

Traub YM, Shapiro AP, Rodnan GP *et al.* Hypertension and renal failure (scleroderma renal crisis) in progressive systemic sclerosis. Report of a 25 year experience with 68 cases. *Medicine* 1984; **62**: 335–52.

Tyndall A, Black C, Finke J *et al.* Treatment of systemic sclerosis with autologous haemopoietic stem cell transplantation. *Lancet* 1997; **349**: 254.

Vancheeswaran R, Black CM, David J *et al.* Childhood-onset scleroderma: is it different from adult onset disease. *Arthritis Rheum* 1996; **39**: 1041–9.

van den Hoogen FH, Boerbooms AM, Swaak AJ *et al.* Comparison of methotrexate with placebo in the treatment of systemic sclerosis: a 24 week randomised double blind trial, followed by a 24 week observational trail. *Br J Rheumatol* 1996; **35**: 364–72.

Varga J. Recombinant cytokine treatment for scleroderma. *Arch Dermatol* 1997; **133**: 637–42.

Weiss S, Stead Jr, EA, Warren JV *et al.* Scleroderma heart disease with a consideration of certain other visceral manifestations of scleroderma. *Arch Intern Med* 1943; **71**: 749–76.

Whiteside TL, Medsger TA Jr, Rodnan GP. HLA-DR antigens in progressive systemic sclerosis (scleroderma). *J Rheumatol* 1983; **10**: 128–31.

Zanelli E, Gonzalez-Gay MA, Davis CS. Could HLA-DRB2 be the protective locus in rheumatoid arthritis? *Immunol Today* 1995; **16**: 274–8.

9 | *Primary anti-phospholipid antibody syndrome*

Introduction

The first edition of this book included references to the clinical association of the anti-phospholipid antibodies within the chapter on systemic lupus erythematosus. Since then the primary anti-phospholipid antibody syndrome (PAPS) has emerged as a distinct entity. This condition has generated enormous interest and clearly deserves this separate chapter.

The condition may be thought of as a disorder in which the presence of anti-phospholipid antibodies is associated closely with a tendency to develop venous and/or arterial occlusion, recurrent fetal loss, and thrombocytopenia (Asherson *et al.* 1989b). The phospholipid antibodies most commonly measured are those binding to cardiolipin and the so-called 'lupus anticoagulant'. These are discussed in detail later. The full range of clinical features that have been linked to these antibodies is shown in Table 9.1 and several are illustrated in Fig. 9.1. As with all the other autoimmune rheumatic diseases, women are more commonly affected, about five times as frequently as men.

Milestones in the history of anti-phospholipid syndrome

1952   Conley and Hartmann described an association between a circulating anticoagulant and systemic lupus erythematosus.

Mid-1950s   Beaumont (1954) and Laurell and Nelson (1957) reported a link between a circulating anticoagulant and recurrent fetal death, spontaneous abortions, and intrauterine growth development.

1963   Bowie and colleagues linked the presence of a circulating anticoagulant with arterial and venous thrombosis.

1972   Feinstein and Rapaport suggested the term 'lupus anticoagulant' to describe the circulating anticoagulants found in

Table 9.1 Clinical features of the anti-phospholipid antibody syndrome

Thrombosis	Venous	Recurrent deep venous
	Arterial	Cerebrovascular accidents
		Transient ischaemic attack
		Coronary occlusion
		Retinal occlusion
		Renal occlusion
Abortion	Recurrent interuterine death	
	Placental thrombosis and infarction	
Thrombocytopaenia		
Others	Livedo reticularis	
	Migraine	
	Chorea	
	Positive Coombs' test	
	? Chronic leg ulcers	

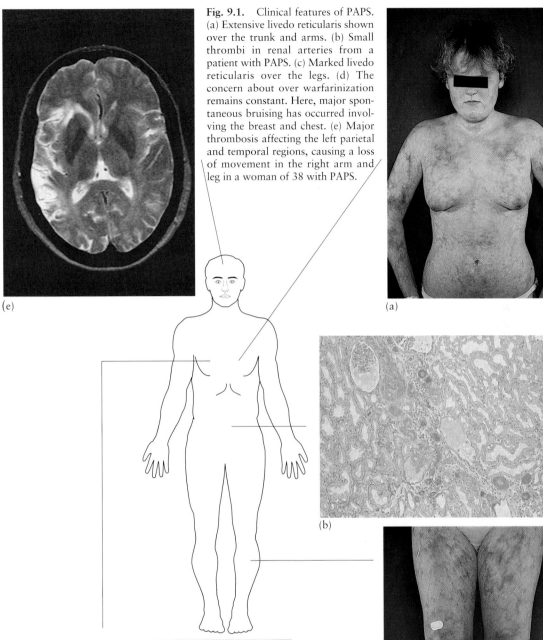

Fig. 9.1. Clinical features of PAPS. (a) Extensive livedo reticularis shown over the trunk and arms. (b) Small thrombi in renal arteries from a patient with PAPS. (c) Marked livedo reticularis over the legs. (d) The concern about over warfarinization remains constant. Here, major spontaneous bruising has occurred involving the breast and chest. (e) Major thrombosis affecting the left parietal and temporal regions, causing a loss of movement in the right arm and leg in a woman of 38 with PAPS.

(e)

(a)

(b)

(c)

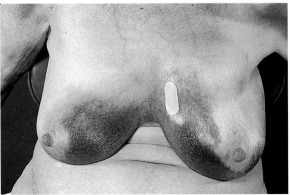

(d)

patients with SLE (a name that has stuck, although most patients with these inhibitors do not have SLE).

1983   Colaco and Elkon described the first solid-phase RIA (radioimmunoassay) for detecting anti-cardiolipin antibodies. The use of this assay (and the development of an ELISA) was extended greatly by Harris, Gharavi, and Asherson, all working in Hughes' laboratory. Criteria for the diagnosis of lupus anticoagulant proposed by the Working Party on Acquired Inhibitors of Coagulation of the International Committee on Thrombosis and Haemostasis (these have proved too stringent). Hughes *et al.* link thrombosis, recurrent abortion and antiphospholipid antibodies.

1984   First international symposium on anti-phospholipid antibodies.

1990 β_2-glycoprotein-I identified as a co-factor for the binding of certain antibodies to anionic phospholipids, by three independent groups.

1991–3   Several animal models of the different aspects of the anti-phospholipid antibody syndrome described.

Clinical features

Thrombosis within the venous or arterial circulation is a major clinical feature of this syndrome. Any size of vessel may be affected. In the venous circulation, deep or superficial vein thrombosis of the legs is particularly common, may be recurrent, and, as with thrombosis due to other causes (e.g. the oestrogen pill), other larger veins, including axillary, renal, hepatic, and inferior vena cava, have all been identified as sites of thrombosis, although less frequently.

Arterial occlusion due to thrombus has been recognized in patients presenting with transient ischaemic attacks or cerebrovascular accidents (Asherson *et al.* 1989a) (Fig. 9.1e). Much less frequently, multiple small thrombi may be associated with a form of multi-infarct dementia. Clearly, the overwhelming majority of

patients presenting over the age of 60 with a stroke will not have anti-phospholipid antibodies. However, these antibodies should be measured in women under 40 who present with a cerebrovascular accident. It has been suggested (Nencini *et al.* 1992) that approximately one-fifth of these patients will have such antibodies. Likewise, patients presenting at a young age with myocardial infarction should certainly be tested for these antibodies as approximately the same proportion will turn out to be positive (Hamsten *et al.* 1986). Rather less frequently, arterial thrombosis involving the renal (Leaker *et al.* 1991), retinal, and mesenteric arteries (Asherson *et al.* 1986) are associated with the syndrome.

Renal thrombosis may be associated with malignant hypertension, though in most patients with renal involvement there is disease in the smaller vessels (microangiopathy) leading to a fall in the glomerular filtration rate (on occasions to 30–50% of normal), mild proteinuria, and modest hypertension (Fig. 9.1b).

Fetal loss

Most investigators consider that a particularly striking feature of PAPS is the development of recurrent, spontaneous fetal loss. However, in a meta-analysis Love and Santoro (1990) struck a note of caution. Most such losses occur in the second or third trimester. In contrast, fetal loss due to other causes (e.g. chromosomal abnormalities) usually occurs during the first trimester. The frequencies of anti-phospholipid antibodies in women with a range of obstetric histories are shown in Table 9.2.

It seems generally agreed that screening normal pregnant women with two or fewer miscarriages for anti-phospholipid antibodies is a waste of time (Harris and Spinato 1991). However, any woman with a history of three or more miscarriages should be tested for these antibodies. Rai *et al.* (1995) have reported that 15% of women with a history of three or more consecutive miscarriages have persistently positive anti-phospholipid antibody results. Several centres have reported that the presence of high titre anti-phospholipid antibodies is an important predictor of poor fetal outcome (Branch *et al.* 1992; Buchanan *et al.* 1992).

The presence of a lupus anticoagulant is a better predictor of thrombotic complications than anti-phospholipid antibodies measured by ELISA (Lockshin 1992). However, high sustained levels of IgG, as opposed to IgM, anti-phospholipid antibodies certainly warrant careful follow-up of the patient. High titre IgG anti-phospholipid antibodies are more sensitive for

Table 9.2 Frequencies of moderate to high titre-positive IgG anti-phospholipid antibodies

Group	% of individuals with raised levels
Healthy controls (non-pregnant)	< 1
Normal pregnant women	0.2–2
Normal pregnant women with a history of one unexplained intrauterine death	< 2
Normal pregnant women with a history of two or more intrauterine deaths	10
Women with SLE	≃ 25

identifying pregnancies at increased risk of premature termination.

Other clinical features

Thrombocytopenia is present in up to half of the patients with the anti-phospholipid antibody syndrome, though the level rarely falls below $25 \times 10^9/l$ and thus haemorrhage is uncommon (Khamashta and Machin 1991). The low platelet count may remain relatively constant for many years or in a few patients may fall precipitously, necessitating the use of corticosteroids and/or other immunosuppressive drugs, or possibly splenectomy. We have recently reviewed our own records (Hakim *et al.* 1998) and found three (now four) patients with PAPS and 9 patients with lupus and features of the APS who required a splenectomy for significant thrombocytopaenia. It should be noted that up to 15% of patients with so-called idiopathic thrombocytopenia purpura go on to develop systemic lupus erythematosus (Karpatkin 1985). It has not yet been established whether determining the anti-cardiolipin antibody levels in patients presenting with so-called idiopathic thrombocytopaenia purpura will provide prognostic information about those likely to go on to develop lupus or the anti-phospholipid antibody syndrome.

Occasionally, patients with anti-phospholipid antibodies and thrombocytopaenia also develop a form of haemolytic anaemia with a direct positive Coombs test (Evans syndrome) (Asherson *et al.* 1989b).

Among other complications of this syndrome, heart valve disease, particularly mitral valve involvement, is a recognized association (Khamashta *et al.* 1990, Galve *et al.* 1992). Using echocardiography, up to one-third of patients with either systemic lupus erythematosus or the anti-phospholipid antibody syndrome had mitral valve involvement, though the majority were asymptomatic.

A skin rash known as livedo reticularis, whose severity varies enormously from a confined area of skin to large parts of the arms or legs, is a recognized complication of this condition (Asherson *et al.* 1989c) (Figs 9.1 and 9.2). These lesions are characterized by thrombi in the intradermal vessels (Fig. 9.3).

Within the central nervous system, and depending on the precise site of the known complications of small thrombi, a variety of conditions have been recognized, including epilepsy, chorea, and transverse myelitis (Alarcon-Segovia *et al.* 1989; Herranz *et al.* 1994).

Between 20 and 50% of patients with lupus have anti-phospholipid antibodies (Isenberg and Horsfall 1998), i.e. a lupus anticoagulant and/or anti-

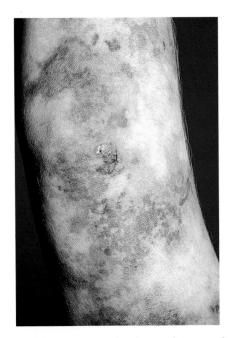

Fig. 9.2.   Close-up of major livedo reticularis over the arm.

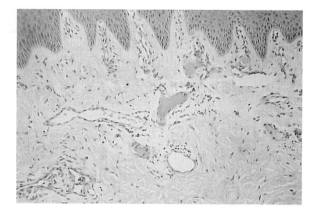

Fig. 9.3. Skin. Dermal vessels are occluded by hyaline thrombi.

cardiolipin antibodies. However, based on our own observation of managing over 200 patients with SLE in a dedicated clinic at UCH/Middlesex for over 15 years, only approximately 10% will develop the clinical features that are associated with the primary APS. Anti-phospholipid antibodies have been reported in a variety of conditions, especially infections but there are important differences with those antibodies found in patients with autoimmune disease (see Table 9.3).

Anti-phospholipid antibody syndrome in children

The number of reports of anti-phospholipid antibody syndrome occurring in children is small. With the obvious absence of the obstetric manifestations, the clinical features of thrombotic and neurological disease are broadly similar. As reviewed elsewhere (Tucker 1994), severe digital ischaemia and myocardial infarc-

tion have been described, as have deep venous thromboses, strokes, and chorea. A recent report has linked thrombotic events in a paediatric population to non-cardiolipin-binding anti-phospholipid antibodies, notably anti-phosphatidic acid and anti-phosphatidylglycerol antibodies (Beaman *et al.* 1995). In contrast, Gattorno *et al.* (1995) emphasized that the combination of a lupus anticoagulant and high titre anti-cardiolipin antibodies identified those paediatric lupus patients at greatest risk of developing deep venous thromboses, autoimmune haemolytic anaemia, pulmonary hypertension, and neurological abnormalities. There are rare reports of a neonatal anti-phospholipid antibody syndrome equivalent to the neonatal lupus syndrome (Silver *et al.* 1992).

Immunogenetics

Early reports suggested a genetic contribution to antiphospholipid antibody production because of the description of families with multiple affected members (Exner *et al.* 1980). A number of studies have examined HLA antigens in patients with the primary antiphospholipid antibody syndrome and APLA associated with other diseases (see Table 9.4). Most studies have utilized serological techniques and investigated relatively small numbers of patients. Among 13 Caucasian patients with PAPS from the UK HLA-DR4 and DR53 were found to be increased (Asherson *et al.* 1992a). A study of 20 patients with lupus anticoagulant from the USA utilized DNA typing techniques and found the strongest HLA association was with DQB1*0301 (Arnett *et al.* 1991). Eight of the patients had PAPS, nine SLE, two Sjögren's syndrome and one scleroderma. DQB1*0301 (DQ7) is in linkage disequilibrium with DR4, and also with DR11 both of which were increased to a lesser extent than DQB1*0301. In

Table 9.3 Differences between autoimmune-associated and infection-induced anti-phospholipid antibodies

Autoimmune	Infection induced
IgG predominates	IgM predominates
IgG$_2$, IgG$_4$ unusually frequent	–
High avidity	Low avidity
Anticoagulant activity often present	Anticoagulant activity invariably absent
Co-factor (β_2-GPI) enhances binding	Co-factor inhibits binding
Clinical features (clotting, miscarriage, etc.) often present	Clinical features not associated

Table 9.4 HLA associations with the primary anti-phospholipid antibody syndrome and with anti-phospholipid antibodies in association with other diseases

First author (Country)	HLA associations (≠ unless otherwise noted)	Disease
Asherson RA (UK)	DR53, DR4, no DQB1 association	PAPS
Arnett FC (USA)	DQB1*0301 (DQ7)	PAPS, SLE, SS, SSc, with LAC
Trabace S (Italy)	DR7	Rsab with aCL
Savi M (Italy)	DR7	SLE with aCL
McHugh NJ (UK)	DR4 (p corrected = ns)	SLE with aCL
Hartung K (Pan-European)	DR53, no DQ no C4 association	SLE with aCL
Sebastiani GD (Italy)	No DR association	SLE with aCL
Wilson WA*	C4A null	SLE with aCL
Petri M (USA)†	C4A negative association	SLE with aCL
Galeazzi M (Italy)	DPB1*1401, DPB1*0301	SLE with aCL
Gulko PS (USA)	No DR, no DQ association	SLE with aCL
Stephansson EA (Sweden)	C4A null	JCA with CBFP
Malleson PN (Canada)	No class I or DR association	SLE with aCL
Asherson RA (UK)	No HLA-DR association	Sjögren's with aCL

* African-Americans.
† African-Americans and Caucasians.
aCL: anti-cardiolipin; Rsab: recurrent spontaneous abortion; SLE: systemic lupus erythematosus; JCA: juvenile chronic arthritis; CBFP: chronic biologically false positive for syphilis; LAC: lupus anticoagulant.

a study from Italy, DR7 was increased among 25 women with recurrent pregnancy loss who had aCL antibodies (Trabace *et al.* 1991).

Some studies of patients with SLE have found no HLA association with aCL antibodies (Sebastiani 1991; Gulko 1993). Other reports have described associations with DR4, DR7 and DR53. A small study of SLE patients from the UK included eight with aCL and found an increase of DR4 (p corrected non significant) (McHugh *et al.* 1989). Much larger studies of SLE patients with aCL from Italy (Savi *et al.* 1988) and in a combined European study (Hartung *et al.* 1992) found significant increases of DR7 and DR53 respectively. No association with DQ was found in the latter study. The HLA antigens that are increased among unselected patients with SLE are DR2 and DR3 (see Chapter 4) and it is noteworthy that no study of APLA among patients with SLE found an increase in these HLA antigens.

Galeazzi *et al.* (1992) utilized DNA typing techniques to determine HLA-DPB1 alleles and found an increase of DPB1*1401 and DPB1*0301 alleles among patients with SLE with aCL antibodies, although a minority of patients with aCL had these alleles. These DPB1 alleles share a common sequence in three hypervariable regions and differ only slightly in a fourth hypervariable region.

Alleles encoding for components of the complement family have also been investigated in patients with SLE with antiphospholipid antibodies. An association of aCL antibodies with null alleles at C4A and C4B was found among African-American patients (Wilson *et al.* 1988). C4 null alleles were also found more frequently among individuals with a false positive test for syphilis in another study (Stephansson *et al.* 1993). In another study, aCL antibodies were less common among SLE patients who were homozygous for C4A deficiency, although the result did not reach statistical significance (Petri *et al.* 1993).

Other than SLE, two studies examined patients with juvenile chronic arthritis (Malleson *et al.* 1992) and with Sjögren's syndrome (Asherson *et al.* 1992b). No significant HLA association with aCL antibodies was found in either study.

It remains to be established which locus most strongly determines susceptibility, or whether particular alleles at several class II loci are important and function to synergistically increase risk. DR4 and DR7 are products of genes at the DRB1 locus and are in virtual 100% linkage disequilibrium with DR53, a product of the DRB3 locus. Therefore, one consideration is whether the DR53 is the underlying primary association. In addition to DR4 and DR7, DR9 is in linkage disequilibrium with DR53. DR9 is relatively uncommon in Caucasian populations; however, DR9 has an antigen frequency in Japanese of more than 25% (Tsjui *et al.* 1992) so that studies among Japanese should be particularly informative to address this possibility. Finally, most of the studies described included relatively small numbers of patients and most did not use molecular typing techniques. The importance of APL antibodies has only recently been appreciated and further studies will be necessary to determine which MHC alleles and/or combination so alleles are of primary importance in PAPS and APL associated with other diseases.

Animal models of anti-phospholipid antibody syndrome

Models of the APS have been recognized in a variety of lupus-prone mice. The details of these models are shown in Table 9.5. In most instances the MRL/*lpr* mouse has been studied. From approximately three months of age these mice develop IgG anti-cardiolipin antibodies. Gharavi *et al.* (1989) reported that pregnancy outcome was affected in these animals (compared with the congenic strain MRL/+/+) and they had a smaller litter size. Smith *et al.* (1990) reported that this model shows histological evidence of an occlusive vasculopathy associated with brain thrombosis and a perivascular lymphocytic infiltrate in the choroid plexus. Hess *et al.* (1993) extended these observations to demonstrate cognitive impairment and neurological abnormalities. A cross between NZB and BXSB F$_1$ male mice has been shown to develop a high incidence of degenerative coronary vascular disease and death apparently as a result of myocardial infarction, at approximately six months of age. These mice were found to have varying levels of IgG anti-cardiolipin antibodies, which were co-factor β_2-GPI dependent.

In the past decade there have been a large number of attempts to induce the anti-phospholipid syndrome in normal mice by the passive infusion of relevant antibodies (see Table 9.6) or by active immunization with different agents (see Table 9.7).

A variety of polyclonal and monoclonal anti-phospholipid antibodies have been passively infused, either intravenously or intraperitoneally, into healthy strain mice with varying consequences. In the first report by Branch *et al.* (1990) polyclonal human anti-phospholipid antibodies taken from women with the APS caused fetal loss in pregnant BALB/c mice on day eight of pregnancy. Examination of the interface between the uterus and the placenta revealed decidual necrosis as well as intravascular deposition of IgG and fibrin. The authors proposed that fetal loss was indeed mediated by this immunoglobulin binding.

In a series of studies by Blank *et al.* (1991, 1994), human polyclonal anti-phospholipid antibodies and mouse monoclonal anti-cardiolipin antibodies have been injected intravenously through the tail vein into pregnant ICR mice. These animals subsequently demonstrated fetal resorption with a reduced number of embryos and lowered placental weight.

Passive infusion of anti-phospholipid antibodies has not reproduced the widespread clotting tendency in other organs, however. Harris and colleagues (Pierangeli and Harris 1994; Pierangeli *et al.* 1995) have developed a model of thrombosis that was achieved by the passive injection of CD-1 mice, intraperitoneally, with immunoglobulins from patients who had APS followed by damaging the femoral vein by pinch injury. The authors noted that eight out of nine immunoglobulin fractions from patients with APS (or affinity purified anti-cardiolipin antibodies of the IgG and IgM isotypes) significantly enhanced the thrombotic area when injected into these mice, suggesting that the antibodies at least play a role in the longevity of the thrombus.

Table 9.5   Anti-phospholipid antibody syndrome occurring in lupus-prone mice

Strain	Serum antibodies reported	Main clinical findings	References
MRL/*lpr*	IgG–anti-CDL/PS/PI/dsDNA	Reduced litter size Thrombocytopaenia	Gharavi *et al.* (1989)
MRL/*lpr*	Anti-CDL	Brain thrombi Choroid plexus infiltrate	Smith *et al.* (1990)
MRL/*lpr*	Anti-CDL/phospholipids	Cognitive and Neurological defects	Hess *et al.* (1993)
NZBX BXSB	Anti-CDL/phospholipids (β_2-GPI dependent)	Myocardial infarction Infarction. Thrombocytopaenia	Hashimoto *et al.* (1992)

CDL = cardiolipin; PS = phosphatidylserine; PI = phosphatidylinositol.

Table 9.6 Selection of APS models induced by passive infusion of anti-phospholipid antibodies in naive mice

Strain	Immunizing antibody	Mode of administration	Clinical manifestations	References
BALB/c	Human polyclonal IgG-anti-PL (15 μg)	IP	Fetal abortions (with decidual necrosis, intravascular IgG, and fibrin deposits)	Branch et al. (1990)
ICR	Human polyclonal IgG-anti-CDL/PS	IV	Fetal resorption. Reduced number of embryos and placental weight	Blank et al. (1991, 1994)
BALB/c	Mouse monoclonal anti-CDL (10 μg) Human monoclonal IgG-anti-PC from primary APS and normal subjects	IV	Fetal resorption. Reduced number of embryos and placental weight	Meroni et al. (1997)
CD-1	Human polyclonal IgG/IgM/IgA Human polyclonal IgG/IgM/IgA anti-PL	IP	Model of thrombosis using a pinch injury to the femoral vein	Pierangeli and Harris (1994) Pierangeli et al. (1995)

IV = intravenous; IP = intraperitoneal; CDL = cardiolipin; PL = phospholipid; PS = phosphatidylserine.

Table 9.7 Selection of models of APS induced in naive mice by active immunization

Strain (mouse except where stated)	Immunizing Agent	Mode of Injection	Manifestations	References
BALB/c	Human monoclonal anti-CL (H3) (1 μg)	ID	Fetal resorption. Reduced number of fetuses and placental weight; TCP	Bakimer et al. (1992)
BALB/c	Mouse monoclonal anti-CL (2C42)	ID	Reduced pregnancy rate, ([as for Bakimer et al. (1992)])	Sthoeger et al. (1993)
BALB/c	Mouse anti CL scFv	ID	Antibodies only	Blank et al. (submitted) Pierangeli and Harris (1993)
NZW (rabbit)	β₂-GPI (150 μg)	SC	Anti-CL/β₂-GPI	
BALB/c	Anti-CL (1 μg)	SC	Accelerated APS clinical manifestations and anti-CL	Aron et al. (1995)
MRL/++	β₂-GPI (20 μg)	Not stated		
BALB/c	β₂-GPI	SC	Antibodies only anti-β₂-GPI	Silver et al. (1995)

ID = intradermal; TCP = thrombocytopenia; SC = subcutaneous; CL = cardiolipin; scFv = single chain Fv.

Active induction

Rather more controversial have been attempts to induce the clinical features as well as the serology of the anti-phospholipid syndrome by active immunization. Bakimer *et al.* (1992) have reported that intradermal injection of a human monoclonal anti-cardiolipin antibody (H3) led to fetal resorption and a reduced number of embryos and lowered placental weight, together with thrombocytopaenic purpura. Sthoeger *et al.* (1993) reported much the same effect using a mouse monoclonal anti-cardiolipin antibody. This too was given by intradermal injection. In contrast, Pierangeli and Harris (1993) and Silver *et al.* (1995), when injecting β_2-GPI into rabbits or mice subcutaneously, were able to produce anti-phospholipid antibodies but no evidence of any clinical disease. A variety of attempts to improve the outcome of animal models, including the use of low dose aspirin, low molecular weight heparin, and intravenous gammaglobulin, have met with some success (Ziporin *et al.* 1997).

Immunopathology, including laboratory tests

There are two broad categories of phospholipids. The neutrally charged phospholipids include phosphatidyl ethanolamine, phosphatidyl choline, platelet-activating factor, and sphingomyelin. Negatively charged phospholipids include phosphatidyl glycerol, phosphatidyl serine, phosphatidyl acid, phosphatidyl inositol, and cardiolipin. Although antibodies to each of these structures can be identified (Ravirajan *et al.* 1995), in practice, anti-phospholipid antibodies are detected conventionally by identifying anti-cardiolipin antibodies, usually by ELISA, or a lupus anticoagulant. While there is clearly some overlap between these populations of antibodies, they may also be distinct. Thus some patients may have a strongly positive lupus anticoagulant but lack IgG or IgM anti-cardiolipin antibodies, and vice versa. More recently the importance of co-factors, in particular β_2-glycoprotein-I (β_2-GPI), which may complex with cardiolipin, has been recognized (see below) and there is an increasing interest in detecting antibodies to β_2-GPI.

The original test for detecting anti-cardiolipin antibodies involved a radioimmunoassay. This test has now been superseded by anti-cardiolipin ELISA kits, which are very popular. These assays may be idotype specific or use polyvalent detecting reagents. As dis-

cussed below, it is evident that the IgG anti-cardiolipin antibodies are those most likely to be truly pathogenic.

Lupus anticoagulants are immunoglobulins (usually IgG, IgM, or a mixture) which interfere with the *in vitro* phospholipid-dependent tests of coagulation (including the prothrombin time, activated partial thromboplastic time APTT), and dilute Russell Viper venom time). These antibodies are directed against phospholipid epitopes and act as an inhibitor of the prothrombinase complex, prolonging the *in vitro* assays that measure coagulation by the extrinsic pathway. In the past decade there have been a number of attempts to compare the various assays which are thought to detect the lupus anticoagulant and a number of interlaboratory comparative studies (discussed by Bick 1993). It is evident that careful plasma preparation with avoidance of platelet contamination and use of a suitable test in addition to the APTT, and attention to methodological detail, are essential for the reliable identification of a lupus anticoagulant.

Anti-phospholipid antibodies in other conditions

Both anti-phospholipid antibodies and the lupus anticoagulant are found in a wide variety of other conditions (Bick 1993). These conditions range from infectious diseases (bacterial and viral, including HIV) to other autoimmune diseases. Treatment with a number of drugs may induce these antibodies. Examples of such drugs include chlorpromazine, hydralazine, procainamide, quinidine, and phenytoin. With the exception of some patients with SLE the presence of these anti-phospholipid antibodies is not associated with thrombosis or fetal loss.

Co-factors and associated autoantibodies

In 1990 three groups (Galli *et al.* 1990, Matsuura *et al.* 1990, McNeil *et al.* 1990) showed that β_2-glycoprotein-I (β_2-GPI) was a co-factor for the binding of certain antibodies to anionic phospholipids, at least as detected in solid-phase ELISAs. Its main features are shown in Table 9.8. β_2-GPI is a protein of approximately 50 kDa that is found at a concentration of approximately 200 μg/ml in plasma. It is a highly glycosylated, single-chain polypeptide of 326 amino acids containing a high proportion of proline and cysteine residues. It has five common repeating motifs/domains of about 60 amino acids, with a highly conserved pattern of cysteine residues. Although its physiological

Table 9.8 Main features of co-factor β_2-glycoprotein-I

Also known as apolipoprotein H

50 kDa glycoprotein (326 amino acids)

Plasma concentration $\sim$ 200 μg/ml

Inhibits
1.   The intrinsic blood coagulation pathway
2.   ADP-mediated platelet aggregation
3.   Prothrombinase activity of activated platelets

Binding of β_2-GPI to cardiolipin induces a change in phospholipid conformation from bilayer to hexagonal form

---

role remains uncertain, *in vitro* it has been shown to inhibit thrombin formation. Attempts to link β_2-GPI levels to disease manifestations in patients with the anti-phospholipid antibody syndrome have produced conflicting results (see Table 9.9) (Inanc *et al.* 1997). Further suggestions that raised β_2-GPI levels in patients with lupus who have hyperlipidaemia may be at greater risk of developing thrombosis have not been confirmed (Ichikawa *et al.* 1992). There is similarly conflicting information about whether a correlation exists between lupus anticoagulant activity and β_2-GPI levels. However, it does seem likely that total β_2-GPI levels are increased in lupus patients who are anti-phospholipid antibody-positive (McNally *et al.* 1995). β_2-GPI may therefore play a role in the pathogenesis mechanism of the thrombus formation that is associated with anti-phospholipid antibodies. Gharavi *et al.* (1992) reported the development of both antiphospholipid and anti-B$_2$-GP1 antibodies in healthy mice and rabbits following immunization with purified human B$_2$-GP1.

Arvieux *et al.* (1991) described an ELISA to detect anti-β_2-GPI antibodies and showed a good correlation between anti-cardiolipin and anti-β_2-GPI antibodies. Viard *et al.* (1992) reported that anti-β_2-GPI anti-bodies were associated with thrombosis and lupus anti-coagulant in patients with lupus. It is now generally agreed, following irradiation of ELISA plates, that β_2-GPI binds plastic better and becomes more reactive to antibodies even in the absence of phospholipid. Recent studies have focused on the value of anti-β_2-GPI antibody as a marker for the clinical features of the anti-phospholipid antibody syndrome. Thus, Roubey *et al.* (1996) and Tsutsumi *et al.* (1996), in retrospective studies, found a positive predictive value for anti-β_2-GPI antibodies for a history of thrombosis. In a sequential analysis of seven lupus patients for whom serum samples were available both prior to as well as after their thrombotic or neurological events, six had IgG anti-β_2-GPI levels raised several months before the advent of clinical disease (Inanc *et al.* 1997).

Several attempts (e.g. Galli and Bevers 1994; Alarcón-Segovia and Cabral 1996) have been made to classify the various types of anti-phospholipid anti-bodies. In Table 9.10 a synthesis of these previous attempts is shown. It seems likely that relatively few of these antibodies will be truly pathogenic but never-theless they may be useful markers for different diseases.

Table 9.9 Studies on β_2-GPI levels in SLE and APS

Patients studied	β_2-GPI levels	Association between	Reference
SLE, $n = 10$	$\uparrow^*$	No data provided	Cohnen (1970)
SLE, $n = 36$	$\downarrow^*$ ($p < 0.005$)	No	Ichikawa *et al.* (1994)
APS, $n = 12$	$\uparrow$($p < 0.05$)	No data provided	Vlachoyiannopoulos *et al.* (1992, 1993)
SLE, $n = 25$			
Lupus anticoagulant-positive patients, $n = 34$	$\uparrow^*$ ($p = 0.005$)	No	Galli *et al.* (1992)
SLE/APS, $n = 17$	$\uparrow\dagger$	Yes	McNally *et al.* (1995)

* Compared with normal controls.

$\dagger$ Compared with anti-phospholipid antibody-negative SLE patients.

Table 9.10   Proposed classification of anti-phospholipid antibodies

1.	True anti-phospholipid antibodies (i.e. no co-factor requirement)
	e.g. IgM anti-phosphatidylcholine in mice
	IgM anti-phosphatidylcholine in patients with autoimmune haemolytic anaemia
	Anti-cardiolipin antibodies (usually IgM) in patients with syphilis
2.	Lupus anticoagulant antibodies (recognize prothrombin–phospholipid complex)
3.	Anti-cardiolipin antibodies (recognize β_2-GPI–phospholipid complex), may/may not have anticoagulant activity
4.	Anti-β_2-GPI
5.	Anti-protein S and activated protein C antibodies (which recognize protein S/C after their binding to anionic phospholipid)
6.	Others — including anti-prothrombin

From Alarcón-Segovia and Cabral (1996).

Anti-phospholipid antibodies: mechanisms of action

Although, as indicated above, some of the animal model studies do indicate support for the notion that anti-phospholipid antibodies may be truly pathogenic, definitive evidence in humans does not exist. Triplett (1992) has reviewed the potential antigenicity of protein–phospholipid complexes, which are certainly very heterogeneous (see Table 9.11), and if antibodies are indeed directed against these varying complexes, different clinical effects may result.

The mechanism of pregnancy loss in this syndrome remains uncertain Merani *et al.* 1995. It seems likely that progressive thrombosis of the microvasculature of the placenta, which leads to infarction (Fig. 9.4–9.9)

may cause placental insufficiency, which in turn leads to fetal growth retardation and fetal death in some patients. However, Out *et al.* (1991) reported that not all placentas examined have shown areas of thrombosis or infarction and it is therefore likely that other mechanisms must be effective.

A variety of hypotheses have been proposed to explain how anti-phospholipid antibodies might cause a thrombotic episode associated with PAPS. These include interference with the production and release of prostacyclin by endothelial cells, interference in the regultion of protein-C and protein-S pathways, inhibition of the action of phospholipid placental anticoagulant protein-1 (PAP-1), endothelial cell damage and activation, activation of platelets by the antibodies, impairment of fibrinolytic mechanisms, and inter-

Table 9.11   Potential phospholipid–protein antigen complexes

Protein–phospholipid complex	Physiological role of the protein	Potential pathological effect of altered protein function
β_2-GPI–phospholipid	Anticoagulant inhibits contact phase of coagulation, inhibits prothrombinases; inhibits ADP–platelet activation	Impaired anticoagulant control
Prothrombin–phospholipid	Zymogen precursor of thrombin Vitamin K-dependent protein	Antibody binding this complex may induce activation to thrombin
Placental anticoagulant Prothrombin-1/phospholipid	Anticoagulant binds to anionic phospholipids: member of lipocortin family	Loss of anti-coagulant properties
Thrombomodulin–phospholipid	Endothelial membrane co-factor for activation of protein C	Loss of protein C's role in anticoagulant regulation
Phospholipase A2–phospholipid	Initiates prostaglandin pathway with the generation of arachidonic acid	Decreased prostaglandin production in endothelial cells

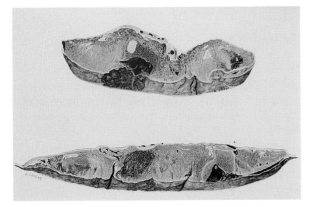

Fig. 9.4. Small thrombi in placental vessels, which are invariably found in women with multiple miscarriages. (This figure and 9.5 to 9.9 are courtesy of Lorin Lakasing)

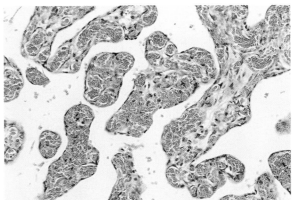

Fig. 9.7. Placental intravascular thromboses in a patient with primary APS delivered at 36 weeks gestation. This patient had suffered 3 second trimester losses and one first trimester loss previously, and had no live children. She was put on aspirin and heparin preconceptually but warfarinised antenatally following a CVA at 14 weeks gestation. She was admitted at 36 weeks gestation and put on an IV heparin infusion with the intention to deliver by Caesarean section at 37 weeks gestation. However, she developed recurrent TIAs on the 3rd day of heparin therapy and was therefore delivered later that evening. The baby was *normally* developed with a birthweight on the 50th centile for gestational age.

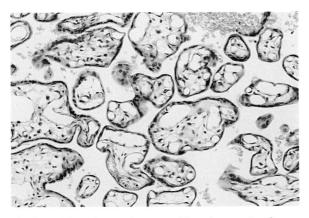

Fig. 9.5. Normal term placenta at 38 weeks gestation from a patient used as a control for the study. Specimen shows mature terminal villi and normal placental architecture.

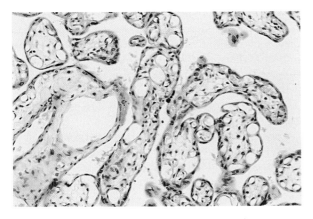

Fig. 9.6. Normal preterm placenta at 32 weeks gestation from a patient delivered electively for treatment of maternal malignancy. Also a control for the study. Specimen shows immature intermediate villi and normal architecture for this gestation.

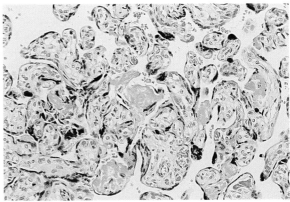

Fig. 9.8. Placenta from a patient with SLE with renal involvement showing syncitial knotting and fibrin deposition, changes seen in hypoxia. This patient developed early-onset, rapidly progressing pre-eclampsia and required delivery at 29 weeks gestation for deteriorating maternal condition. The baby's birthweight was on the 15th centile for gestational age. This patient has suffered from 2 previous third trimester intrauterine deaths and a neonatal death following delivery of a 26 weeks gestation infant the year before. She was treated with aspirin and a range of antihypertensives in this pregnancy. Interestingly, the same changes are seen in high altitude pregnancies.

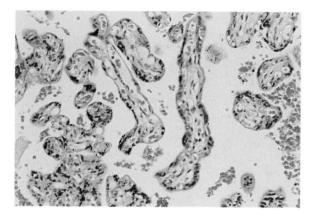

Fig. 9.9. Long placental villi showing unbranched villous vasculature in a patient with primary APS delivered at 31 weeks gestation for pre-eclampsia and intrauterine growth restriction (IUGR). This patient was a primagravida with a previous CVA. She was put on aspirin and heparin preconceptually but warfarinised antenatally following a cerebellar artery thrombosis at 12 weeks gestation. Serial ultrasound scans showed abnormal uterine artery Doppler waveforms and subsequently abnormal umbilical artery waveforms with a poor biophysical profile. Delivery was expedited for deteriorating maternal and fetal condition. The baby was·on the 8th centile for gestational age. These placental findings are typical of IUGR.

ference with the activity of antithrombin III (for review see Santoro 1994). The recent work of Shibata *et al.* (1994) has supported the notion that anti-phospholipid antibodies are able to bind heparin/heparan sulphate which could in turn lead to the elevation of prothrombin fragments and fibrinopeptide A that are known to be associated with increased thrombin activity. Thrombin is known to have multiple actions in promoting coagulation and by this somewhat circuitous route anti-phospholipid antibodies may be linked to vascular thrombosis.

Although, as indicated previously in this chapter, there is considerable interest in the precise targets to which anti-phospholipid antibodies bind, it is generally agreed that the β_2-GPI co-factor increases the binding of the autoimmune anti-phospholipid antibodies to phospholipid, and combines with the phospholipid itself, whereupon both undergo conformational change. This change seems likely to create a neoantigen that is almost certainly the epitope recognized by the anti-phospholipid antibody. However, as with many aspects of PAPS, the relationship of this new antigen with the normal coagulation and pathogenesis of PAPS is not well understood.

Management of anti-phospholipid antibody syndrome

Patients with anti-phospholipid antibodies are at high risk of thrombosis. Other risks for vascular disease should be reduced or removed. Treatment of hypertension and hypercholesterolaemia is necessary, together with advice about weight control, cessation of smoking, and exercise. Female patients should be counselled against the use of oestrogen-containing contraceptive pills.

Thrombosis

The immediate management of arterial or venous thrombotic events follows standard methods of anticoagulation using heparin initially, followed by warfarin. These patients are at high risk of recurrent events and the optimal long-term strategy for these patients is unknown. At present, prolonged (possibly lifelong) prophylaxis is recommended. In the largest retrospective study, of 147 patients, recurrent thrombosis occurred in 69% of patients. Intensive warfarin anticoagulation (INR >3.0) was the most effective secondary prevention of arterial and venous thrombosis (Khamashta *et al.* 1995). A smaller prospective study suggested that patients with venous thrombosis and lupus anticoagulant, but no other features of the anti-phospholipid antibody syndrome, may respond to less intensive anticoagulation with warfarin (INR 2.0–3.0) (Ginsberg *et al.* 1995). The potential benefits of long-term anticoagulation must be balanced against the risks, particularly of major haemorrhage (Fig. 9.1d).

A few patients develop progressive and catastrophic thrombosis despite anticoagulation, affecting many organs (Asherson 1992a). In these patients immunosuppression with high dose corticosteroids combined with either cyclophosphamide or azathioprine is necessary, possibly with plasmapheresis (Neuwelt *et al.* 1997).

The optimum treatment of patients with anti-phospholipid antibodies but no history of thrombosis is controversial. Many clinicians use low dose aspirin (75 mg/day) in patients with no history of thrombosis but persistently high IgG anti-cardiolipin antibodies and/or positive lupus anticoagulant. These patients should be monitored carefully as they are at greatest risk of thrombosis. In addition, consideration should be given to prophylactic anticoagulation with heparin in high risk situations, such as surgery.

Hydroxychloroquine has an anti-platelet effect and SLE patients taking hydroxychloroquine have fewer thrombotic complications (Wallace 1987). A prospective study from Johns Hopkins University has confirmed this observation (reviewed in Petri 1997).

Recurrent fetal loss

The management of women with recurrent fetal loss in the primary anti-phospholipid antibody syndrome is controversial. Options include low dose aspirin (Silver *et al.* 1993), prednisolone (Lockshin *et al.* 1989; Cowchock *et al.* 1992) or anticoagulation with subcutaneous heparin (Cowchock *et al.* 1992). Prednisolone alone is not effective in preventing fetal death (Lockshin *et al.* 1989) and is associated with increased fetal and maternal complications (Cowchock *et al.* 1992; Silver *et al.* 1993). Subcutaneous heparin and low dose aspirin are equally effective in terms of fetal outcome (Cowchock *et al.* 1992). The combination of heparin and aspirin is more effective than aspirin alone in women with cardiolipin antibodies (Kutteh 1996; Rai *et al.* 1997). Recently, prednisolone and aspirin were shown not to be effective in preventing fetal loss in patients with autoantibodies (including ANA and DNA) and also increased the risk of prematurity (Laskin *et al.* 1997). This study only included a small number of patients with cardiolipin antibodies. Other experimental therapies include intravenous immunoglobulin (Wapner *et al.* 1990) but the role of this modality remains uncertain.

Patients with cardiolipin antibodies or lupus anticoagulant and no history of fetal loss do not require treatment. The use of aspirin (75 mg/day) in pregnant women with high titres of anti-phospholipid antibodies and no previous pregnancy loss has not been prospectively tested.

Thrombocytopaenia

Many (perhaps 30%) of anti-phospholipid antibody syndrome patients have thrombocytopaenia, despite which they are at risk of thrombosis. Corticosteroids should be used to increase the platelet count to above $50 \times 10^9/l$. Splenectomy is beneficial in at least some of these patients (Hakim *et al.* 1998).

Treatment in experimental models

In experimental models, particularly the active immunization model, a number of different therapies have been tried with promising results for reduction in fetal loss and increase in embryo weights, these include: low dose aspirin, recombinant IL-3, low molecular weight heparin, intravenous immunoglobulin, thromboxane receptor antagonist, anti-CD4 monoclonal antibodies, bone marrow transplantation, bromocriptine, ciprofloxacin, and anti-idiotypic antibodies (reviewed in Ziporen *et al.* 1997).

Summary

While coagulopathies associated with anti-phospholipid antibodies have been recognized for some time, particularly in association with SLE, it is only relatively recently that the primary anti-phospholipid antibody syndrome has been recognized as a distinct disease entity. The condition manifests clinically as blood clots in veins or arteries, thrombocytopenia, and recurrent fetal loss. Antibodies to cardiolipin and its associated co-factor, β_2-glycoprotein are evident and it may be that anti-co-factor antibodies are better markers of thrombotic disease than anti-cardiolipin antibodies. The long-term outcome of the syndrome is still uncertain. The clotting aspects of the syndrome can be managed by oral anticoagulants, while the recurrent fetal loss can be controlled by aspirin and low molecular weight heparin subcutaneous injections.

References

Alarcón-Segovia D, Cabral AR. The anti-phospholipid/cofactor syndromes. *J Rheumatol* 1996; **23**: 1319–32.

Alarcón-Segovia D, Deleze M, Oria CV *et al.* Antiphospholipid antibodies and the anti-phospholipid syndrome in systemic lupus erythematosus: a prospective analysis of 500 consecutive patients. *Medicine* 1989; **68**: 353–65.

Arnett FC, Olsen ML, Anderson KL *et al.* Molecular analysis of major histocompatibility complex alleles associated with the lupus anticoagulant. *J Clin Invest* 1991; **87**: 1490–5.

Aron AL, Cuellar ML, Brey RL *et al.* Early onset of autoimmunity in MRL/++ mice following immunization with β_2 glycoprotein. *Clin Exp Immunol* 1995; **101**: 78–81.

Arvieux J, Roussel B, Jacob MC *et al.* Measurement of anti-phospholipid antibodies by ELISA using β_2 glycoprotein-1 as an antigen. *J Immunol Meth* 1991; **143**: 223–9.

Asherson RA. The catastrophic anti-phospholipid syndrome. *J Rheumatol* 1992; **19**: 508–12.

Asherson RA, Morgan SH, Harris EN *et al.* Arterial occlusion causing large bowel infarction in SLE? Reflection of clotting diathesis. *Clin Rheumatol* 1986; **5**: 102–6.

Asherson RA, Khamashta MA, Gil A *et al.* Cerebrovascular disease and anti-phospholipid antibodies in systemic lupus erythematosus, 'lupus-like' disease and the 'primary' anti-phospholipid syndrome. *Am J Med* 1989a; **86**: 391–9.

Asherson RA, Khamashta MA, Ordi-Ros J *et al.* The 'primary' antiphospholipid syndrome–major clinical and serological features. *Medicine* 1989b; **68**: 366–74.

Asherson RA, Mayou SC, Merry P *et al.* The spectrum of livedo reticularis and anticardiolipin antibodies. *Br J Dermatol* 1989c; **120**: 215–21.

Asherson RA, Doherty DG, Vergnai D *et al.* Concise communication: Major histocompatibility complex associations with primary anti-phospholipid syndrome. *Arthritis Rheum* 1992a; **35**: 124–5.

Asherson RA, Fei H-M, Staub HL *et al.* Antiphospholipid antibodies and HLA associations in primary Sjögren's syndrome. *Ann Rheum Dis* 1992b; **51**: 495–8.

Bakimer R, Fishman P, Blank M *et al.* Induction of primary anti-phospholipid syndrome in mice by immunizing with a human monoclonal anticardiolipin antibody (H3). *J Clin Invest* 1992; **89**: 1558–63.

Beaman KD, Gilman-Sachs A, Cifuentes D *et al.* Presence of multiple anti-phospholipid antibody specificities in a pediatric population. *Autoimmunity* 1995; **21**: 99–106.

Bick RL. The anti-phospholipid-thrombosis syndromes. Fact, fiction, confusion and controversy. *Am J Clin Pathol* 1993; **100**: 477–80.

Blank M, Tincani A, Shoenfeld Y. Induction of anti-phospholipid syndrome in naive mice with purified IgG anti-phosphatidylserine antibodies. *J Rheumatol* 1994; **21**: 100–4.

Branch DW, Dudley DJ, Mitchell MD *et al.* Immunoglobulin G fractions from patients with anti-phospholipid antibodies cause fetal death in BALB/c mice. A model for autoimmune fetal loss. *Am J Obstet Gynecol* 1990; **163**: 210–16.

Branch DW, Silver RM, Blackwell JL *et al.* Outcome of treated pregnancies in women with anti-phospholipid syndrome: an update of the Utah experience. *Obstet Gynecol* 1992; **80**: 614–20.

Buchanan NMM, Khamashta MA, Morton KE *et al.* A study of 100 high risk lupus pregnancies. *Am J Reprod Immunol* 1992; **28**: 192–4.

Cohnen G. Immunochemical quantitation of β_2-glycoprotein-1 in various diseases. *J Lab Clin Med* 1970; **75**: 212–16.

Cowchock FS, Reece EA, Balaban D *et al.* Repeated fetal losses associated with anti-phospholipid antibodies: a collaborative randomised trial comparing prednisone to low-dose heparin treatment. *Am J Obstet Gynecol* 1992; **166**: 1318–23.

Exner T, Barber S, Kronenberg H *et al.* Familial association of the lupus anticoiagulant. *Br J Haematol* 1980; **45**: 89–96.

Galeazzi M, Sebastiani GD, Passiu G *et al.* HLA-DP genotyping in patients with systemic lupus erythematosus: correlations with autoantibody subsets. *J Rheumatol* 1992; **19**: 42–6.

Galli M, Bevers EM. Inhibition of phospholipid dependent coagulation reactions by anti-phospholipid antibodies: possible modes of action. *Lupus* 1994; **3**: 223–8.

Galli M, Comfurius P, Masson C *et al.* Anticardiolipin antibodies (ACA) directed not to cardiolipin but to a plasma protein cofactor. *Lancet* 1990; **336**: 1544–7.

Galli M, Cortelazza S, Daldossi M *et al.* Increased levels of β_2-glycoprotein 1 (aca-cofactor) in patients with lupus anticoagulant. *Thromb Haemostat* 1992; **67**: 386.

Galve E, Ordi J, Barquinero J *et al.* Valvular heart disease in primary anti-phospholipid syndrome. *Ann Int Med* 1992; **116**: 293–8.

Gattorno M, Buoncompagni A, Molinari AC *et al.* Antiphospholipid antibodies in paediatric systemic lupus erythematosus, juvenile chronic arthritis and overlap syndrome: SLE patients with both lupus anticoagulant and high titre anticardiolipin antibodies are at risk for clinical manifestations related to the anti-phospholipid syndrome. *Br J Rheumatol* 1995; **34**: 873–81.

Gharavi AE, Mellors RC, Elkon KB. IgG anti-cardiolipin antibodies in murine lupus. *Clin Exp Immunol* 1989; **78**: 233–8.

Gharavi AE, Sammaritano LR, Wen J *et al.* Induction of antiphospholipid autoantibodies by immunization with β-2 glycoprotein 1 (apolipoprotein H). *J Clin Invest* 1992; **90**: 1105–9.

Ginsberg JS, Wells PS, Brill-Edwards P *et al.* Anti-phospholipid antibodies and venous thromboembolism. *Blood* 1995; **86**: 3685–91.

Gulko PS, Reveille JD, Koopman WJ *et al.* Anticardiolipin antibodies in systemic lupus erythematosus: clinical correlates, HLA associations, and impact on survival. *J Rheumatol* 1993; **20**: 1684–93.

Hakim A, Machin SJ, Isenberg DA. Autoimmune thrombocytopenia in primary anti-phospholipid syndrome and systemic lupus erythematosus. The response to splenectomy. *Semin Arthritis Rheum* 1998; **28**: 20–5.

Hamsten A, Norberg R, Bjorkholm M *et al.* Antibodies to cardiolipin in young survivors of myocardial infarction: an association with recurrent cardiovascular events. *Lancet* 1986; **i**: 113–16.

Harris EN, Spinnato JA. Should anticardiolipin tests be performed in otherwise healthy pregnant women? *Am J Obstet Gynecol* 1991; **165**: 1272–7.

Hartung K, Coldewey R, Corvetta A *et al.* MHC gene products and anticardiolipin antibodies in systemic lupus erythematosus: results of a multicenter study. SLE study group. *Autoimmunity* 1992; **13**: 95–9.

Hashimoto Y, Kawamura M, Ichikawa K *et al.* Anticardiolipin antibodies in NZW × BcSB F1 mice. *J Immunol* 1992; **149**: 1063–8.

Herrantz MT, Rivier G, Khamashta MA *et al.* Association between anti-phospholipid antibodies and epilepsy in patients with systemic lupus erythematosus. *Arthritis Rheum* 1994; **37**: 568–71.

Hess DC, Taormina M, Thompson J *et al.* Cognitive and neurologic deficits in the MRL/*lpr* mouse: a clinico-pathologic study. *J Rheumatol* 1993; **20**: 610–17.

Ichikawa K, Takamatsu K, Shimizu H *et al.* Serum apolipoprotein H levels in systemic lupus erythematosus are not influenced by anti-phospholipid antibodies. *Lupus* 1992; **1**: 45–9.

Ichikawa K, Khamashta M, Koike T *et al.* β_2-glycoprotein-1 reactivity of monoclonal anticardiolipin antibodies from patients with the anti-phospholipid syndrome. *Arthritis Rheum* 1994; **37**: 1453–61.

Inanc M, Radway-Bright EL, Isenberg DA. β_2-glycoprotein-1 and anti-β_2-glycoprotein-1 antibodies: where are we now? *Br J Rheumatol* 1997; **36**: 1247–57.

Inanc M, Donohoe S, Ravirajan CT *et al*. Anti β_2-glyco-protein-I and anti prothrombin antibodies in patients with SLE before and after thrombotic neurological events. *Brit J Rheumatol* (In press).

Isenberg DA, Horsfall A. Systemic lupus erythematosus — adult onset. In: eds *Oxford Textbook of Rheumatology*, 2nd edn, Maddison P, Isenberg DA, Woo P, Glass D. Oxford University Press, Oxford. 1998; 1146–80.

Karpatkin S. Autoimmune thrombocytopenia purpura. *Sem Haematolo* 1985; **22**: 260–88.

Khamashta MA, Machin SJ. Hematological immune cytopenias and anti-phospholipid antibodies. In: *Phospholipid Binding Antibodies*, eds Harris EN, Exner T, Hughes GRV, Asherson RA. CRC Press, Boca Raton, Florida, 1991; 247–54.

Khamashta MA, Cervera R, Ascherson RA *et al*. Association of anti-phospholipid antibodies with heart valve disease in systemic lupus erythematosus. *Lancet* 1990; **335**: 1541–4.

Khamashta MA, Cuadrado MJ, Mujic F *et al*. the management of thrombosis in the anti-phospholipid antibody syndrome. *N Eng J Med* 1995; **332**: 993–7.

Kutteh WH. anti-phospholipid antibody associated recurrent pregnancy loss: treatment with heparin and low dose aspirin is superior to low dose aspirin alone. *Am J Obstet Gynecol* 1996; **174**: 1584–9.

Laskin CA, Bombardier C, Hannah ME *et al*. Prednisolone and aspirin in women with autoantibodies and unexplained recurrent fetal loss. *N Eng J Med* 1997; **337**: 148–53.

Leaker B, McGregor A, Griffiths M *et al*. Insidious loss of renal function in patients with anti-cardiolipin antibodies and absence of overt nephritis. *Ann Rheum Dis* 1991; **30**: 422–5.

Lockshin MD. Antiphospholipid antibody syndrome. *JAMA* 1992; **268**: 1451–3.

Lockshin MD, Druzin ML, Qamar T. Prednisone does not prevent recurrent fetal death in women with anti-phospholipid syndrome. *Am J Obstet Gynecol* 1989; **160**: 439–43.

Love PE, Santoro SA. Antiphospholipid antibodies: anti-cardiolipin and the lupus anticoagulant in systemic lupus erythematosus (SLE) and in non-SLE disorders. *Ann Intern Med* 1990; **112**: 682–98.

Malleson PN, Fung MY, Petty RE *et al*. Autoantibodies in chronic arthritis of childhood: Relationship with each other and with histocompatibility antigens. *Ann Rheum Dis* 1992; **51**: 1301–6.

Matsuura E, Igareshi Y, Fujimoto M *et al*. Anticardiolipin co-factor(s) and differential diagnosis of autoimmune disease. *Lancet* 1990; **336**: 177–8.

McHugh NJ, Maddison PJ. HLA-DR antigens and anti-cardiolipin antibodies in patients with systemic lupus erythematosus. *Arthritis Rheum* 1989; **32**: 1623–24.

McNally T, Mackie I, Machin SJ *et al*. Elevated levels of β_2 glycoprotein-1 (β_2 GPI) in anti-phospholipid antibody syndrome are due to increased amounts of β_2 GPI in association with other plasma constituents. *Blood Coag Fibrin* 1995; **6**: 411–16.

McNeil HP, Simpson RJ, Chesterman CN *et al*. Anti-phospholipid antibodies are directed against a complex antigen that includes a lipid-binding inhibitor of coagulation: β_2 glycoprotein 1 (apolipoprotein H). *Proc Natl Acad Sci USA* 1990; **87**: 4120–4.

Meroni PL, Piona A, La Rosa L *et al*. Antiphospholipid antibodies and fetal loss: clinical association and possible pathogenic role in experimental models. *Reg Immuno* 1995; **6**: 344–9.

Nencini P, Baruffi MC, Abbati R *et al*. Lupus anticoagulant and anticardiolipin antibodies in young adults with cerebral ischemia. *Stroke* 1992; **23**: 189–93.

Neuwelt CM, Daikh DI, Linfoot JA *et al*. Catastrophic anti-phospholipid syndrome–response to repeated plasma-pheresis over ten years. *Arthritis Rheum* 1997; **40**: 1534–9.

Out HJ, Kooijman CD, Bruinse HW *et al*. Histopathological findings in placentae from patients with intra-uterine fetal death and anti-phospholipid antibodies. *Eur J Obst Gynaecol Reprod Biol* 1991; **341**: 179–86.

Petri M. Pathogenesis and treatment of the anti-phospholipid antibody syndrome. *Med Clin North Am* 1997; **81**: 151–77.

Petri M, Watson R, Winkelstein JA *et al*. Clinical expression of systemic lupus erythematosus in patients with C4A deficiency. *Medicine* 1993; **72**: 236–44.

Pierangeli SS, Harris EN. Induction of phospholipid binding antibodies in mice and rabbits by immunization with human β_2 glycoprotein 1 or anticardiolipin antibodies alone. *Clin Exp Immunol* 1993; **93**: 269–72.

Pierangeli S, Harris EN. Antiphospholipid antibodies in an in vivo thrombosis model in mice. *Lupus* 1994; **3**: 247–51.

Pierangeli S, Wei Liu X, Barker JH *et al*. Induction of thrombosis in a mouse model by IgG, IgM and IgA immuno-globulins from patients with the anti-phospholipid syndrome. *Thromb Haemost* 1995; **74**: 1361–7.

Rai RS, Regan L, Clifford K *et al*. Antiphospholipid antibodies and β_2 glycoprotein-I in 500 women with recurrent miscarriage: results of a comprehensive screening approach. *Hum Reprod* 1995; **10**: 101–5.

Rai R, Cohen H, Dave M *et al*. Randomised controlled trial of aspirin and aspirin plus heparin in pregnant women with recurrent miscarriage associated with phospholipid antibodies. *Br Med J* 1997; **314**: 253–7.

Ravirajan CT, Harmer I, McNally T *et al*. Phospholipid binding specificities and idiotype expression of hybridoma derived monoclonal autoantibodies from splenic cells of patients with systemic lupus erythematosus. *Ann Rheum Dis* 1995; **S4**: 471–6.

Roubey RAS, Maldonado MA, Byrd S. Comparison of an enzyme-linked immunosorbent assay for antibodies to β_2-glycoprotein-1 and a conventional anti-cardiolipin immuno-assay. *Arthritis Rheum* 1996; **79**: 1606–7.

Santoro SA. Antiphospholipid antibodies and thrombotic pre-disposition: underlying pathogenetic mechanisms. *Blood* 1994; **83**: 2389–91.

Savi M, Ferraccioli GF, Teri TM *et al*. HLA-DR antigens and anticardiolipin antibodies in northern Italian systemic lupus erythematosus patients. *Arthritis Rheum* 1988; **311**: 1568–70.

Sebastiani GD, Lulli P, Passiu G *et al*. Anticardiolipin anti-bodies: their relationship with HLA-DR antigens in systemic lupus erythematosus. *Br J Rheumatol* 1991; **30**: 156–7.

Shibata S, Harpel PC, Gharavi A *et al*. Autoantibodies to heparin from patients with anti-phospholipid antibody syndrome inhibit formation of antithrombin III-thrombin complexes. *Blood* 1994; **83**: 2532–40.

Silver RK, MacGregor SN, Pasternak JF *et al.* Fetal stroke associated with elevated maternal anticardiolipin antibodies. *Obstet Gynecol* 1992; **80**: 497–9.

Silver RK, MacGregor SN, Sholl JS *et al.* Comparative trial of prednisone plus aspirin versus aspirin alone in the treatment of anticardiolipin positive obstetric patients. *Am J Obstet Gynecol* 1993; **169**: 1411–17.

Silver RN, Pierangeli SS, Gharavi AE *et al.* Induction of high levels of anticardiolipin antibodies in mice by immunization with β_2-glycoprotein 1 does not cause fetal death. *Am J Obstet Gynecol* 1995; **173**: 1410–15.

Smith HR, Hansen CL, Rose R *et al.* Autoimmune MRL-lpr/lpr mice are an animal model for the secondary anti-phospholipid syndrome. *J Rheumatol* 1990; **17**: 911–15.

Stephansson EA, Koskimies S, Lokki ML. HLA antigens and complement C4 allotypes in patients with chronic biologically false positive (CBFP) seroreactions for syphilis. A follow-up study of SLE patients and CBFP reactors. *Lupus* 1993; **2**: 77–81.

Sthoeger ZM, Mozes E, Tartakovsky B. Anti-cardiolipin antibodies induce pregnancy failure by impairing embryonic implantation. *Proc Natl Acad Sci USA* 1993; **90**: 6464–7.

Trabace S, Nicotra M, Cappellacci S *et al.* HLA-DR and DQ antigens and anticardiolipin antibodies in women with recurrent spontaneous abortions. *Am J Reprod Immunol* 1991; **26**: 147–9.

Triplett DA. Antiphospholipid antibodies: proposed mechanisms of action. *Am J Reprod Immunol* 1992; **28**: 211–15.

Tsuji K, Aizawa M, Sasazuki T. (eds). *HLA 1991. Proceedings of the Eleventh International Histocompatibility Workshop and Conference*, held in Yokohama Japan 6–13 November 1991. Oxford University Press, New York, 1992.

Tsutsumi A, Matsuura E, Ichikawa K *et al.* Antibodies to β_2 glycoprotein-1 and clinical manifestations in patients with systemic lupus erythematosus. *Arthritis Rheum* 1996; **39**: 1466–74.

Tucker LB. Antiphospholipid syndrome in childhood: the great unknown. *Lupus* 1994; **3**: 367–9.

Viard JP, Amoura Z, Bach JF. Association of anti-β_2 glycoprotein-I antibodies in lupus-type circulating anticoagulant and thrombosis in systemic lupus erythematosus. *Am J Med* 1992; **93**: 181–6.

Vlachoyiannopoulos PG, Krilis SA, Hunt JE *et al.* Patients with anticardiolipin antibodies with and without anti-phospholipid syndrome: their clinical features and anti-β_2 glycoprotein-I plasma levels. *Eur J Clin Invest* 1992; **22**: 482–7.

Vlachoyiannopoulos PG, Beigbeder G, Dueymes M *et al.* Antibodies to phosphatidyl ethanolamine in anti-phospholipid syndrome and systemic lupus erythematosus: their correlation with anticardiolipin antibodies and anti-β_2 glycoprotein-I plasma levels. *Autoimmunity* 1993; **16**: 245–9.

Wallace DJ. Does hydroxychloroquine sulphate prevent clot formation in systemic lupus erythematosus. *Arthritis Rheum* 1987; **30**: 1435–6.

Wapner RJ, Cowchock FS, Shapiro SS. successful treatment in two women with anti-phospholipid antibodies and refractory pregnancy losses with intravenous immunoglobulin infusions. *Am J Obstet Gynecol* 1990; **162**: 1271–2.

Wilson WA, Perez MC, Michalski JP. Cardiolipin antibodies and null alleles of C4 in Black Americans with systemic lupus erythematosus. *J Rheumatol* 1988; **15**: 1768–72.

Ziporen L, Blank M, Shoenfeld Y. Animal models for antiphospholipid syndrome in pregnancy. *Rheum Dis Clin North Am* 1997; **23**: 99–117.

10 | *Overlap syndromes*

Introduction

As is evident from the preceding chapters, the auto-immune rheumatic diseases are a group of distinct conditions of unknown aetiology whose diagnosis is dependent on accepted criteria. Many patients, how-ever, at presentation cannot be readily pigeon-holed into any single disease category. This difficulty has led to the development of the concept of 'overlap syn-drome' or undifferentiated autoimmune rheumatic disease (UARD). Attempts to distinguish overlap syndromes have been undertaken in two ways:

(i) identification of a specific pattern of clinical features, e.g. myositis, interstitial lung disease (tRNA synthetase syndrome), or

(ii) detection of unique autoantibodies, e.g. U1 RNP antibody associated specific clinical findings (mixed connective tissue disease, MCTD).

There are, in addition, a group of patients who simultaneously fulfil criteria for more than one autoimmune rheumatic diseases, for example 'rhupus' (a hybrid of RA and SLE), scleroderma/polymyositis overlap. Sjögren's syndrome overlaps with several diseases, most typically SLE and RA.

Milestones in the history of overlap syndromes

1972   Sharp described 'mixed connective tissue disease' and claimed distinctive clinical and serological features including anti-RNP antibodies.

1979   Lerner and Steitz showed that the RNP antigen is bound to the U1 RNP complex.

1980   Nimelstein reviewed the original patients with MCTD and concluded that the original claims for a distinct disease were not substantiated during follow-up.

1983   Jo-1 antigen identified by Mathews and Bernstein as tRNA–histidyl synthetase.

1990   Marguerie described features associated with anti-tRNA synthetase antibodies.

Mixed connective tissue disease

With one exception, the emergence of diagnostic criteria to define the individual autoimmune rheumatic diseases have always been based upon the recognition of combinations of clinical features, followed later by the development of diagnostic investigations, notably autoantibody tests. Consider, for example, systemic lupus erythematosus (for details, see Chapter 4). In 1852 Pierre Cazenave, recognizing its dermatological manifestations, first coined the term 'lupus erythèma-teux'. Its systemic features were recognized clinically between 1870 and 1900. Tests of end-organ dysfunc-tion, e.g. serum biochemistry, radiology, renal, and cardiac tests, were incorporated from 1900 onwards and then in 1948 the LE test and, subsequently in 1957, the anti-dsDNA antibody assay were utilized in the initial criteria of the American Rheumatism Association (1971). This sort of pattern has also been followed for Sjögren's syndrome, rheumatoid arthritis, scleroderma, and myositis. In contrast, so-called mixed connective tissue disease (MCTD) resulted from the identification of anti-U1 and RNP autoantibodies, and an attempt to link (perhaps force together is better!) a number of clinical features in the presence of these antibodies. Thus, in 1972 Sharp and colleagues proposed that MCTD was defined as follows.

- A syndrome clinically identifiable by a particular group of features.
- Associated with the presence of high titre antibodies to U1 RNP, a unique and perhaps diagnostic serological test.
- Cerebral, pulmonary, and renal involvement virtually never occurred.
- Its outcome was benign and that the patients responded to a very small dose of corticosteroids.

However, none of these four points has stood the test of time. Indeed, doubts about the existence of MCTD as a real entity emerged within a few years of the original claim, when Nimelstein *et al.* (1980) re-evaluated 22 of the original 25 patients on whom the identification of the syndrome had been based. They made the following observations: 'Features of the MCTD patients originally thought to make them clinically distinct have not held true over time'. Furthermore, they noted that a few of Sharp's original patients with high titres of anti-U1 RNP antibodies 'never displayed a clear overlap syndrome'.

A significant number of reports reviewed elsewhere (Black and Isenberg 1992) make it very clear that the syndrome, as originally identified, is untenable. Although high titres of antibodies to U1 RNP may be associated with problems such as Raynaud's phenomenom, swollen hands, and myositis, many patients have been identified with these clinical features but who lack these autoantibodies. Likewise, patients with autoantibodies have been identified who lack the so-called distinctive features. Furthermore, many of the clinical and serological features initially thought to be associated with, or never present in, MCTD have apparently changed dramatically (Table 10.1). For example, pulmonary disease, which was not noted at all in 1972, was, according to the study of Sullivan *et al.* (1984), present in 85% of patients. It is also clear that the con-

Table 10.1   The MCTD 'leopard' changes its spots!

Feature	1972(%)	1984(%)
Arthritis/arthralgia	96	85
Swollen hands	88	85
Raynaud's	84	91
Oesophagus	77	74
Myositis	72	79
Lymphadenopathy	68	50
Fever	32	–
Hepatomegaly	28	–
Serositis	24	35
Splenomegaly	21	–
Renal	2	26
Cardiac	0	26
Pulmonary	0	85
Alopecia	0	41
Malar flush	0	29
Trigeminal neuralgia	0	6
Anaemia	48	24
Leucopaenia	52	21
Hypergammaglobulinaemia	80	32

From Sharp *et al.* (1972) and Sullivan *et al.* (1984).

dition, what ever it may be, is not benign. The published mortality figures shown in Table 10.2 indicate that approximately 15% of patients diagnosed with MCTD died of the disease. The figure is remarkably similar to the experience we have had in the Bloomsbury lupus clinic where 30 of the first 265 (11%) patients with lupus to be followed up for a minimum of two years (or until death) had died. Soriano and McHugh (1997), having reviewed the evidence, have concluded that 'virtually all patients with MCTD will fulfil criteria for another autoimmune disease at some stage in their illness'. In their experience, patients with anti-U1 RNP antibodies who fulfil criteria for MCTD without fulfilling criteria for SLE or systemic sclerosis are extremely rare. It is thus evident that in 1972 MCTD may have stood for 'mixed con-

Table 10.2   Mortality figures in 'MCTD'

Patients studies (*n*)	Deaths (*n*)	Mean duration of disease (if stated) (years)	
20	4	–	Bennett *et al.* (1980)
22	8	12	Nimelstein *et al.* (1980)
23	5	–	Grant *et al.* (1981)
34	4	11	Sullivan *et al.* (1984)
81	6	–	Prakash *et al.* (1985)
30	4	–	Kitridov *et al.* (1986)
Totals 210	31(15%)		

Table 10.3   Classification criteria for mixed connective tissue disease (MCTD)

Serological
>   Positive anti-nRNP at a haemagglutination titre of 1:1600 or higher

Clinical
>   Oedema of both hands
>   Synovitis
>   Myositis (laboratory or biopsy proven)
>   Raynaud's phenomenon
>   Acrocyanosis (with or without proximal scleroderma)

Requirements for the diagnosis: serological criterion plus at least three clinical. If oedema, Raynaud's phenomenon, acrocyanosis are combined then four clinical criteria are required.

From Alarçon-Segovia (1994).

nective tissue disease', but in 1998 it stands for 'muddled concept to be discarded'!

It may still be possible to reconcile the conflicting views that are evident in the literature. Several classification criteria of what we would prefer to think of as undifferentiated autoimmune rheumatic disease have emerged since the original criteria were published. Of these, those by Alarçon-Segovia (1994) are perhaps the most practical (Table 10.3). As discussed in the first

edition of this book, conceptually, one may think of a group of patients who have antibodies to U1 RNP with particular accompanying features as being in the eye of 'an autoimmune rheumatic disease storm'. This is a relatively calm and mild state, but one that is prone to be followed or buffeted into a more severe though more recognizable condition. Some patients may be lucky enough to stay in the eye of the storm (see Fig. 10.1). The following section thus refers essentially

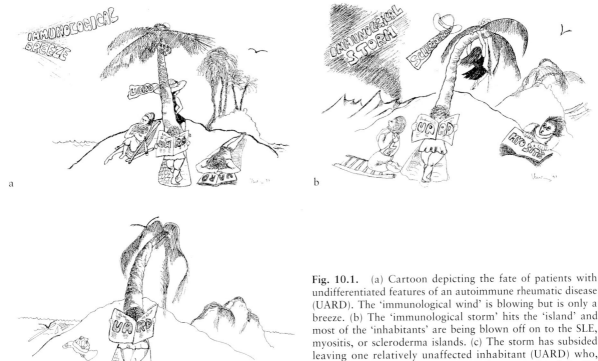

a

b

c

Fig. 10.1.   (a) Cartoon depicting the fate of patients with undifferentiated features of an autoimmune rheumatic disease (UARD). The 'immunological wind' is blowing but is only a breeze. (b) The 'immunological storm' hits the 'island' and most of the 'inhabitants' are being blown off on to the SLE, myositis, or scleroderma islands. (c) The storm has subsided leaving one relatively unaffected inhabitant (UARD) who, being in the eye of the storm, was only aware of a slight disturbance. (Reproduced with the permission of Dr Lesley Isenberg.)

to patients with undifferentiated rheumatic disease that do not meet the criteria for scleroderma or myositis, the conditions they are most likely to differentiate into in time.

Epidemiology

Undifferentiated autoimmune rheumatic disease (UARD) has a mean age at diagnosis of 35 years (Sharp *et al.* 1972; Prakash *et al.* 1985) with women more frequently affected. The annual incidence of all the overlap syndromes in adults is unknown. In Finland the annual incidence of childhood MCTD was 0.1 in 100 000, which is approximately one-third the rate for SLE or polymyositis/dermatomyositis (Pelkonen *et al.* 1994).

The clinical picture

Patients, predominately female, present aged 20–30 years with Raynaud's phenomenom, arthralgias/arthritis, swollen hands, and/or puffy fingers (Table 10.1), in association with a high titre ANA showing a speckled pattern.

Vascular involvement

Raynaud's phenomenom occurs almost universally in patients with UARD and is often the presenting feature. Loss of finger tip pulp is uncommon, nailfold capillaroscopy shows capillary dilatation and loss in 50–90% of patients. Only a small proportion of patients with Raynaud's phenomenom have an underlying autoimmune disorder (Table 10.4).

Cutaneous involvement

Oedema and swelling of the hands, particularly of the fingers, results in a sausage appearance. The skin of the hands may be taut and thick and resemble scleroderma histologically. Other cutaneous features include alopecia, depigmentation, telangectasia, erythema nodosum, and chronic discoid lesions.

Musculoskeletal

Polyarthralgia is a common and early feature. Polyarthritis is usually symmetrical but not typically erosive. However, ulnar deviation, swan-neck deformities, and atlantoaxial subluxation have been described, together with small, punched-out erosions. Multiple small peritendonous nodules can occur along the flexor and extensor tendons of the forearms. Myalgias are a common feature and around two-thirds of patients develop a myopathy that is clinically and histologically identical to polymyositis.

Gastrointestinal tract involvement

Involvement of the gastrointestinal tract is similar to that seen in systemic sclerosis, with oesophageal reflux and dysphagia the most common symptoms. Hepatosplenomegaly occurs in a quarter of patients.

Pulmonary disease

The most frequent clinical findings are shortness of breath, pleuritic pain, and bibasal crackles, but these may be mild and not clinically apparent. Pulmonary function tests show a restrictive pattern, and chest radiography shows interstitial fibrosis, pleural effusion, infiltrates, and pleural thickening. Pulmonary hypertension is frequent and causes significant morbidity and mortality. The presence of scleroderma-like capillary changes on microscopy may be predictive of pulmonary hypertension.

Cardiovascular disease

Significant cardiovascular involvement is uncommon but pericarditis may occur in up to 20% of patients.

Neurological disease

Trigeminal neuralgia may be an early feature of the disease and can occur in up to 10% of patients. Central nervous system involvement is, however, rare.

Table 10.4   Features suggestive of an underlying autoimmune rheumatic disease in patients with Raynaud's phenomenon

1. Scleroderma-like nailfold capillary abnormalities
2. Positive anti-nuclear antibody (titre > 1/100)
3. Anti-centromere or anti-topoisomerase-I (Scl-70 antibody)
4. Digital pitting scars
5. Evidence of acute phase response

Renal disease

As discussed in the original description of MCTD by Sharp *et al.* (1972), lack of renal disease was one of the defining features. Subsequent reports have recorded renal disease in up to 26% of patients (Sullivan *et al.* 1984). Nephrotic syndrome associated with a membranous nephropathy is most common. Renal crisis is rare. Renal disease, as in SLE, can be detected on biopsy in patients with minimal clinical evidence of renal involvement.

Aetiopathogenesis

The U1 RNP particle is one of a series of uridine-rich RNA particles that are involved in the splicing of mRNA. It comprises eight polypeptides of which the 68 and 33 kDa peptides carry the epitopes recognized by sera from patients with UARD. The other polypeptides, principally the 16 and 28 kDa ones, react with anti-Sm antibodies.

Over 80% of sera positive for Sm (virtually always from patients with SLE) also contain antibodies to nRNP. Antibodies to nRNP alone occur in UARD. Both Sm and nRNP polypeptides bind to uridine-rich RNA species, termed U1, and Sm was present on U4, U5, and U6 RNAs (Lerner and Steitz 1979). The concordance of the antibody response suggests that the autoimmune response is driven by the whole U1 RNP complex.

There is evidence of B cell hyperactivity with polyclonal hypergammaglobulinaemia and spontaneous *in vitro* production of IgG (Kallenberg *et al.* 1988). The antibody response to the U1 RNP particle seems to be antigen driven rather than as a result of non-specific polyclonal activation. The question is, how is immunological tolerance overcome? Recognition of one protein on Sn RNP could allow processing presentation of other proteins on the same B cell complex by B cells (Fatenjad *et al.* 1993). Molecular mimicry is one possible mechanism, based on sequence similarities between the 33 kDa polypeptide of U1 RNP and a consensus sequence common to a number of retrovirus proteins (Query and Keene 1987). Bcl-2 transgenic mice, with the transgene in B cells (not T cells), develop an autoimmune disease with immune complex glomerulonephritis (Strasser *et al.* 1991). Among the serological abnormalities is the appearance of Sm RNP antibodies together with dsDNA and histone antibodies.

T cell clones reactive to the sn RNP A protein show restricted usage of TCR β chain genes (Okubo *et al.*

1994) and sn RNP-reactive oligoclonal T cell may accumulate in patients with UARD.

Patients with UARD are reported to have a higher frequency of HLA-DR4 than controls (Genth *et al.* 1987; Ruuska *et al.* 1992) but this seems to be restricted to the subgroup of patients with polyarthritis. The presence of 70 kDa anti-U1 RNP antibodies is associated with HLA-DR4/HLA-DR53 or HLA-DR2 (Kaneoka *et al.* 1992). In one study, evolution into systemic sclerosis was associated with HLA-DR5 and non-evolution with HLA-DR1 or DR4 (Gendi *et al.* 1995).

Environmental factors are the most likely triggers for UARD in genetically predisposed individuals. Such agents include drugs such as procainamide, polyvinyl chloride, and silicone implants (see Chapter 8).

Clinical investigations

The assessment and investigation of a patient with a suspected overlap syndrome should be similar to that of patients with SLE or other autoimmune rheumatic disease. The diagnosis of UARD is dependent on the demonstration of high titre antibodies against U1 RNP. U1 RNP antibodies are associated with a speckled pattern of nuclear staining on indirect immunofluorescence using HEp-2 cells. However, other autoantibodies particularly anti-Sm and anti-La also give rise to a speckled pattern. Immunodiffusion or ELISA assays are more usually used in place of the original haemagglutination assay and have different sensitivity and specificity.

Prognosis and mortality

As already discussed, the original claim that MCTD was associated with a better prognosis than SLE has not been borne out by subsequent studies. In addition to the studies on adults, Tiddens *et al.* (1993) reviewed 14 children followed for nearly 10 years, observing that features of SLE and polymyositis became less prominent but that scleroderma-like features and arthritis became more prominent.

Van den Hoogen *et al.* (1994) followed 46 patients with anti-U1 RNP antibodies for at least five years after initial presentation. At presentation 33 (72%) patients were classified as having MCTD, during the follow-up 18 patients were reclassified: SLE (5 patients), systemic sclerosis (7), RA (3), and combination (3). At the end of the study 67% of patients fulfilled the criteria for another connective tissue disease.

Overlap syndromes in children

Overlap syndromes with RNP antibodies are rare in children. The spectrum of disease manifestations is similar to that in adults (Tiddens *et al.* 1993). Arthritis occurs in more than 90% of patients, Raynaud's phenomenom in greater than 80%, together with features of more than one autoimmune rheumatic disease. A recent long-term follow-up study (five years) reported a wide variety of outcomes which cast doubt as to whether MCTD was a unique and distinctive disorder in children (Mier *et al.* 1996).

Management and treatment

The treatment of UARD is determined by the clinical features present. As for patients with SLE, myalgias, arthralgias, and cutaneous disease are treated initially with NSAIDs and antimalarials. Pulmonary, neurological, and renal involvement need treatment with corticosteroids and immunosuppressives. Raynaud's phenomenom is treated with vasodilators as described in the chapter on scleroderma. Therapy of myositis usually requires corticosteroids.

Specific assessment instruments have not been developed for use in the overlap syndromes, however, the same basic principles apply as in lupus. BILAG, SLEDAI, and other systems have not been formally validated in the overlap syndromes.

tRNA synthetase syndrome

The tRNA syndrome is characterized by myositis (83–100%), interstitial lung disease (50–80%), and Raynaud's phenomenom (60–93%) (Marguerie *et al.* 1990). Interstitial lung disease is found more frequently than in patients with myositis without antibodies to the tRNA synthetases and is a greater cause of morbidity than the myositis. Mechanics finger is a typical cutaneous feature, with hyperkeratosis and fissuring along the lateral aspects of the fingers. Arthritis is more frequent in patients with Jo-1 antibodies which were first identified 15 years ago (Mathews and Bernstein 1983). Myositis is indistinguishable from idiopathic myositis but may occur at a younger age and have a more rapid onset.

This syndrome is characterized by the presence in serum of antibodies against aminoacyl–tRNA synthetases. The tRNA synthetases are a series of 20 cytoplasmic enzymes that attach tRNA to its corresponding amino acid during the assembly of polypeptides. Antibodies against five different aminoacyl–tRNA synthetases have been described: anti-Jo-1 (histidyl), PL-7 (threonyl), PL-12 (alanyl), OJ (isoleucyl), and EJ (glycyl). Of these, anti-Jo-1 is the most common. The clinical features are similar in patients with histidyl–tRNA synthetase antibodies to those with antibodies against the other tRNA synthetases (Marguerie *et al.* 1990). A serological association between Jo-1 and Ro52 has recently been described (Rutjes *et al.* 1997). Anti-Jo-1 antibodies do not cross-react with Ro52, nor do they precipitate related RNA species or interact together. The mechanism for this has not yet been adequately explained (Venables 1997).

Diagnosis of the tRNA synthetase overlap syndromes is also dependent on detection of the appropriate autoantibodies. The tRNA synthetases are located in the cytoplasm and hence are often not detected routinely on ANA testing, although a perinuclear pattern may be a clue to their presence.

Treatment

Myositis requires treatment with corticosteroids. Additional immunosuppression is required in patients with the anti-synthetase syndrome since the associated pulmonary involvement is associated with a poor outcome. As with other forms of inflammatory myositis there is a paucity of controlled trials to guide therapy (see Chapter 7).

Scleroderma/polymyositis overlap

Polymyositis occurs infrequently in systemic sclerosis and resembles idiopathic polymyositis. Bohan *et al.* (1977) reported that 21% of patients with polymyositis had another autoimmune disorder, most frequently scleroderma (36%). Anti-PM/Scl antibodies occur in patients with polymyositis overlap. Anti-PM/Scl antibodies are found in 8% of myositis patients, and 3% of scleroderma patients (Targoff 1992). In patients with anti-PM/Scl antibodies, polymyositis/dermatomyositis alone was present in 55%, scleroderma without polymyositis/dermatomyositis in 5%, and myositis/scleroderma overlap in 40% (Reichlin *et al.* 1984). The clinical features of these last patients is similar to that seen in the anti-synthetase syndrome but the myositis and fibrosing alveolitis are less frequent, less severe, and respond better to treatment.

SLE/Sjögren's syndrome overlap

Although Sjögren's syndrome may occur in patients with any of the other autoimmune rheumatic diseases it is mainly found in those with SLE or RA. Antibodies against La/SS-B occur in patients with SLE and Sjögren's syndrome and in particular when both conditions occur together. Sjögren's syndrome patients with anti-La have systemic features resembling SLE. The most characteristic feature is a purpuric hypergammaglobulinaemic rash (in 30%) and a relatively low frequency of nephritis compared with classical SLE. Renal tubular acidosis may occur in up to 30% of patients (Venables 1997).

Rhupus

The existence of patients with a combination of features of RA and SLE has been observed for many years. The arthropathy of lupus is typically non-erosive and not associated with nodules. Occasional patients with SLE develop nodules or an erosive arthropathy suggesting an overlap between the two conditions, and the term 'Rhupus' was coined to describe such patients (Panush *et al.* 1988). However, whether this is a genuine overlap or chance occurrence of both conditions in the same patient is debatable (Panush *et al.* 1988).

Immunogenetics

Studies that have examined patients categorized by the prior criteria for MCTD found an increase of DR4, including Caucasians from England (Black *et al.* 1988), from Finland (Ruuska *et al.* 1992), and Japanese (Dong *et al.* 1993). The subtype of DR4 was identified as 'Dw4' (cellular equivalent of DRB1*0401) in Finns and DRB1*0401 in Japanese, although only 19% of all Japanese patients had this HLA allele and 45% of Finns. However, as discussed previously, the criteria for so called 'MCTD' required antibodies to RNP and it is likely that the primary HLA association is with antibodies to U1-RNP. Studies that have begun with patient populations that exhibit antibodies to U1-RNP, inclusive of patients with systemic lupus, scleroderma, undifferentiated connective tissue disease, and overlap have found that antibodies to RNP are associated with DR4 (Genth *et al.* 1987; Hoffman *et al.* 1990). One study described an increase of DR4 and DR2 (Kaneoka *et al.* 1992), however a later report from the same group did not show a difference of DR2 between patients with and those without antibodies to U1-RNP (Hoffman *et al.* 1995). In another study of patients categorized by antibodies to U1-RNP, DR4 was associated with hand swelling and the DRB1*0405 allele with arthritis (Kuwana *et al.* 1996). No significant HLA association with DQ antigens was found in one study (Kaneoka *et al.* 1992). However, alleles of DQA1 and DQB1 and combinations of alleles have not been thoroughly investigated for correlation with antibodies to U1-RNP.

Another antibody that has been investigated in patients with overlap of myositis and scleroderma is to the nucleolar antigen PM-Scl, also found in patients with myositis alone and scleroderma without myositis. An increase of DR3 and DQ2 was found in a study of 20 patients with antibodies to PM-Scl, the majority of whom had overlap with features of myositis and scleroderma (Oddis *et al.* 1992). HLA associations have been found with antibodies to Ro and La in patients with SLE and with Sjögren's syndrome (see Chapters 3 and 6). The HLA associations of myositis specific antibodies are described in Chapter 7.

Summary

The clinical features present in many patients do not permit easy or early classification. Patients with UARD typically evolve into a more recognizable syndrome (most commonly SLE, myositis, or scleroderma). The concept of MCTD has become discredited primarily because the clinical features identified with the disease have changed significantly and also it is difficult to accept the notion that U1 RNP antibodies are pathogenic or merely linked to sets of clinical features when the same features can be found in patients who do not express these antibodies. There are patients, however, who fulfil criteria for more than one ARD at the same time and they can be considered to have a genuine overlap syndrome.

References

Alarcon-Segovia D. Mixed connective tissue disease and overlap syndromes. *Clin Dermatol* 1994; **12**: 309–16.

Bennett RM, O'Connell DJ. Mixed connective tissue disease. a clinico-pathologic study of 20 cases. *Sem Arthritis Rheum* 1980; **10**: 25–52.

Black C, Isenberg DA. Mixed connective tissue disease — goodbye to all that. *Br J Rheum* 1992; **31**: 695–700.

Black CM, Maddison PJ, Welsh KI et al. HLA and immunoglobulin allotypes in mixed connective tissue disease. *Arthritis Rheum* 1988; **31**: 131–4.

Bohan A, Peter JB, Bowman RL et al. A computer assisted analysis of 153 patients with polymyositis and dermatomyositis. *Medicine* 1977; **56**: 255–86.

Dong RP, Kimura A, Hashimoto H et al. Difference in HLA-linked genetic background between mixed connective tissue disease and systemic lupus erythematosus. *Tissue Antigens* 1993; **41**: 20–5.

Fatenjad S, Mamula MJ, Craft J. Role of intermolecular/intrastructural B- and T-cell determinants in the diversification of autoantibodies to ribonuclearprotein particles. *Proc Natl Acad Sci USA* 1993; **90**: 12010–14.

Gendi NST, Welsh KI, van Venrooij WJ et al. HLA type as predictor of mixed connective tissue disease differentiation. *Arthritis Rheum* 1995; **38**: 259–66.

Genth E, Zarnowski H, Mierau R et al. HLA-DR4 and Gm (1,3; 5,21) are associated with U1-nRNP antibody positive connective tissue disease. *Ann Rheum Dis* 1987; **46**: 189–96.

Grant KD, Adams LE, Hess EV. Mixed connective tissue disease — a subset with sequential clinical and laboratory features. *J Rheumatol* 1981; **8**: 587–98.

Hoffman RW, Rettenmaier LJ, Takeda Y et al. Human autoantibodies against the 70-kD polypeptide of U1 small nuclear RNP are association with HLA-DR4 among connective tissue disease patients. *Arthritis Rheum* 1990; **33**: 666–73.

Hoffman RW, Sharp GC, Deutscher SL. Analysis of anti-U1-RNA antibodies in patients with connective tissue disease. Association with HLA and clinical manifestations of disease. *Arthritis Rheum* 1995; **38**: 1837–44.

Kallenberg CG, van. Dissel Emiliani F, Huitema MG et al. B cell proliferation and differentiation in systemic lupus erythematosus and mixed connective tissue disease. *J Clin Lab Immunol* 1988; **26**: 55–61.

Kaneoka H, Hsu K, Takeda Y et al. Molecular genetic analysis of HLA-DR and HLA-DQ genes among anti-U1-70-Kd autoantibody positive connective tissue disease patients. *Arthritis Rheum* 1992; **35**: 83–94.

Kitridou RC, Akmal M, Turkel SB et al. Renal involvement in mixed connective tissue disease: a longitudinal clinicopathological study. *Sem Arthritis Rheum* 1986; **16**: 135–45.

Kuwana M, Okano Y, Kaburaki J, et al. Clinical correlations with HLA type in Japanese patients with connective tissue disease anti-U1 small nuclear RNP antibodies. *Arthritis Rheum* 1996; **39**: 939–42.

Lerner MR, Steitz JA. Antibodies to small nuclear RNAs complexed with proteins are produced by patients with systemiclupus erythematosus. *Proc Natl Acad Sci USA* 1979; **76**: 5495–9.

Marguerie C, Bunn CC, Beynon HLC et al. Polymyositis, pulmonary fibrosis and autonatibodies to aminoacyl-tRNA synthetase enzymes. *Q J Med* 1990; **77**: 1019–38.

Mathews MB, Bernstein RM. Myositis autoantibody inhibits histidyl-tRNA synthetase: a model for autoimmunity. *Nature* 1983; **304**: 177–9.

Mier R, Ansell BM, Hasson N et al. Long term follow up of children with mixed connective tissue disease. *Lupus* 1996; **5**: 221–6.

Nimelstein SH, Brody S, McShane D, Holman HR. Mixed connective tissue disease: subsequent evaluation of the original 25 patients. *Medicine* 1980; **59**: 239–48.

Oddis CV, Okano Y, Rudert WA et al. Serum autoantibody to the nuclear antigen PM-Scl. *Arthritis Rheum* 1992; **35**: 1211–17.

Okubo M, Kurokawa M, Ohto H et al. Clonotype analysis of peripheral blood T cells and autoantigen-reactive T cells from patients with mixed connective tissue disease. *J Immunol* 1994; **153**: 3784–90.

Panush RS, Edwards L, Longley S et al. 'Rhupus' syndrome. *Arch Int Med* 1988; **148**; 1633–6.

Pelkonen PM et al. Incidence of systemic connective tissue diseases in children: a nationwide prospective study in Finland. *J Rheumatol* 1994; **21**: 2143–6.

Prakash UBS, Luthra HS, Divertie MB. Intrathoracic manifestations in mixed connective tissue disease. *Mayo Clin Proc* 1985; **60**: 813–21.

Query CC, Keene JD. A human autoimmune protein associated with U1RNP contains a region of homology that is cross reactive with retroviral p30^{gag} antigen. *Cell* 1987; **51**: 211–20.

Reichlin M, Maddison P, Targoff I et al. Antibodies to a nuclear/nucleolar antigen in patients with polymyositis overlap syndromes. *J Clin Immunol* 1984; **4**: 40–4.

Rutjes SA, Vree Ebberts WTM, Jongen P et al. Anti-Ro-52 antibodies frequently co-occur with anti-Jo-1 antibodies in sera from patients with idiopathic inflammatory myopathy. *Clin Exp Immunol* 1997; **109**: 32–40.

Ruuska P, Hämeenkorpi R, Forsberg S et al. Differences in HLA antigens between patients with mixed connective tissue disease and systemic lupus erythematosus. *Ann Rheum Dis* 1992; **51**: 52–5.

Sharp GC, Irwin WS, Tan EM et al. Mixed connective tissue disease — an apparently distinct rheumatic disease syndrome associated with a specific antibody to an extractable nuclear antigen. *Am J Med* 1972; **52**: 148–59.

Soriano ER, McHugh NJ. Overlap syndromes in adults and children. In: *Oxford Textbook of Rheumatology*, (eds Isenberg DA, Woo P, Glass D, Maddison P). Oxford University Press, Oxford, 1998; 1413–32.

Strasser A, Whittingham S, Vaux DL et al. Enforced bcl-2 expression in B lymphoid cells prolongs antibody responses and elicits autoimmune disease. *Proc Natl Acad Sci USA* 1991; **88**: 8661–5.

Sullivan WD, Hurst DJ, Harman CE et al. A prospective evaluation emphasizing pulmonary involvement in patients with mixed connective tissue disease. *Medicine* 1984; **63**: 92–8.

Targoff LN. Autoantibodies in polymyosits. *Rheum Dis Clin North Am* 1992; **18**: 455–82.

Tiddens HAWM, van der Nett JJ der Grueff Maeder ER et al. Juvenile onset mixed connective tissue disease: longitudinal follow-up. *J Paediatr* 1993; **122**: 191–7.

van den Hoogen FH, Spronk PE, Boerbooms AM *et al.* Long-term follow up of 46 patients with anti-(U1)snRNP antibodies. *Br J Rheumatol* 1994; **33**: 1117–20.

Venables PJW. Overlap syndromes. In: *Rheumatology*, eds Klippel J, Dieppe P. Mosby, St Louis, pp 28.1–28.8.

Venables PJW. Antibodies to Jo-1 and Ro-52: Why do they go together? *Clin Exp Immunol* 1997; **109**: 403–5.

11 | *Vasculitis*

Introduction

The vasculitides are a mixed group of uncommon diseases characterized by inflammation and necrosis of blood vessels. Vasculitis can either be primary (e.g. Wegener's granulomatosis, polyarteritis nodosa), occurring in the absence of a recognized precipitating cause or associated disease, or secondary to established disease (e.g. rheumatoid arthritis or systemic lupus erythematosus) or infection (such as hepatitis B, C, or HIV) (Somer and Finegold 1995).

The consequence of vascular inflammation depends on the size, location, and number of blood vessels involved. Involvement may be relatively indolent, with disease isolated to a single organ or vessel, or a rapidly fulminant, life-threatening, multisystem disease. Muscular arteries may develop segmental or focal lesions. Segmental lesions (affecting the whole vessel circumference) lead to stenosis or occlusion, with infarction of distal organs. Focal lesions are less common and may lead to aneurysm formation, followed by possible rupture. Haemorrhage into or infarction of vital internal organs are the most serious complications of vasculitis. Untreated disease has a poor prognosis with a five-year survival of 10% (Frohnert and Sheps 1967). Advances in treatment have dramatically improved the survival of systemic vasculitis, but there is still significant mortality and morbidity from the disease (or its treatment).

Milestones in the history of systemic vasculitis

1755   Michaelis and Matani recognized the systemic vasculitides (referred to by Lamb 1914).

1837   Schönlein described a childhood illness characterized by acute purpura and arthritis.

1874   Henoch described the features of colicky abdominal pain and nephritis in patients with Schönlein purpura.

1866   Kussmaul and Maier described periarteritis nodosa in a patient with a severe systemic illness. At necropsy, numerous nodules were found along the course of small muscular arteries.

1903   Ferrari introduced the term polyarteritis nodosa but this has only been used more generally since the 1950s.

1908   Takayasu presented a case of a 21-year-old woman with an unusual arteriovenous malformation in the retina associated with blindness due to cataract formation. Colleagues pointed out the association between ocular abnormalities and the absence of radial pulses.

1936   Wegener described a disease characterized by necrotizing granulomata of the upper and lower respiratory tract, focal glomerulonephritis, and necrotizing systemic vasculitis (Godman and Churg 1954).

1950   Bagentoss and colleagues reported the effect of cortisone on polyarteritis nodosa.

1950   Wainwright and Davson introduced the concept of microscopic polyarteritis.

1951   Churg and Strauss described, in a post-mortem series, a form of vasculitis characterized by asthma, eosinophilia, fever, systemic upset, and a granulomatous necrotizing vasculitis.

1952   Zeek classified vasculitis into different groups mainly based on vessel size, and this has formed the basis of most subsequent classification schemes.

1967   Kawasaki described an acute vasculitis of unknown aetiology which predominately affects infants and young children (mucocutaneous lymph node syndrome).

1970s   Cyclophosphamide introduced for treatment of systemic vasculitis (Novak and Pearson 1971).

1982   Davies described anti-neutrophil cytoplasmic antibodies (ANCA) in association with vasculitis.

1985   van der Woude showed that a specific immunofluorescence pattern for ANCA was highly specific for Wegener's granulomatosis.

1990   American College of Rheumatology criteria for the classification of the systemic vasculitides developed.

1994   Chapel Hill Consensus Conference described definitions for the systemic vasculitides.

Systemic vasculitis in humans

Classification

The classification of systemic vasculitis is confusing and controversial. There is considerable overlap in the clinical expression of different vasculitic syndromes and in most cases the underlying cause is unknown. Even when infection such as hepatitis B virus is found it may be associated with several types of vasculitis, such as polyarteritis nodosa, cutaneous vasculitis, cryoglobulinaemic vasculitis, and glomerulonephritis.

We advocate classification of patients on the basis of the size of the dominant vessels involved, known aetiological factors, and ANCA (Table 11.1). Wegener's granulomatosis, Churg–Strauss syndrome, and microscopic polyangiitis are placed together because they have some common features, namely: (i) involvement of small and sometimes medium-sized arteries; (ii) most frequently associated with ANCA; (iii) associated with a high risk of glomerulonephritis; and (iv) respond best to immunosuppression with cyclophosphamide.

Diagnostic criteria for individual diseases

In 1990, the American College of Rheumatology addressed the classification of individual types of vasculitis (Hunder *et al.* 1990). They proposed classi-

Table 11.1 Classification of systemic vasculitis

Dominant vessel involved	Primary	Secondary
Large arteries	Giant cell arteritis Takayasu arteritis	Aortitis associated with RA Infection (e.g. syphilis, TB)
Medium arteries	Classical PAN Kawasaki disease	Hepatitis B-associated PAN
Small vessels and medium arteries	Wegener's granulomatosis[*] Churg–Strauss syndrome[*] Microscopic polyangiitis[*]	Vasculitis secondary to RA, SLE Sjögren's Drugs Infection (e.g. HIV)
Small vessels (leucocytoclastic)	Henoch–Schönlein purpura Essential mixed cryoglobulinaemia Cutaneous leucocytoclastic angiitis	Drugs[†] Hepatitis C-associated cryoglobulinaemia Infection

PAN = polyarteritis nodosa.
[*] Diseases most commonly associated with ANCA (anti-myeloperoxidase and anti-proteinase-3 antibodies), a significant risk of renal involvement and which are most responsive to immunosuppression with cyclophosphamide.
[†] e.g. sulphonamides, penicillins, thiazide diuretics, and many others.

fication criteria for seven types of systemic vasculitis: Takayasu arteritis, giant cell arteritis, polyarteritis nodosa, Churg–Strauss syndrome, Wegener's granulomatosis, hypersensitivity vasculitis, and Henoch–Schönlein purpura (Hunder *et al.* 1990). The sensitivity and specificity rates varied considerably: 71.0–95.3% for sensitivity and 78.7–99.7% for specificity (Fries *et al.* 1990). The most sensitive and specific criteria were found in Churg–Strauss syndrome, giant cell arteritis, and Takayasu arteritis; hypersensitivity vasculitis was the least well-defined condition. It should be remembered that these criteria were designed to facilitate epidemiological and clinical studies but not the diagnosis of individual patients.

In 1993 an international consensus conference was convened in Chapel Hill, North Carolina, USA (CHCC).

Table 11.2 Names and definitions of vasculitides adopted by the Chapel Hill Consensus Conference on the nomenclature of systemic vasculitis[*]

Name	Definition
Large vessel vasculitis	
Giant cell (temporal) arteritis	Granulomatous arteritis of the aorta and its major branches, with a predilection for the extracranial branches of the carotid artery. *Often involves the temporal artery. Usually occurs in patients older than 50 and often is associated with polymyalgia rheumatica.*
Takayasu arteritis	Granulomatous inflammation of the aorta and its major branches. *Usually occurs in patients younger than 50.*
Medium-sized vessel vasculitis	
Polyarteritis nodosa[†] (classic polyarteritis nodosa)	Necrotizing inflammation of medium-sized or small arteries without glomerulonephritis or vasculitis in arterioles, capillaries, or venules.
Kawasaki disease	Arteritis involving large, medium-sized, small arteries, and associated with mucocutaneous lymph node syndrome. *Coronary arteries are often involved. Aorta and veins may be involved. Usually occurs in children.*
Small vessel vasculitis	
Wegener's granulomatosis[††]	Granulomatous inflammation involving the respiratory tract, and necrotizing vasculitis affecting small to medium-sized vessels (e.g. capillaries, venules, arterioles, and arteries). *Necrotizing glomerulonephritis is common.*
Churg–Strauss syndrome[††]	Eosinophil-rich and granulomatous inflammation involving the respiratory tract, necrotizing vasculitis affecting small to medium-sized vessels, and associated with asthma and eosinophilia.
Microscopic polyangiitis[†] (microscopic polyarteritis)[††]	Necrotizing vasculitis, with few or no immune deposits, affecting small vessels (i.e. capillaries, venules, or arterioles). *Necrotizing arteritis involving small and medium-sized arteries may be present. Necrotizing glomerulonephritis is very common. Pulmonary capillaritis often occurs.*
Henoch–Schönlein purpura	Vasculitis, with IgA-dominant immune deposits, affecting small vessels (i.e. capillaries, venules, or arterioles). *Typically involves skin, gut, and glomeruli, and is associated with arthralgia or arthritis.*
Essential cryoglobulinaemic vasculitis	Vasculitis, with cryoglobulin immune deposits, affecting small vessels (i.e. capillaries, venules, or arterioles), and associated with cryoglobulins in serum. *Skin and glomeruli are often involved.*
Cutaneous leucocytoclastic angiitis	Isolated cutaneous leucocytoclastic angiitis without systemic vasculitis or glomerulonephritis.

[*] Large vessel refers to the aorta and the largest branches directed towards the major body regions (e.g. to the extremities and the head and neck); medium-sized vessel refers to the main visceral arteries (e.g. renal, hepatic, coronary, and mesenteric arteries); small vessel refers to venules, capillaries, arterioles, and the intraparenchymal distal arterial radicals that connect with arterioles. Some small and large vessel vasculitides may involve medium-sized arteries, but large and medium-sized vessel vasculitides do not involve smaller arteries. Essential components are represented by normal type; italicized type represents usual, but not essential, components.
[†] Preferred term.
[††] Strongly associated with anti-neutrophil cytoplasmic antibodies.
Reproduced from Jeanette *et al.* (1994) with permission.

The objective of this conference was to develop definitions for the nomenclature of different systemic vasculitides based on clinical and laboratory features (Table 11.2) (Jeanette *et al.* 1994). Microscopic polyangiitis was distinguished from classical polyarteritis nodosa. Cutaneous leucocytoclastic angiitis is a separate entity; the term hypersensitivity vasculitis was abandoned because it had previously been used to describe patients with microscopic polyangiitis or cutaneous leucocytoclastic vasculitis.

Epidemiology

The overall annual incidence of systemic vasculitis is around 40 per million (Watts and Scott 1997), which represents an increase from the 1970s, when the incidence was estimated to be 10 per million (Scott *et al.* 1982). Whether this figure represents a true increase or better case recognition is unknown. Giant cell arteritis is the most common form of vasculitis, with an annual incidence of 180 per million adults aged over 50 years (Salvarani *et al.* 1995). Wegener's granulomatosis, microscopic polyangiitis, and Churg–Strauss syndrome have a similar incidence of 3–8 per million (Table 11.3). Takayasu arteritis and classical polyarteritis nodosa are very rare in the United Kingdom. There are believed to be geographical and ethnic variations, with giant cell arteritis being common in northern Europe but rare in Asia. Takayasu arteritis is considered to be more common in Asia, particularly in women.

The clinical picture

The major causes of primary large vessel vasculitis, Takayasu arteritis and giant cell arteritis (GCA), involve predominately large vessels, occasionally medium-sized vessels (i.e. renal, hepatic, coronary, mesenteric arteries), but almost never involve vessels smaller than arteries.

Takayasu arteritis

Takayasu arteritis (TA) is a chronic granulomatous panarteritis affecting large elastic arteries such as the aorta and its major branches, and, less frequently, the pulmonary arteries. The classic description of TA is a triphasic illness characterized by pre-pulseless inflammation, followed by painful ischaemic vessels, and ending in 'burnt-out disease' (Lupi-Herrera *et al.* 1977; Hall *et al.* 1985). More recent studies suggest that 20% of patients have a single phase illness not requiring therapy, and 57% of patients never have constitutional (fever, weight loss) symptoms (Kerr *et al.* 1994).

The hallmark of the disease is vascular ischaemic symptoms with bruit, claudication, or decreased pulses. Disease is often extensive, involving the aorta and its branches. The most common vascular abnormality (> 90% of cases) is a bruit occurring most frequently in the carotid vessels (70%) and in multiple sites in 33% of cases. Claudication and a diminished or absent pulse is more common in the arms than in the legs. Carotodynia (tenderness of carotid arteries) occurs in 33% of patients and a similar proportion complain of light-headedness or dizziness. Hypertension occurs in 30–70% of patients as a consequence of renal artery stenosis, which may be either unilateral or bilateral (Lupi-Herrera *et al.* 1977; Kerr *et al.* 1994).

Musculoskeletal symptoms occur in 50% of patients, with arthralgias occurring in one-third to one-half of patients. Peripheral synovitis is less common, occurring in 18% of patients. Myalgia occurs infrequently but can be severe.

Cardiac lesions occur in 40%, with aortic incompetence (20%) resulting from aortitis, which may also involve the proximal coronary arteries. Congestive

Table 11.3   Incidence of vasculitis in the Norwich Health Authority (1988–1994)

Condition	Annual incidence (95%CI) per million
Wegener's granulomatosis	8.5 (5.2-12.9)
Microscopic polyangiitis	3.6 (1.7–6.9)
Classic polyarteritis nodosa	0.0 (0.0–1.5)
Churg–Strauss syndrome	3.3 (1.7–5.9)
Henoch–Schönlein purpura (adult)	3.4 (1.4–6.9)
Cutaneous leucocytoclastic angiitis	15.4 (10.6-21.8)
Systemic rheumatoid vasculitis	12.5 (8.5–17.7)

Data from Watts and Scott (1997).

cardiac failure may result from aortic incompetence or systemic hypertension and accounts for the majority of fatal outcomes. Hypertension contributes to left ventricular hypertrophy and myocardial failure, but coronary arteritis results in myocardial infarction and fibrosis. Pulmonary artery involvement is common (50%) with lesions localized to large and medium pulmonary vessels (Lupi-Herrera *et al.* 1977).

Cutaneous manifestations are uncommon and include erythema nodosum (8%), leg ulcers, hypocomplementaemic vasculitis, and pyoderma gangrenosum.

Neurological features occur in all stages of the disease and reflect carotid artery involvement. Non-specific symptoms, such as headache and vertigo, are seen in up to 90% of cases, but sensory loss and aphasia occur infrequently. Strokes are an important contributor to mortality. Visual disturbance occurs in 30% of patients, with either blurring of vision (which may be posturally dependent), diplopia, or amaurosis fugax. Retinal disease with arteriovenous anastomosis occurs late in the disease. Visual disturbances are often related to systemic hypertension and 40% of cases have fundal changes consistent with hypertension. Cataracts and neovascularization, as described by Takayasu, are now uncommon (Hall *et al.* 1985; Kerr *et al.* 1994).

Giant cell arteritis

Giant cell arteritis (also known as temporal arteritis or cranial arteritis) is a granulomatous arteritis of the aorta and its major branches with a predilection for the extracranial branches of the carotid artery (Jeannette *et al.* 1994).

The typical manifestations are headache (often localized around the temporal arteries), scalp tenderness, fever, and malaise. Giant cell arteritis may occur in association with polymyalgia rheumatica, a condition characterized by shoulder and pelvic girdle pain and stiffness. Sudden visual loss due to involvement of the ciliary or ophthalmic arteries is the most feared complication because it may be permanent and bilateral.

The inflammatory process of GCA may involve the aorta and its major branches. This involvement may be minimal and clinically silent; however, extensive inflammation may lead to aortic incompetence, aneurysm formation, aortic rupture, and death. Post-mortem studies demonstrated the extensive nature of the inflammatory process in GCA, but many lesions are clinically silent (Wilkinson and Russell 1972). Clinical

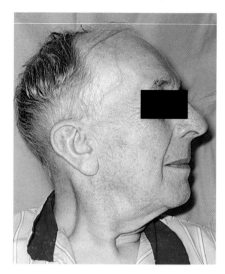

a

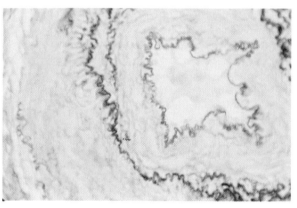

(b)

Fig. 11.1. (a) Swollen temporal artery in giant cell arteritis. (b) Destruction of internal elastic lamina in giant cell arteritis (elastic stain).

studies suggest that aortic involvement is present in around 14% of patients with GCA (Klein *et al.* 1975).

Clinical examination reveals tenderness and/or enlargement of the temporal and, occasionally, the occipital arteries (Fig. 11.1). There may be evidence of ophthalmic involvement with visual field defects. In patients with extracranial involvement there may bruits audible over large arteries and/or decreased pulses.

Wegener's granulomatosis

Wegener's granulomatosis is characterized by necrotizing granulomata of the upper and lower respiratory tract, necrotizing vasculitis, and focal glomerulo-

Table 11.4 ACR 1990 criteria for the classification of Wegener's granulomatosis (traditional format)

1. Nasal or oral inflammation
2. Abnormal chest radiograph
3. Urinary sediment
4. Granulomatous inflammation on biopsy

For purposes of classification, a person shall be said to have Wegener's granulomatosis if at least two of these four criteria are present. The presence of any two or more criteria yields a sensitivity of 88.2% and a specificity of 92.0%.
From Leavitt *et al.* (1990).

nephritis. A more limited form, with lesions limited to the upper and lower respiratory tract, can occur.

The ACR 1990 classification criteria for the diagnosis of Wegener's granulomatosis are shown in traditional format in Table 11.4 (Leavitt *et al.* 1990).

Upper airway disease is the most common presenting feature of Wegener's granulomatosis. It occurs in more than 70% of patients at onset, and develops in 90% or more of patients. Nasal disease presents with obstruction, crusted nasal ulcers and septal perforation, serosanguinous discharge, or epistaxis. Destruction of the nasal cartilage by granulomatous inflammation results in perforation of the nasal septum and development of the typical saddle nose deformity (Fig. 11.2f). Sinusitis is present in up to 85% of patients at some time during the disease. Deafness may occur as a result of serous otitis media. Laryngotracheal disease in Wegener's granulomatosis may be asymptomatic, but clinical presentation may range from hoarseness to stridor and life-threatening upper airway obstruction, the most characteristic lesion being subglottic stenosis.

Renal disease is a feature of Wegener's granulomatosis, occurring in 18% of patients at presentation and in 77% subsequently (Hoffman *et al.* 1992a), but may not be clinically apparent and therefore must be sought and monitored carefully. Patients may present with life-threatening acute renal failure owing to rapidly progressive glomerulonephritis requiring urgent dialysis and immunosuppression. At the other end of the spectrum are patients with proteinuria or haematuria with no evidence of impairment of renal function. The typical histological appearance is a focal segmental necrotizing vasculitis (Fig. 11.2b). The presence or absence of renal disease defines the subsets of generalized or limited Wegener's granulomatosis, respectively (Carrington and Liebow 1966). Limited disease may occasionally become generalized. Renal disease is a stong predictor of a poor prognosis; particularly oliguric renal failure.

Cutaneous manifestations occur in up to 50% of patients with Wegener's granulomatosis and occur at presentation in up to 25% (Fig. 11.2a). The cutaneous manifestations include ulcers, palpable purpura, subcutaneous nodules, papules and vesicles and reflect involvement of small vessels.

Pulmonary involvement is one of the principle features of Wegener's granulomatosis, occurring in 45% of patients at presentation and 87% during the course of disease (Hoffman *et al.* 1992a). Cough, haemoptysis, and pleuritis are the most common pulmonary symptoms. The most common radiographic findings are pulmonary infiltrates, granuloma (Fig. 11.2d) and nodules. Pleural effusions, diffuse pulmonary haemorrhage, and hilar lymphadenopathy are less common.

Neurological involvement is a less common presenting feature of Wegener's granulomatosis but occurs in up to 50% of patients during the course of the disease.

Ocular disease occurs in up to 50% of patients with Wegener's granulomatosis. Any compartment of the eye may be affected: keratitis, conjunctivitis, scleritis, episcleritis, nasolachrymal duct obstruction, uveitis, retro-orbital pseudo-tumour with proptosis, retinal vessel occlusion, and optic neuritis have all been described. Visual loss may occur in 8% of patients.

Cardiac involvement occurs in about 10% of Wegener's granulomatosis patients. The most frequent cardiac manifestation is pericarditis, presenting with pericardial pain or friction rub. Coronary vasculitis is uncommon but should be considered in patients developing angina or myocardial infarction.

Musculoskeletal symptoms are common in patients with Wegener's granulomatosis, with most patients only experiencing arthralgias and myalgias, but a true arthritis may occur in a quarter of patients. The arthritis of Wegener's granulomatosis is usually non-deforming and non-erosive. The joint disease usually parallels other disease manifestations.

Microscopic polyangiitis

Kussmaul and Maier's (1866) original description of periarteritis nodosa was of a condition with inflammation and necrosis of medium-sized arteries, leading to aneurysm formation and organ infarction. Wainwright and Davson (1950) described patients with segmental necrotizing glomerulonephritis who also had features of polyarteritis nodosa with involvement of extrarenal small and medium arteries. He used the term microscopic polyarteritis to describe these patients in whom

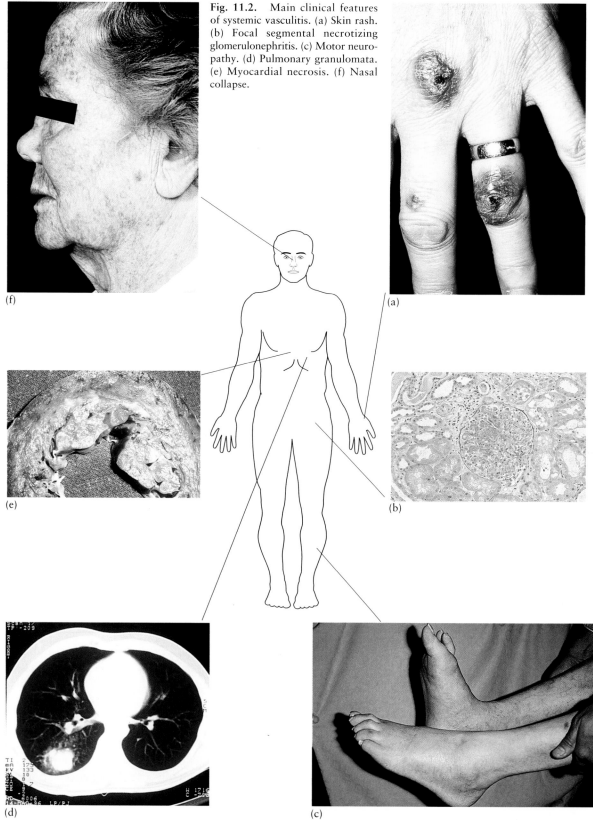

Fig. 11.2. Main clinical features of systemic vasculitis. (a) Skin rash. (b) Focal segmental necrotizing glomerulonephritis. (c) Motor neuropathy. (d) Pulmonary granulomata. (e) Myocardial necrosis. (f) Nasal collapse.

(f)

(a)

(e)

(b)

(d)

(c)

Table 11.5 Differences between classical polyarteritis nodosa (PAN) and microscopic polyangiitis (MPA) [from Guillevin *et al.* (1995)]

Criteria	PAN	MPA
Histology		
Type of vasculitis	Necrotizing with mixed cells, rarely granulomatous	Necrotizing with mixed cells, not granulomatous
Size of vessels	Medium- and small-sized muscular arteries, sometimes arterioles	Small vessels (i.e. capillaries, venules, or arterioles)
		Small- and medium-sized arteries may also be affected
Distribution and localization		
Kidney		
Renal vasculitis with renovascular hypertension, renal infarcts, and microaneurysms	Yes	No
Rapidly progressive glomerulnephritis	No	Very common
Lung		
Lung haemorrhage	No	Yes
Peripheral neuropathy	50–80%	10–20%
Relapses	Rare	Frequent
Laboratory data		
pANCA	Rare (< 20%)	Yes (50–80%)
HBV infection	Yes (uncommon)	No
Abnormal angiography	Yes	No

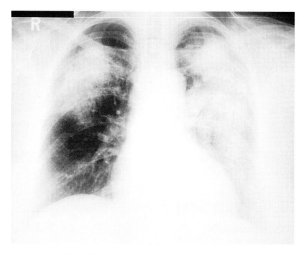

Fig. 11.3. Pulmonary haemorrhage.

the dominant feature is rapidly progressive renal failure. This group is now termed microscopic polyangiitis. In polyarteritis nodosa, the dominant feature is organ infarction (e.g. gut, nerve, bowel) as a result of involvement of medium-sized arteries. This group of patients are now termed 'classical' polyarteritis nodosa. Classical polyarteritis is not associated with ANCA. Orchitis is a typical feature. Microscopic polyangiitis is characterized by rapidly progressive glomerulonephritis, cutaneous involvement, and ANCA. Visceral angiography is usually normal (Guillevin *et al.* 1996) (Table 11.5).

Microscopic polyangiitis shares some features with Wegener's granulomatosis (Savage *et al.* 1985) and in early disease the distinction may be difficult. Renal disease is a very common feature, with microscopic haematuria, proteinuria, and impairment of renal function. The typical histological appearance is a focal segmental necrotizing vasculitis (Fig. 11.2b) but other appearances can occur. Hypertension is less common than in classical polyarteritis nodosa. Lung haemorrhage occurs in up to 29% of patients with microscopic polyangiitis and is an important contributor to morbidity and mortality (Fig. 11.3). Haemoptysis varies from blood-streaked sputum to expectoration of frank blood. Severe lung haemorrhage is characterized by dyspnoea and anaemia, which precedes diffuse alveolar damage. Mononeuritis multiplex is uncommon. Ocular and nasopharyngeal symptoms are less frequent compared with Wegener's granulomatosis.

Polyarteritis nodosa

The typical features of classical polyarteritis nodosa are organ infarction, haemorrhage, and myalgia. Mono-

neuritis multiplex is a common feature of polyarteritis nodosa at diagnosis, when it is observed in 70% of patients (Guillevin *et al.* 1992). Motor and sensory nerve involvement is asymmetrical and affects predominately the legs, especially the sciatic nerve (Fig. 11.2c). The radial, ulnar, and median nerves are less commonly affected. Orchitis is typical but an uncommon feature. Gastrointestinal disease is uncommon but carries a significant morbidity and mortality, and abdominal pain occurs in up to 34% of patients (Guillevin *et al.* 1993). Ischaemia usually affects the small bowel, and intestinal bleeding and perforation can occur.

Churg–Strauss syndrome

The characteristic features of Churg–Strauss syndrome (CSS) are: asthma, eosinophilia, fever and a systemic illness (Churg and Strauss 1951). Asthma in particular distinguishes Churg–Strauss syndrome from Wegener's granulomatosis, microscopic polyangiitis, and classical polyarteritis nodosa. Histologically there is a granulomatous necrotizing vasculitis. Renal involvement is relatively uncommon (Chumbley *et al.* 1977). Lanham provided a clinical definition: asthma, eosinophilia (> 1×10^9/l), and a systemic vasculitis involving two or more extrapulmonary organs (Lanham *et al.* 1984), which in our experience is more useful clinically than either the ACR 1990 criteria or the CHCC definition (Reid *et al.* 1998). In Lanham's experience, extravascular granulomata were not essential for the diagnosis of Churg–Strauss syndrome. They also noted a triphasic pattern of illness with allergic rhinitis, evolving into asthma; followed by peripheral blood eosinophilia and eosinophilic tissue infiltrates; and, finally, a systemic vasculitic phase. The necrotizing vasculitis may be indistinguishable from that found in classical polyarteritis nodosa and microscopic polyangiitis.

Asthma is the cardinal manifestation of Churg–Strauss syndrome and precedes the systemic features in virtually all cases. Asthma usually starts relatively late in life and becomes progressively severe until the onset of systemic vasculitis. Chest radiographs are often abnormal with pulmonary infiltrates in up to 77% of patients. Upper airways changes may include sinusitis, allergic rhinitis, and nasal polyps.

Cardiac disease is common and is a major cause of mortality, with congestive heart failure, pericardial effusion, and restrictive cardiomyopathy (Fig. 11.2e) Reid *et al.* 1998. Fifty per cent of patients in Lanham's series had abnormal electrocardiographs and 25% developed heart failure. Histologically, the most

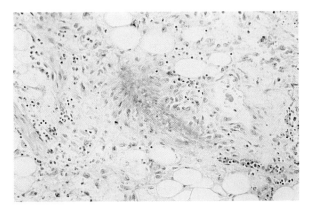

Fig. 11.4. Histology of myocardium in Churg–Strauss syndrome showing eosinophilic infiltrate with necrosis and granulomata.

common lesions are granulomatous infiltration of the myocardium and coronary vessel vasculitis (Fig. 11.4).

Skin lesions occur in approximately two-thirds of patients with CSS, nodules are the most distinctive but occur in other types of vasculitis.

Mononeuritis multiplex is a common (70%) feature of both polyarteritis nodosa and Churg–Strauss syndrome at diagnosis (Guillevin *et al.* 1992), but less frequently than Wegener's granulomatosis. Blindness has also been described in patients with CSS, though this is rare (Sutcliffe *et al.* 1997).

Renal disease is uncommon, but a necrotizing glomerulonephritis can occur.

Cryoglobulinaemic vasculitis

Cryoglobulins are plasma proteins that reversibly precipitate or gel in the cold, and were first described by Wintrobe and Beuell (1933). Waldenström first reported that cryoglobulins contained immunoglobulin and, in 1962, Lospalluto observed that cryoglobulins may contain more than one type of immunoglobulin and possess rheumatoid factor activity (Lospalluto *et al.* 1962). Cryoglobulins have been classified into three types on the basis of the type of immunoglobulin contained within the cryoprecipitate (Brouet *et al.* 1974). Type I cryoglobulins are monoclonal immunoglobulin (usually IgM), whereas types II and III are mixed, containing more than one class of immunoglobulin. Type II cryoglobulins are a mixture of a polyclonal component (usually IgG) and a monoclonal component (IgMκ with antiglobulin activity). Type III cryoglobulins are a mixture of two types of polyclonal immunoglobulin, one of which has rheumatoid factor activity.

Type I cryoglobulins may be found in a wide variety of conditions, including myeloma, macroglobulinaemia, and lymphoproliferative disorders. Type III are found in patients with autoimmune disorders and infections (e.g. hepatitis A, B, C). Types II and III may occur in the absence of an underlying disease — essential mixed cryoglobulinaemia (Meltzer *et al.* 1966). Recent studies have demonstrated an association between type II cryoglobulinaemia and hepatitis C virus infection (Agnello *et al.* 1992) and it has been proposed that immune complexes formed after hepatitis C virus infection stimulate the production of monoclonal IgM with rheumatoid factor activity (Miescher *et al.* 1995).

Vascular purpura is more common in types II and III, while skin necrosis, necrotic purpura, and severe Raynaud's phenomenon are features of type I cryoglobulinaemia. Arthralgias are a common feature of mixed cryoglobulinaemia and an arthropathy with erosions can occur. Renal involvement ranges from isolated proteinuria, with microscopic haematuria, to an acute nephritis. Histologically, there is a mesangiocapillary glomerulonephritis with a monocytic infiltrate and inflammation of small and medium-sized vessels. Renal disease is an important cause of morbidity and mortality, with a mortality exceeding 60% (Frankel *et al.* 1992).

The demonstration of cryoglobulins requires that the blood sample should be kept at 37°C until analysis (Fig. 11.5). There may be a cryoglobulin concentration of greater than 1 g/l, however levels do not reflect disease activity or degree of renal involvement.

The pathogenesis of the vasculitis of cryoglobulinaemia is poorly understood. A murine model has been described in which monoclonal IgG with rheumatoid factor activity is injected. Five to ten days later glomerulonephritis and leucocytoclastic vasculitis develops. A specific monoclonal IgG anti-idiotypic antibody can prevent cryoprecipitation and inhibit cutaneous vasculitis and glomerulonephritis (Spertini *et al.* 1989).

Hypocomplementaemic urticarial vasculitis

Hypocomplementaemic urticarial vasculitis syndrome (HUVS) is an uncommon vasculitic syndrome initially described as a triad of hypocomplementaemia, cutaneous vasculitis, and arthritis (McDuffie *et al.* 1973). The rash resembles urticaria, on biopsy there is a leucocytoclastic vasculitis with involvement of post-capillary venules. Patients may have associated angioedema, arthralgias, arthritis, abdominal pain, chest pain, renal disease (proteinuria, haematuria, and impairment of function), episcleritis, and uveitis.

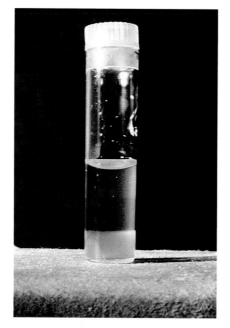

Fig. 11.5. Cryoglobulinaemia. Cryoglobulins are proteins that precipitate on exposure to cold.

Hypocomplementaemia is only present in one-third of patients and they are more likely to have systemic features (Mehregan *et al.* 1992). Eleven per cent of patients fulfil the ACR criteria for the diagnosis of SLE. The pathogenesis is believed to be a type III hypersensitivity reaction, but the antibody is at present unknown, with circulating immune complexes being reported in up to 75% of patients with urticarial

vasculitis. Alternatively, there may be an intrinsic abnormality of the complement system. There is an IgG precipitin that binds to C1q through its Fc portion. Autoantibodies to C1q in patients with HUVS are similar to the C1-binding autoantibodies found in SLE.

Behçet's disease

Behçet's disease is a chronic inflammatory disease. The classical triad of features are recurrent orogenital ulceration and uveitis. The first modern description was by Behçet in 1937, but the condition has been known since the time of Hippocrates. The condition is more common in the Mediterranean and Japan than in Europe or North America. It occurs in young adults and more commonly in males. Japanase and eastern Mediterranean patients have more severe uveitis.

The major clinical features of Behçet's disease are recurrent oral and genital aphthous ulceration. These ulcers are often painful, 3–10 mm in diameter, and take several weeks to heal. The uveitis may be severe and lead to blindness (Fig. 11.6). The arthralgia is usually a mild synovitis and in general affects hands, knees, and ankles. Erosive disease is rare. Vascular involvement occurs in up to 35% of patients (Lie *et al.* 1992). Venous involvement is more common than arterial disease, with deep venous thrombosis of extremities, trunk, and intracranial sinuses, and may be accompanied by superficial thrombophlebitis. Arterial aneurysm formation is more common than arterial occlusion and may lead to death following rupture. Small vessel vasculitis is common in Behçet's disease

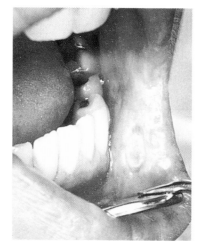

(a)

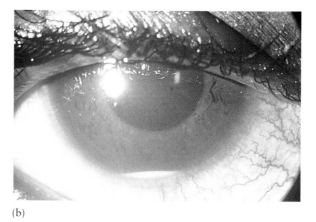

(b)

Fig. 11.6. (a) Oral ulceration in Behçet's syndrome. (b) Hypopyon occuring in Behçet's syndrome.

Table 11.6   Criteria for diagnosis of Behçet's disease (International Study Group)

Diagnosis requires recurrent aphthous stomatitis* plus two of the following:

Genital aphthae
  Aphthous ulcer or scarring

Eye lesions
  Anterior or posterior uveitis
  Cells in vitreous humour on slit lamp examination
  Retinal vasculitis observed by ophthalmologist

Skin lesions
  Erythema nodosum
  Pseudo-folliculitis
  Papulopustular lesions
  Acneiform nodules (absence of steroid treatment in post-adolescent patient)
Positive pathergy test results†

---

* Three times in one year. Diagnosis excludes other clinical syndromes (e.g. inflammatory bowel disease, relapsing polychondritis, infections, and sarcoidosis).
† Method: subcutaneous injection of a small volume of sterile normal saline. Test results less commonly positive in USA and UK than in the Mediterranean and Japan.
From: International Study Group on Behçet's Disease (1990).

and vascular necrosis and a lymphocytic infiltrate have been found in most organs involved. Central nervous system involvement occurs in 20% of patients, with aseptic meningitis, hemiparesis, cerebellar disease, and an altered emotional state.

There is no diagnostic test for Behçet's disease and the diagnosis is based on clinical criteria (Table 11.6).

Secondary vasculitis

Vasculitis may be secondary to established auto-immune rheumatic disease, malignancy, or to other exogenous antigens such as drugs and infections.

The clinical and pathological features of vasculitis occurring secondary to autoimmune rheumatic disease are similar to the primary form of vasculitis. Large vessel lesions can be morphologically indistinguishable from giant cell arteritis, whereas medium-sized vessel involvement is akin to polyarteritis nodosa. Small vessel involvement leads to a leucocytoclastic vasculitis or predominately hyperplasia of the intima with endarteritis obliterans. Response to treatment is similar to that seen in primary vasculitis.

Many cases of vasculitis are considered to have an infectious cause, although frequently a causal relationship is not established. A wide variety of organisms have been implicated, including bacterial, fungal, spirochaetal, and viral infections (Somer and Finegold 1995). Two mechanisms have been proposed: (i) direct microbial toxicity, either by endothelial invasion or the effect of microbial toxins on endothelium; and

(ii) immune-mediated either by humoral (immune complex) or by cellular responses. Hepatitis B virus infection is recognized as a cause of systemic vasculitis that is histologically indistguishable from polyarteritis nodosa, while hepatitis C virus infection is associated with cryoglobulinaemia.

Vasculitis in children

Vasculitis occurring in childhood has a different spectrum of disease from adults. Wegener's granulomatosis, microscopic polyangiitis, Behçet's syndrome, Churg–Strauss syndrome, Takayasu arteritis, and leucocytoclastic angiitis all occur in childhood, albeit rarely. Kawasaki disease occurs almost entirely in childhood, while Henoch–Schönlein purpura, post-streptococcal cutaneous vasculitis, and the vasculitis of familial meditteranean fever are more common in children.

Kawasaki disease

Kawasaki disease (mucocutaneous lymph node syndrome) is an acute vasculitis of unknown aetiology that primarily affects infants and young children, and was first described in Japan in 1967 (Kawasaki 1967). In Japan the annual incidence is 150 per 100 000 in children under five years, but it is much less common in the USA (10 per 100 000) and the UK (3.4 per 100 000). The aetiology is generally thought to be infective but the nature of the organism is obscure.

Table 11.7   Clinical features of Kawasaki disease

Fever
Bilateral non-exudative conjunctival injection
Oropharynx: injected or fissured lips, injected pharynx, or 'strawberry tongue'
Erythema of the palms or soles
Oedema of the hands or feet
Periungual desquamation
Rash: primarily polymorphous but not vesicular
Acute non-suppurative cervical lymphadenopathy

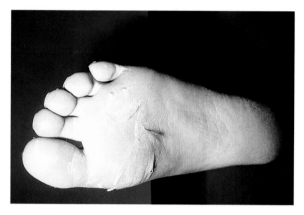

Fig. 11.7.   Desquamating skin rash in Kawasaki syndrome.

The principal features are given in Table 11.7 (see also Fig. 11.7). Coronary vasculitis with development of aneurysms is a major cause of morbidity and mortality. Coronary aneurysms may occur in up to 30% of cases. Other cardiac complications include pericarditis, pericardial effusions, ECG abnormalities, and myocardial infarction (see review by Leung *et al.* 1998).

Henoch–Schönlein purpura

Henoch–Schönlein purpura is the most common form of systemic vasculitis of childhood. The main features are non-thombocytopaenic palpable purpura, arthritis or arthralgia (in two-thirds of patients, especially in the ankles, knees, wrists, and hands), abdominal pain, gastrointestinal haemorrhage, and glomerulonephritis. The palpable purpura occurs in dependent and pressure-bearing areas such as the lower limbs and buttocks (Fig. 11.8a). Glomerulonephritis occurs in 50%, and the spectrum of renal disease varies from isolated microscopic haematuria to a nephritic/nephrotic syndrome with renal failure. Renal biopsy may demonstrate deposits of IgA. Histologically there is a small vessel vasculitis with predominately IgA deposition and this has been considered to be diagnostic (Jeanette *et al.* 1994). In the skin there may be a leucocytoclastic vasculitis with IgA deposition (Fig. 11.8b).

Henoch–Schönlein purpura is very much less common in adults and there is often difficulty in distinguishing Henoch–Schönlein purpura from a hypersensitivity vasculitis.

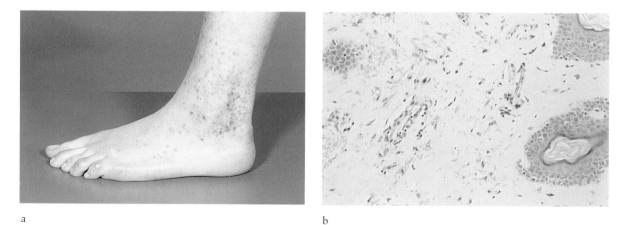

a   b

Fig. 11.8.   (a) Purpuric skin rash in Henoch–Schönlein purpura. (b) Leucocytoclastic vasculitis in Henoch–Schönlein purpura with nuclear dust formation (leucocytoclasis) and red cell extravasation.

Table 11.8 Investigation patients with vasculitis

Assessment of inflammation
- Urine analysis (proteinuria, haematuria, casts)
- Renal function tests (creatinine clearance, 24 hour protein excretion)
- Blood count (total, white cells, eosinophils)
- Acute phase response (erythrocyte sedimentation rate, C-reactive protein)
- Liver function tests

Immunological tests
- Autoantibodies (rheumatoid factor, anti-nuclear antibodies, anti-neutrophil cytoplasmic antibodies, anti-cardiolipin antibodies)
- Complement and immune complexes
- Cryoglobulins

Differential diagnosis
- Blood cultures
- Viral serology (hepatitis B and C, cytomegalovirus)
- Echocardiography

Specific investigations
- Radiographs of chest and sinus
- Biopsy of affected organs (especially kidneys and skin)
- Temporal artery biopsy
- Angiography

Investigation of vasculitis

Laboratory investigations are directed towards establishing the diagnosis, the organs affected, and assessing disease activity (Table 11.8).

Urinalysis is the most important investigation because the overall prognosis is chiefly determined by the extent of renal involvement. The finding of haematuria and/or proteinuria in a patient with systemic illness requires immediate further investigation with renal function tests and possibly a renal biopsy.

A full blood count may show a leucocytosis, which suggests either a primary vasculitis or infection, and neutropaenia or lymphopaenia in an untreated patient suggests vasculitis secondary to a connective tissue disease. Eosinphilia suggests either Churg–Strauss syndrome or a drug reaction.

Abnormalities of liver function may be non-specific but suggest a viral infection (hepatitis A, B, or C).

The presence of rheumatoid factor or anti-nuclear antibodies suggests vasculitis secondary to rheumatoid arthritis or other autoimmune rheumatic disease. Anti-neutrophil cytoplasmic antibodies (ANCA) are associated with vasculitis (see below for detailed discussion). Complement levels are low in SLE and infection, but high in primary vasculitis.

Other more specific investigations include coeliac axis angiography which may reveal aneurysms typical of classical polyarteritis nodosa (Fig. 11.9a). Angiography of the carotid vessels and aorta will show the stenotic lesions of Takayasu arteritis (Fig. 11.9b).

Biopsies of affected organs, in particular skin and kidney, are necessary to confirm the diagnosis, preferably before starting potent immunosuppression. Giant cell arteritis is often diagnosed by temporal artery biopsy.

Blood cultures, viral serology, and echocardiography are important to exclude infection and other conditions that may present as multisystem disease and mimic systemic vasculitis.

Autologous indium-labelled polymorphs demonstrate foci of activity that may be clinically silent (Reuter *et al.* 1995).

Aetiopathogenesis

Autoantibodies

Anti-neutrophil cytoplasmic antibodies

Anti-neutrophil cytoplasmic antibodies (ANCA) were first described by Davies *et al.* (1982) in sera from eight patients with crescentic necrotizing glomerulonephritis using indirect immunofluorescence. It was initially thought that these were a response to arbovirus infection. In 1985, van der Woude demonstrated that ANCA were present in sera from 90% of patients with Wegener's granulomatosis (van der Woude *et al.* 1985). Two main staining patterns are recognized using indirect immunofluorescence on human neutrophils — a cytoplasmic (cANCA) and a perinuclear (pANCA) — and these result from binding of

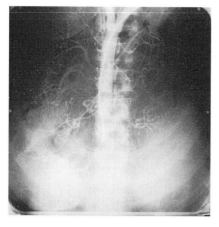

a

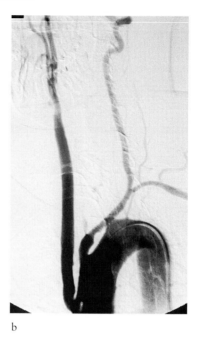

b

Fig. 11.9. (a) Classical polyarteritis nodosa. Aortic angiogram showing typical renal artery aneurysms. (b) Arch aortogram from a patient with aortic arch syndrome, showing a long tapering stenosis of the left subclavian artery.

autoantibodies to primary granule enzymes (see also Chapter 2). The pANCA pattern is an effect of the ethanol fixation of human neutrophils which solubilizes granule membranes allowing cationic granule enzymes to redistribute to the anionic nucleus. This effect can be prevented by using formalin fixation. It can be difficult to distinguish pANCA from ANA and formalin fixation can be used to confirm granular rather than nuclear staining. An atypical pattern is sometimes seen in patients with non-vasculitic conditions (discussed in Hoffman and Spechs, 1998).

There is a close association between cANCA and serine proteinase-3 (located in azurophilic granules) reactivity in patients with vasculitis (Lüdemann *et al.* 1990). Approximately 90% of vasculitis sera with cANCA activity recognize PR3 (Hagan *et al.* 1996). In patients with pANCA and vasculitis, about 70% recognize myeloperoxidase (MPO), an enzyme (MW 140 kDa) from azurophilic granules of neutrophils that catalyses the peroxidation of chloride to hypochlorite (Falk and Jeanette 1988). Anti-MPO antibodies occur in necrotizing glomerulonephritis (65%), microscopic polyangiitis (45%), Churg–Strauss syndrome (60%), and Wegener's granulomatosis (10%) (Hagan *et al.* 1996). pANCA occur in conditions other than vasculitis, including rheumatoid arthritis (16% of patients) (Braun *et al.* 1996), malignancy, inflammatory bowel disease, infection, and other autoimmune rheumatic

disorders, but the target antigen is rarely MPO. The autoantibodies recognize other antigens in the primary and secondary neutrophil granules, including lactoferrin, bacterial permeability-inducing protein (BPI) (Zhao *et al.* 1995), cathepsin G, azurocidin (Zhao and Lockwood 1996), glucuronidase, and lysozyme. BPI appears to be associated with inflammatory bowel disease but not with renal vasculitis (Yang *et al.* 1996). The clinical associations of the minor antigens are less well clarified.

Rao *et al.* (1995), in a meta-analysis, have confirmed the specificity of cANCA for active Wegener's granulomatosis (98%); however, the sensitivity was much lower (66%), although in the studies reviewed sensitivity ranged from 34 to 92%. In patients with limited Wegener's granulomatosis the sensitivity is lower at around 50%.

Anti-endothelial cell antibodies

Anti-endothelial cell antibodies (AECA) occur in many types of vasculitis in varying proportions, with high prevalences in Wegener's granulomatosis (50–80%), microscopic polyangiitis (50%), rheumatoid vasculitis (80%), Behçet's disease (18–80%), and Kawasaki disease (65%) (Meroni and Youinou 1996). In Wegener's granulomatosis and microscopic polyangiitis, AECA titres decrease during remission, correlate with clinical and laboratory parameters of disease activity, as well as endothelial damage, and are predictors of relapse (Chan *et al.* 1993).

AECA may cause vessel damage by several possible mechanisms, including antibody-dependent, cell-mediated cytotoxicity (ADCC), complement fixation with formation of membrane attack complexes, enhanced intravascular thrombosis, and recruitment of neutrophils to sites of inflammation. ADCC is probably not a major mechanism in vascular damage (del Papa *et al.* 1994). AECA of IgG isotype from Wegener's granulomatosis patients can upregulate adhesion molecule expression and increase secretion of pro-inflammatory cytokines (IL-1β, IL-6) and chemoattractants (IL-8, MCP-1). IL-1 can, in turn, stimulate expression of ELAM-1, VCAM-1, and ICAM-1 by endothelial cells.

AECA of IgG isotype have been found in 59% of Wegener's granulomatosis/microscopic polyangiitis patients with 68% IgM isotype (Savage *et al.* 1991), other studies have reported much lower prevalences (19 and 2%, respectively) (Varagunam *et al.* 1993). Antigenic characterization of AECA has proved difficult, the clinical significance of AECA in the follow-up of patients is doubtful.

Adhesion molecules

Leucocyte and endothelial cell adhesion molecules mediate a three-stage process for migration of leucocytes from the intravascular space into tissues (Springer 1994). During step 1, selectins (endothelial P- and E-selectin, and leucocyte L-selectin) are important during leucocyte rolling, and members of the integrin family (e.g. leucocyte LFA-1, MAC-1, and VLA-4) and the immunoglobulin superfamily (e.g. endothelial ICAM-1, ICAM-2, and VCAM-1) are involved in tighter adhesion, de-adhesion, and transmigration.

Increases in serum VCAM-1, ICAM-1, and LFA-3 have been reported in 22 patients with Wegener's granulomatosis (Stegeman *et al.* 1994). VCAM-1 was increased prior to clinical relapse. Increased levels of various adhesion molecules have been described in other types of vasculitis, but the specificity for active disease is questionable (reviewed in Cohen-Tervaert and Kallenberg 1997). Peripheral blood lymphocyte expression of ICAM-1 and LFA-3 have been reported. In the skin, enhanced E-selectin expression occurs in dermal vessels and is associated with a neutrophilic infiltrate, while in the kidney, enhanced VCAM-1 has been found in capillary loops of glomeruli with focal segmental necrosis (Pall *et al.* 1996).

Cytokine and growth factors

Fever, malaise, and weight loss in vasculitis may be attributable to the systemic effects of pro-inflammatory cytokines (IL-1, TNF-α, and IL-6). Serum interferon-α and IL-2 are elevated in polyarteritis nodosa and decrease with treatment (Grau *et al.* 1989). IL-1β and TNF-α have been shown to be produced locally by *in situ* hybridization and reverse transcriptase PCR in the renal lesions of Wegener's granulomatosis and microscopic polyangiitis (Noronha *et al.* 1993).

The vasculitic lesions of GCA are characterized by *in situ* production of IL-1β, IL-6, and TGF-β1 mRNA (indicative of macrophage activation) and IFN-γ and IL-2 mRNA (indicative of T cell activation) (Weyand *et al.* 1994). Both macrophage and T cell-derived cytokines were also detected in temporal artery biopsy specimens from patients with polymyalgia rheumatica. However, in polymyalgia rheumatica-derived specimens only IL-2 was detected, suggesting that IFN-γ may be important in progression to arteritis. This is supported by subsequent observations that the presence of IFN-γ mRNA was associated with jaw claudication and/or visual symptoms. Formation of giant cells in the granulomatous infiltrates was associated with local synthesis of IFN-γ mRNA (Weyand *et al.* 1997).

PR3–ANCA interaction

Cytokines (e.g. TNF-α, IL-8, TGF-β) are capable of inducing translocation of PR3 to the surface neutrophils. PR3 then becomes accessible to interact with ANCA (Mayet *et al.* 1993; Csernok *et al.* 1994, 1996) (Fig. 11.10). Several consequences of the PR3–ANCA interaction can be envisaged.

(i) Activation of primed neutrophils by ANCA resulting in production of reactive oxygen species and degranulation via binding of PR3 and engaging FCγRII.

(ii) ANCA may inhibit binding of PR3 to its physiological inhibitors α1-antitrypsin and α1-macroglobulin and thus prevent inactivation of PR3. This could be where α1-antitrypsin is functionally impaired. In a study of 105 patients with PR3–ANCA-positive vasculitis, 17 were heterozygous for α1-antitrypsin deficiency and one homozygous (El Zouki *et al.* 1994). Severe α1-antitrypsin deficiency is characterized by multiorgan involvement and a fatal outcome (Mazodier *et al.* 1996).

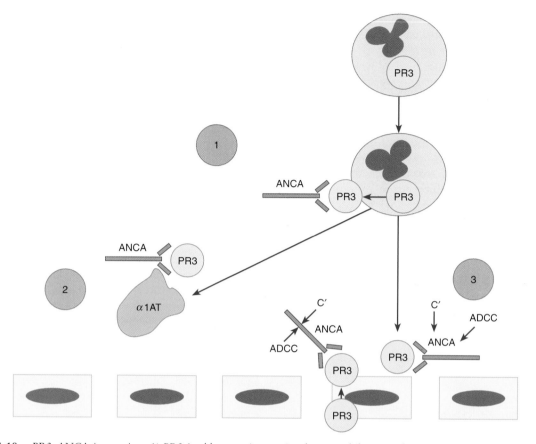

Fig. 11.10. PR3–ANCA interaction. 1) PR3 is able to activate primed neutrophils to produce reactive oxygen species, and to degranulate by binding to PR3 and engaging Fcγ RII; 2) inhibition of PR-3 inactivation by ANCA; 3) endothelial cell activation/lysis by ANCA. Modified from Gross and Csernok (1995).

(iii) ANCA binding to membrane PR3 is able to enhance adhesion molecule expression (E-selectin, ICAM-1, VCAM-1) and IL-8 production by endothelial cells (Mayet *et al.* 1993, 1996). Activated endothelial cells express PR3 and binding of ANCA is followed by complement activation and ADCC resulting in endothelial cell lysis.

(iv) Anti-PR3 have cytokine-like effects on human endothelial cells and ANCA are able to modulate the interaction of T cells and endothelium and contribute to the regulation of T cell migration from blood (Mayet *et al.* 1996).

Animal models

There are few good animal models for systemic vasculitis (Reviewed in Heeringa *et al.* 1998). Spontaneous

vasculitis occurs in some rodents, dogs, horses, and lupus mice, with ageing. Vasculitis occurs in serum sickness, murine models of lupus, in association with infection (particularly chronic viral infections), and after certain drugs. None of these models feature antibodies analogous to ANCA.

In genetically susceptible rodents, gold salts, D-penicillamine, and mercuric chloride induce an auto-immune syndrome characterized by IgE production (Piesch *et al.* 1989). In the brown Norway (BN) rat these agents also induce lymphoproliferation, T cell-dependent polyclonal B cell activation, hypergamma-globulinaemia with IgG autoantibodies against a number of antigens such as glomerular basement membrane, and mild tissue injury with glomerulonephritis and pro-teinuria (Hirsch *et al.* 1982). Mercuric chloride-treated BN rats develop a necrotizing leucocytoclastic vasculitis predominantly affecting the caecum, with milder tissue injury in the lung, liver, pancreas, and skin

(Mathieson *et al.* 1992), together with production of anti-myeloperoxidase antibodies (Esnault *et al.* 1992). Organ damage occurs at the peak of the antibody response. More recently, gold and D-penicillamine have been shown to induce a similar but less intense necrotizing leucocytoclastic vasculitis in the BN rat (Qasim *et al.* 1997). Possible mechanisms include chemical modification of MHC class II molecules such that modified epitopes are recognized as foreign by T cells; the T cell receptor could be chemically modified either by binding at the T cell surface or by an effect on the T cell receptor gene; or cell membrane molecules such as adhesion molecules could be chemically modified resulting in enhanced but non-specific interaction between T and B cells (Qasim *et al.* 1997).

Recently a model for PR3–ANCA-associated pauci-immune necrotizing crescentic glomerulonephritis has been established in Lewis rats (Gross *et al.* 1997). Immunization with human PR3 induced proliferation of cANCA. Following renal perfusion with purified human PR3, a proliferative crescentic glomerulonephritis developed within 4–10 days only in cANCA-positive rats. The lesions resemble rapidly progressive glomerulonephritis in patients with cANCA-positive Wegener's granulomatosis.

Mice (BALB/c) immunized with human ANCA develop mouse ANCA with specificity for both PR3 and MPO as well as anti-endothelial cell antibodies (Blank *et al.* 1995). The mice develop pulmonary lesions with mononuclear cell infiltrates resembling human vasculitis.

MHC immunogenetics

Takayasu arteritis

Most HLA studies in patients with Takayasu arteritis have come from Asian populations. Dong *et al.* (1992) utilized DNA-typing methods to determine HLA class II alleles and serological methods to determine HLA class I antigens. Statistically significant associations were found with both class II alleles and with a class I HLA antigen. The haplotype that was increased in patients with Takayasu arteritis included HLA-B52, DRB1*1502, DRB5*0102, DQA1*0103, DQB1*0601, DPA1*02, and DPB1*0901. The strongest association was with the class I antigen B52 (relative risk 3.6). HLA class II alleles DRB1*1502, DRB5*0102, and DPB1*0901 were also significantly associated, although the relative risk was lower than that found with B52.

A protective effect was also observed for a haplotype including HLA-B54, DRB1*0405, DRB4*0101, DQA1*0301, and DQB1*0401.

The association of Takayasu arteritis with the class I antigen B52 has been found in other populations. As summarized by Yajima *et al.* (1994) an increase of B52 was found in patients with Takayasu arteritis from Korea, Japan, and an increase of B5 in patients from India (B52 is one subtype of B5). Yoshida *et al.* (1993) applied DNA-typing techniques to provide somewhat greater discrimination of class I antigens (although specific class I alleles were not determined) and found an increase of B39.2 and B52. The authors proposed that positions 63 and 67 of the HLA-B class I molecule may be particularly important because B39.2 and B52 both encode glutamic acid and serine (respectively), whereas B51 and B39.1 differ at positions 63 and 67 and are not associated with Takayasu arteritis.

Studies in other racial populations are limited. A small study of patients with mixed racial composition was reported from the US and suggested that DR4 and DQ3 might be increased in patients with Takayasu arteritis (Volkman *et al.* 1982). No significant HLA association was found in a somewhat larger study that included 21 Caucasian patients with Takayasu arteritis (Khraishi *et al.* 1992).

Giant cell arteritis

Early reports utilizing serological techniques described an increase of HLA-DR4 in patients with giant cell arteritis (GCA) (Barrier *et al.* 1981). Other reports also described an increase of DR4, but found that the association was limited to patients with GCA who also had symptoms of polymyalgia rheumatica (Calamia *et al.* 1981; Cid *et al.* 1988). The most common DQB1 alleles associated with DR4 in Caucasian populations are DQB1*0301 and *0302. DQB1 was examined using RFLP techniques that are capable of distinguishing 'DQ3.1' and '3.2', which correspond to DQB1*0301 and DQB1*0302, but no difference was observed in patients with GCA compared with controls (Bignon *et al.* 1988).

The largest and most extensive study has been described by Weyand *et al.* (1992b). Forty-two patients with biopsy-proven GCA were studied for DRB1 alleles using allele-specific oligonucleotide primers and compared with 63 controls. A significant increase of HLA-DR4 was observed and found to be due to the DRB1*0401, *0404, and *0408 alleles. These allelic variants of DR4 are also associated with susceptibility to rheumatoid arthritis. However, the 'shared epitope' sequence that is associated with rheumatoid arthritis is in the third hypervariable region of the DRβ1 chain and is also encoded by DRB°0101, which was not increased in patients with GCA. The authors therefore examined all DRB1 alleles in GCA patients (including those not in the DRB°04 family) for shared amino acid sequences. Alleles that encode for a shared amino acid sequence in the second hypervariable region of DRβ1 chains from position 28 to 31 were increased. The sequence aspartic acid, arginine, tyrosine, and phenyl-alanine, was found to be encoded in DRB1°401, °0404, °0408, as well as °0301, °1301, °0801, and °1501. However, this is a consensus sequence that is also encoded by numerous other DRB1 alleles including those in the DRB1°16 and DRB1°11 families as well as some DRB1°14 alleles and no test of statistical significance in comparison to controls was given. Concomitant symptoms of polymyalgia rheumatica were not examined with respect to this shared sequence.

Wegener's granulomatosis and microscopic polyarteritis

There is no general agreement among studies regarding HLA class II antigen associations with Wegener's granulomatosis. An early study of a limited number of patients described an increase of DR2 (Elkon et al. 1983). However, other studies have not confirmed this observation. One report described a significant increase of DR1 and DQ1 (and no increase of DR2) (Papiha et al. 1992). Another somewhat larger study described an increase of DQ7 in patients with Wegener's and microscopic polyarteritis (Spencer et al. 1992). Differences in race or ethnic origin seem unlikely to explain the observed differences since all of theses studies were conducted in England and with Caucasian populations. The largest study was reported from the Netherlands and examined 224 Dutch Caucasoid patients and 2443 controls; 181 patients studied had a diagnosis of Wegener's granulomatosis, 25 had microscopic polyangiitis, and 18 idiopathic, rapidly progressive glomerulonephritis. No significant increase of any HLA class II antigen was observed (Hagan et al. 1995). A protective effect was found for DR13 that remained significant after correction for multiple comparisons (11% of patients vs. 28% of controls). A significant decrease of DQ1 was also found (which is in linkage disequilibrium with DR13).

A consistent association of any HLA class II antigen is also not apparent if patients are categorized according to autoantibody. HLA-DR9 was increased in Japanese patients with positive tests for cANCA and Wegener's granulomatosis (Nakamura et al. 1996) and DR8 in Scottish patients with cANCA and systemic vasculitis (most with Wegener's granulomatosis or microscopic polyarteritis) (Thomson et al. 1994) although only a minority of patients had DR8 in the latter study. Wegener's granulomatosis and microscopic polyarteritis patients with persistently positive ANCA tests were reported to have DR2 more frequently in a study of Caucasians from the UK (Spencer et al. 1992).

In summary, there is no consensus that any class II antigen is associated with susceptibility to Wegener's granulomatosis (WG). As noted above, the largest study found a protective effect of DR13. None of the above studies utilized PCR-based DNA-typing techniques, which discriminate specific class II alleles, so it remains possible that a shared amino acid sequence of otherwise different HLA class II molecules could be important. However, this possibility appears unlikely, since DR1 and DR2 allelic variants do not share amino acid sequences, and DQ7 is uncommon on DR1- and DR2-containing haplotypes. It is possible that differences in clinical subsets of patients may have contributed to the differences in study results reported to date, or that there are no specific HLA alleles that result in increased susceptibility to WG.

Behçets disease

There is remarkably uniform agreement that the class I antigen HLA-B51 is associated with risk of Behçet's disease in a multitude of populations world-wide. An increase of HLA-B51 has been described in Japanese (Mizoguchi et al. 1988; Mitzuki 1992), northern Han Chinese (Mineshita et al. 1992), Taiwan Chinese (Chung et al. 1987), Spaniards (Burson et al. 1992), Italians (Baricordi et al. 1986; Balboni et al. 1992), Iraqis (Al-Rawi et al. 1986), and in non-Ashkenazi Jewish and Arab patients (Chajek-Shaul et al. 1987). The relative risk associated with HLA-B51 is substantial and has been reported to be as high as 22.7 (Mitzoguchi et al. 1988). In contrast, when class II antigen associations have been described the relative risks have been less than that with HLA-B51, and no consistent observation has been found in the different ethnic and racial populations. One group from Japan described an increase of DQ3 (Mitzogochi et al. 1988) and another a decrease of DQ1 (DQA1*0103, DQB1*0601 and *0501) (Mizuki *et al.* 1992). An increase of DQ3 was also described in an Italian population (Balboni *et al.* 1992) where the relative risk was substantial but still less than that found with B51 (RR = 14 rs 20). Two studies in northern Han Chinese and in Taiwanese Chinese found no significant association with any HLA class II antigen (Mineshita *et al.* 1992; Chung *et al.* 1987). In Japanese, DRB1*0802 was also increased but accounted for a minority (18%) of patients (Mizuki *et al.* 1992).

Kawasaki disease

A number of reports have described HLA class I antigen associations with Kawaski disease. In Japanese where the number of patients studied is large (>200), an increase of B22 has been reported in Kawasaki's disease (Kato *et al.* 1978). However, only a minority of Japanese patients had B22 and the relative risk was low (25% vs 12% in controls, RR 2.5). The subtype of B22 was also identified and is one that is not found in Caucasians. Consistent with this observation, B22 has not been found in Caucasians with Kawasaki's disease, where instead B51 is increased. Although fewer patients were studied (n=51), the increase of B51 was found in the majority of patients and with a high relative risk, particularly in endemic Kawasaki's disease (70% vs 5%, RR 80) (Krensky *et al.* 1983). An increase of B51 was also found in a small study (n=12) of Israeli patients (Keren *et al.* 1982). In the former study that was based in the USA, a non-significant increase of B44 was observed in epidemic Kawasaki's disease. Other investigators, also from the USA, subsequently reported a significant increase of the class I haplotype A2-B44-Cw5 in epidemic Kawasaki's disease (Kaslow *et al.* 1985). There is no apparent sequence homology between the B alleles that have been described in patients with Kawasaki's disease. Thus there are differences in HLA antigen associations with Kawasaki's disease both according to race/ethnicity and also as to whether the disease is of the endemic or epidemic form.

Henoch–Schönlein purpura (HSP)

No HLA class I association was observed with HSP in a study from Denmark (Ostergaard *et al.* 1990). Possible associations with DQA1*0301 reported (Jin *et al.* 1996), and with DR4 have been suggested (Abe *et al.* 1993). Patients with HSP have been found to have abnormalities of genes that encode for complement components. C4 phenotypes were investigated in 19 patients with HSP (McLean *et al.* 1984) and the presence of two null variants (C4A and/or C4B) was observed significantly more often in patients than in controls (18% vs. 4%). Other investigators reported a seven fold or greater increased risk of HSP associated with gene deletion in the complement 4 locus (Jin *et al.* 1996; Abe *et al.* 1993), although fewer than 20% of patients had the abnormality. Thus a number of groups have described abnormalities of complement genes and a contribution of MHC class III complement genes to HSP is likely, however for a minority of patients. No convincing evidence has emerged of a role for class I or class II HLA antigens in HSP although the number of patients that have been studied is limited.

Rheumatoid vasculitis

Westedt *et al.* (1986) reported a frequency of HLA-DR4 among patients with rheumatoid vasculitis (RV) that was further increased over that found in patients with rheumatoid arthritis. A subsequent study did not find an increase of DR4 in patients with RV, but reported a disproportionate increase of the DR4 'subtype', Dw14 (DRB1*0404 and *0408) (Hillarby *et al.* 1991). This study, however, differs from subsequent studies that examined allelic variants in the DR4 family.

Weyand *et al.* (1992*a*) utilized DNA-typing techniques and determined specific DRB1 alleles. Eighteen patients with extra-articular disease were studied for HLA alleles, 11 of whom had rheumatoid vasculitis (seven cutaneous and four organ system vasculitis). The study by Weyand *et al.* is most often cited as demonstrating an association of disease severity with two DRB1 alleles that encode for the 'shared epitope' sequence. However, in this study the authors have carefully presented the specific phenotypes of patients with extra-articular disease and shown that RV is associated with homozygosity for DRB1*04. Seven of the 11 patients with RV (64%) were DRB1*04,*04. This is greater than that seen among patients with nodular RA without vasculitis (28%) and non-nodular RA (0%). In contrast, when assessed for two DRB1 alleles that encode the 'shared epitope' sequence, no significant difference was found when patients with RV were compared with patients with nodular RA without RV (64% vs. 56%).

Voskuyl *et al.* (1997) utilized DNA-typing techniques to study patients with RV and also found an association with DRB1*04. The authors further analysed patients according to whether vasculitis involved major organ systems or was limited to the skin, and found that homozygosity for DRB1*04 was increased in those patients with only cutaneous vasculitis. They did not find an association with the 'shared epitope' sequence when patients with RV were compared with those with RA without vasculitis. The authors studied DQB1 alleles and found no association with any DQB1 allele. They also reported no association with any DQA1 allele; however, data for DQA1 are not provided in the paper and this conclusion appears unlikely. Because of extremely tight linkage disequilibrium of DR4-containing haplotypes with DQA1*0301, given the description of increased homozygosity for DRB1*04, it is highly likely that an equivalent increased homozygosity of DQA1*0301 would have been observed. Further emphasizing this probability, the authors also report no haplotypes exhibiting unusual class II linkage disequilibrium patterns in their patient population.

An interesting report was described by Hillarby *et al.* (1993) in which patients with RV were found to have haplotypes with highly unusual linkage disequilibrium patterns in the HLA class II region. Among 39 patients with RV the authors observed 20 haplotypes with unusual combinations of class II alleles. A recently proposed model for the role of HLA molecules in the autoimmune pathogenesis of RA is that an HLA peptide derived from one molecule is presented by another HLA molecule. For example, a peptide from the DRβ1 chain might be presented by a DQ molecule (Zanelli *et al.* 1995). In this context, the finding of unusual combinations of DRB1, DQA1, and DQB1 alleles is of interest because an abnormal immune response could be postulated for example due to unusual combinations of DRβ1 peptides and DQ molecules. In this study the DQB1 allele *0302 was somewhat increased in patients with RV when compared with RA patients without RV. However, the difference was not significant when corrected for multiple comparisons, and this DQB1 allele was also not increased in RV patients in the study by Voskuyl *et al.* (1997). One study examined HLA-DPA1 and DPB1 alleles. An increase of DPB1*0801, *1001, and *1801 was found in patients with RV and a decrease of DPB1*0401; however, no finding reached statistical significance (Hutchings *et al.* 1993).

Rheumatoid vasculitis is relatively uncommon and the number of patients that have been studied is modest (at most, 40 patients were studied). Nevertheless, there is general agreement that RV is associated with DRB1*04, particularly homozygosity for DRB1*04. The association appears not to be due to the 'shared epitope' sequence, because RV is not increased among patients who have the 'shared epitope' sequence on non-DR4-containing haplotypes. These observations are consistent with a role for the first and/or second hypervariable region of the DRβ1 chain, or for DQA1*0301, which is in strong linkage disequilibrium with DRB1*04.

Prognosis and mortality

The natural history of vasculitis is very varied, ranging from mild disease limited to a single organ with an excellent prognosis, to rapidly fulminant fatal disease.

Large vessel vasculitis has a good prognosis provided that aortic involvement is adequately controlled. The majority of patients (74%) with Takayasu arteritis have some degree of impairment of activities of daily living, and 47% are permanently disabled (Kerr *et al.* 1994). Mortality is, however, low- and a 15-year survival of 82.9% has been reported (Ishikawa and Maetani 1994). Hypertension, cardiac involvement, aortic or arterial aneurysms, and severe functional disability predict greater morbidity and mortality.

The natural history of systemic necrotizing vasculitis (i.e. Wegener's granulomatosis, Churg–Strauss syndrome, and microscopic polyangiitis) is of a progressive course. Untreated, the five-year survival was 10% (Frohnert and Sheps 1967). The use of corticosteroids improved the five year survival to rate to 55% (Frohnert and Sheps 1967), which was further improved following the introduction of cyclophosphamide to 82% (Fauci *et al.* 1983). In most series, over 80% of patients with Wegener's granulomatosis and classical polyarteritis nodosa survive for over five years, and 75% of Wegener's granulomatosis patients survive for 10 years (Gordon *et al.* 1993). The outcome for microscopic polyangiitis is less good, with a 50–80% five-year survival (Gordon *et al.* 1993).

Relapse occurs in all types of systemic vasculitis and can occur during maintenance therapy or after cessation of treatment. The clinical features of relapse may differ from those at presentation with new organ involvement. The incidence of relapse does not reduce with time, unlike mortality. The highest mortality is seen early and there is relatively little mortality directly attributable to vasculitis after four years (Gordon *et al.* 1993).

Permanent morbidity occurs in 86% of patients with Wegener's granulomatosis — chronic renal impairment (42%), hearing loss (35%), nasal deformity (28%), tracheal stenosis (13%), visual loss (8%) (Hoffman *et al.* 1992a).

Guillevin studied 342 patients with polyarteritis nodosa and related conditions (classical polyarteritis nodosa with and without hepatitis B infection, microscopic polyangiitis, and Churg–Strauss syndrome) showing that the major clinical features associated with a poor outcome are renal insufficiency (creatinine > 140 mmol/l), proteinuria (> 1 g/day), and/or gastrointestinal tract involvement. Other poor prognostic features were cardiomyopathy and central nervous system disease (Guillevin *et al.* 1996).

Management and treatment

Disease assessment

Routine tests of organ function (urinalysis, renal function tests) should be used to monitor the effect of therapy on disease activity and observe for early detection of relapse. Full blood counts should be watched closely as cytopaenia may complicate immunosuppressive therapy. Serial measurements of the acute phase response are useful, but non-specific, and the acute phase response may be elevated during concurrent infection or secondary to other causes of inflammation. Serial ANCA (if initially present) may be helpful but some patients have persistently high ANCA titre despite no detectable disease activity and some patients have active disease without detectable ANCA. A number of studies have addressed this issue. Cohen-Tervaert *et al.* (1996) performed a meta-analysis and found a sensitivity of 48% (94 out of 197 increases in ANCA were followed by a relapse) and a specificity of 52% (81 of 157 relpases were preceded by an increase in ANCA titre).

Several scoring systems have been devised to facilitate the assessment of patients with vasculitis: e.g. the Birmingham vasculitis activity score (BVAS) (Luqmani *et al.* 1994b). Disease attributable to active vasculitis must be distinguished from damage caused by previous active disease. Damage occurs early and is associated with a poor outcome (Exley *et al.* 1997a). Pulmonary and multisystem disease are early indicators of poor outcome in patients with initially non-fatal disease. The vasculitis damage index has been designed to measure the impact of scars from previous disease or treatment (Exley *et al.* 1997b). The BVAS has recently been incorporated into the VITAL score (vasculitis intergrated assessment log) which has three components: activity, damage, and function (Exley and Bacon 1996).

Treatment

Treatment of patients with vasculitis depends on the extent and size of the vessels involved (Table 11.9). Patients with isolated skin disease may require no treatment or only modest doses of prednisolone, whereas patients with fulminant multisystem disease may require intensive immunosuppression combined with plasma exchange.

The large vessel vasculitides are treated initially with prednisolone (60–80 mg/day). Response rates of 20–100% have been reported in Takayasu arteritis with subsequent resolution of symptoms and stabilization of vascular abnormalities (Kerr *et al.* 1994). However, 40% of patients require addition of cytotoxic agents, and 23% have chronic unremitting disease (Hall *et al.* 1985). Hypertension can be difficult to manage in patients with Takayasu arteritis, particularly in those individuals with involvement of subclavian and femoral arteries, making measurement of blood pressure difficult. Wherever possible hypertension should be controlled by angioplasty or surgery. Medical control of hypertension must be cautious because of the risk to organs perfused by stenosed

Table 11.9 Relationship between initial treatment and vessel size

Dominant vessel involved	Corticosteroids alone	Cyclophosphamide + corticosteroids	Others*
Large arteries	+++	–	+
Medium arteries	+	++	++
Small vessels and medium arteries	+	+++	+
Small vessels	+	–	++

* Includes plasmapheresis, methotrexate, antiviral therapy for hepatitis B-associated vasculitis, and intravenous immunoglobulin for Kawasaki disease.

arteries from a fall in blood pressure. Angiotensin-converting enzyme (ACE) inhibitors must be used with caution in patients with renal artery stenosis because such patients have elevated renin levels and may be especially sensitive to the first dose of an ACE inhibitor. Beta-blockers may be used as an alternative. Vasodilators are potentially dangerous in the presence of fixed stenotic lesions. Percutaneous transluminal angioplasty has been reported to restore patency in up to 80% of cases, but restenosis can occur within 1–2 years.

Giant cell arteritis requires similar doses of prednisolone (60–80 mg/day) to prevent blindness. Improvement in blood flow through extremities rapidly occurs following treatment with high dose corticosteroids, rendering reconstructive surgery unnecessary. Angiographically occluded vessels rarely recanalize and in these cases clinical improvement is due to collateral formation. Surgery should be considered in patients with persistent limb ischaemia. This should be after the inflammatory phase has subsided to prevent early thrombosis of the graft (Ninet *et al.* 1990).

The combination of corticosteroids and cyclophosphamide is standard therapy for the systemic necrotizing vasculitides due to medium and small vessel arteritis. Treatment can be divided into three phases: (i) induction of remission; (ii) consolidation of remission; and (iii) maintenance of remission. Corticosteroids and cyclophosphamide are the treatment of choice for induction of remission in patients with active disease (Fauci *et al.* 1983). Cyclophosphamide may be given as continuous, low dose daily oral therapy (2 mg/kg/day) or by intermittent intravenous pulse therapy (10–15 mg/kg, maximum dose 1 g) repeated every 2–4 weeks. Both regimens are probably equally effective at inducing remission and are associated with a one-year survival of 84% (Adu *et al.* 1997). Remission is usually consolidated by continuing cyclophosphamide after remission has been achieved before changing to a combination of azathioprine and prednisolone as maintenance therapy. Prolonged use of cyclophosphamide leads to an uacceptable level of side-effects, particularly haemorrhagic cystitis, bladder malignancy, and lymphoma. The current trend is to reduce the duration of cyclophosphamide therapy and most patients switch from cyclophosphamide to azathioprine between three and 12 months after starting therapy. A multicentre study is currently in progress addressing the question of duration of cyclophosphamide therapy. During the maintenance phase the doses of azathioprine and prednisolone are gradually reduced, depending on the clinical condition. Vigilance must be maintained, as relapse may occur at any time.

Vasculitis localized to the skin may not require any specific treatment other than removal of the precipitating factor (drugs or infection). Prednisolone (20–40 mg/day) may be necessary to control cutaneous disease, and should be considered early in patients with evidence of extracutaneous involvement. Additional immunosuppression with azathioprine may be needed, but cyclophosphamide only rarely.

Other drug therapies

Methotrexate

Weekly, low dose methotrexate has been shown, in an open, uncontrolled trial, to be effective treatment for Wegener's granulomatosis, with 71% of patients achieving remission (Hoffman *et al.* 1992b), but whether methotrexate is as effective as cyclophosphamide in inducing remission is unknown. Methotrexate is effective in preventing relapse with or without the use of concomitant prednisolone (de Groot *et al.* 1996) and may be a useful alternative to azathioprine in maintaining remission. Methotrexate is also effective at inducing remission and minimizing glucocorticod therapy and toxicity in Takayasu arteritis (Hoffman *et al.* 1994).

Antibiotics

Upper and lower respiratory tract disease is present in 90% of Wegener's granulomatosis patients. Chronic nasal carriage of *Staphylococcus aureus* has been associated with relapse. De Remee *et al.* (1985) first reported the use of trimethoprim/sulphamethoxazole (co-trimoxazole) as treatment for of Wegener's granulomatosis. Stegeman *et al.* (1996) reported that the addition of co-trimoxazole to therapy with cyclophosphamide and prednisolone reduced the relapse rate. Co-trimoxazole alone, or combined with prednisolone, is not effective at preventing relapse in patients in remission (de Groot *et al.* 1996).

Antiviral therapy

Vidarabine or interferon-α 2B in addition to prednisolone and plasma exchange are effective in treating hepatitis B-associated polyarteritis nodosa (Guillevin *et al.* 1994). This approach can result in disease cure and elimination of viral replication. The seven-year survival was 83%; in 24% of patients viral clearance was seen and in 56% there was no evidence of viral replication (Gullevin *et al.* 1993). Antiviral therapy is also useful in patients with hepatitis C-associated cryoglobulinaemia (Agnello and Romain 1996).

Dapsone

Dapsone affects various neutrophil functions, including chemotaxis, lysosomal activity, and myeloperoxidase-mediated iodination, as well as cell attachment to IgA and IgG on basement membranes. Dapsone is useful in urticarial vasculitis and some other forms of mild cutaneous vasculitis.

Intravenous immunoglobulin

Intravenous immunoglobulin (IVIg), in combination with other immunosuppression, has been used to treat patients with systemic vasculitis refractory to conventional therapies. Remission at two months has been reported in 50% of such patients maintained for one year (Jayne and Lockwood 1993). In six patients with previously untreated disease IVIg was used as the sole therapy: four patients remained in remission after one year (Jayne and Lockwood 1996). The mechanism is unknown but possible actions include regulation of autoantibody production by B cells through idiotype– anti-idiotype interactions.

Intravenous immunoglobulin is the treatment of choice for Kawasaki disease, preventing development of coronary arteritis (Newburger *et al.* 1986).

Monoclonal antibodies

Humanized monoclonal antibodies directed against lymphocytes (CD4 and CD52) have been used in open studies to treat patients with refractory lymphocytic vasculitis (Lockwood *et al.* 1993) and Wegener's granulomatosis (Lockwood *et al.* 1996). In both groups of patients, prolonged remissions were obtained in some patients permitting reduction or even cessation of corticosteroid therapy. This approach may prove valuable in patients in whom conventional immunosuppression is contraindicated.

Plasma exchange

Plasma exchange has been advocated as an adjunctive therapy to cyclophosphamide and prednisolone in severe necrotizing vasculitis. Guillevin *et al.* (1995) reported a randomized trial of plasma exchange in addition to cyclophosphamide and prednisolone in 62 patients with severe polyarteritis nodosa and Churg–Strauss syndrome, and they showed that there was no additional benefit attributable to plasma exchange. A European Union-sponsored multicentre trial is currently investigating the role of plasma exchange in severe vasculitis with significant renal involvement.

Summary

The systemic vasculitides are a group of inflammatory diseases affecting blood vessels. The clinical features of the major types are increasingly well recognized with the help of defined classification criteria. The immunopathology, particularly of the ANCA-associated vasculitides, is better understood. Following introduction of cyclophosphamide the prognosis for these patients has improved, but further efforts are needed to minimize the morbidity from this therapy.

References

Abe J, Kohsaka T, Tanaka M *et al.* Genetic study on HLA class II and class III region in the disease associated with IgA nephropathy. *Nephron* 1993; **65**: 17–22.

Adu D, Pall A, Luqmani RA *et al.* Controlled trial of pulse versus continuous cyclophosphamide in the treatment of systemic vasculitis. *Q J Med* 1997; **90**: 401–9.

Agnello V, Romain PL. Mixed cryoglobulinaemia secondary to hepatitis C virus infection. *Rheum Dis Clin North Am* 1996; **22**: 1–21.

Agnello V, Chung RT, Kaplan LM. A role of hepatitis C virus infection in type II cryoglobulinaemia. *N Eng J Med* 1992; **327**: 1490–5.

Al-Rawi ZS, Sharquie KE, Khalifa SJ *et al.* Behcet's disease in Iraqi patients. *Ann Rheum Dis* 1986; **45**: 987–90.

Balboni A, Pivetti-Pezzi P, Orlando P *et al.* Serological and molecular HLA typing in Italian Behcet's patients: significant association to B51-DR5-DQ3 haplotype. *Tissue Antigens* 1992; **39**: 141–3.

Baricordi OR, Sensi A, Pivetti-Pezzi P. Behcet's disease associated with HLA-B51 and DRw52 antigens in Italians. *Hum Immunol* 1986; **17**: 297–301.

Barrier J, Bignon JD, Coulilou JP *et al.* Increased prevalence of HLA-DR4 in giant cell arteritis. *N Eng J Med* 1981; **305**: 104.

Bignon JD, Ferec C, Bomier, J. *et al.* HLA class II genes polymorphism in DR4 giant cell arthritis patients. *Tissue Antigens* 1988; **32**: 254–58.

Blank M, Tomer Y, Stein M *et al.* Immunisation with antineutrophil cytoplasmic antibody (ANCA) induces the production of mouse ANCA and perivascular infiltration. *Clin Exp Immunol* 1995; **102**: 120–30.

Braun MG, Csernok E, Schmitt WH *et al.* Incidence, target antigens, and clinical implications of ANCA. *J Rheumatol* 1996; **23**: 826–30.

Brouet JC, Clauvel JP, Danon F *et al.* Biologic and clinical significance of cryoglobulins. A report of 86 cases. *Am J Med* 1974; **57**: 775–88.

Burson JS, Grana GJ, Rodriguez RM *et al*. HLA and Behcet's disease in northern Spain: their lack of correlation with arthritis pattern. *Clin Rheumatol* 1992; **11**: 261–4.

Calamia KT, Moore SB, Elveback LR *et al*. HLA-DR locus antigens in polymyalgia rheumatica and giant cell arteritis. *J Rheumatol* 1981; **8**: 993–6.

Carrington CB, Liebow AA. Limited forms of angiitis and granulomatosis of Wegener's type. *Am J Med* 1966; **41**: 497–527.

Chajek-Shaul T, Pisanty S, Knobler H. HLA-B51 may serve as an immunogenetic marker for a subgroup of patients with Behcet's syndrome. *Am J Med* 1987; **83**: 666–72.

Chan TM, Frampton G, Jayne DRW *et al*. Clinical significance of antiendothelial cell antibodies (AECA) in systemic vasculitis: a longitudinal study comparing AECA and ANCA. *Am J Kidney Dis* 1993; **22**: 387–72.

Chumbley LC, Harrison RA, DeRemee RA. Allergic granulomatous angiitis (Churg Strauss syndrome): report and analysis of 30 cases. *Mayo Clinic Proc* 1977; **52**: 477–84.

Chung Y-M, Tasai S-T, Liao F *et al*. A genetic study of Behcet's disease in Taiwan Chinese. *Tissue Antigens* 1987; **30**: 68–72.

Churg J, Strauss L. Allergic granulomatosis, allergic angiitis and periarteritis nodosa. *Am J Pathol* 1951; **27**: 277–301.

Cid M-C, Ercilla G, Vilaseca J *et al*. Polymyalgia rheumatica: a syndrome associated with HLA-DR4 antigens. *Arthritis Rheum* 1988; **31**: 678–82.

Cohen-Tervaert JW, Kallenberg CGM. Cell adhesion molecules in vasculitis. *Curr Opin Rheumatol* 1997; **9**: 16–25.

Cohen-Tervaert JW, Stegeman CA, Kallenberg CGM. serial ANCA testing is useful in monitoring disease activity of patients with ANCA-associated vasculitides. *Sarcoidosis* 1996; **13**: 241–5.

Csernok E, Ernst M, Schmitt WH *et al*. Activated neutrophils express PR3 on their plasma membrane in vitro and in vivo. *Clin Exp Immunol* 1994; **95**: 244–50.

Csernok E, Szymkowiak CH, Mistry N *et al*. Transforming growth factor-beta (TGF-β) expression and interaction with proteinase 3 (PR3) in anti-neutrophil cytoplasmic antibody (ANCA) associated vasculitis. *Clin Exp Immunol* 1996; **105**: 104–11.

Davies DJ, Moran JF, Niall JF. Segmental necrotising glomerulonephritis with anti-neutrophil antibody: possible arbovirus aetiology. *Br Med J* 1982; **285**: 606.

de Groot K, Reinhold- Keller E, Tatsis E *et al*. Therapy for the maintenance of remission in generalized Wegener's granulomatosis. *Arthritis Rheum* 1996; **39**: 2052–61.

del Papa N, Conforti G, Gambini D *et al*. Characterisation of the endothelial surface proteins recognised by anti-endothelial antibodies in primary and secondary auto-immune vasculitis. *Clin Immunol Immunopathol* 1994; **70**: 211–16.

de Remee RA, McDonald TJ, Weiland LH. Wegener's granulomatosis: observations on treatment with micro-biological agents. *Mayo Clin Proc* 1985; **60**: 27–32.

Dong RP, Kimura A, Numano F *et al*. HLA-DP antigen and Takayasu arteritis. *Tissue Antigens* 1992; **39**: 106–10.

Elkon KB, Sutherland DC, Rees AJ *et al*. HLA antigen frequencies in systemic vasculitis: increase in HLA-DR2 in Wegener's granulomatosis. *Arthritis Rheum* 1983; **26**: 102–5.

ElZouki AN, Segelmark M, Wieslander J *et al*. Strong link between the alpha 1 antitrypsin PiZ allele and Wegener's granulomatosus. *J Intern Med* 1994; **236**: 543–8.

Esnault VLM, Mathieson PW, Thiru S *et al*. Autoantibodies to myeloperoxidase in Brown Norway rats treated with mercuric chloride. *Lab Invest* 1992; **67**: 114–20.

Exley A, Bacon PA. Assessment of vasculitis. *Cur Opin Rheumatol* 1996; **8**: 12–18.

Exley AR, Carruthers DM, Luqmani RA *et al*. Damage occurs early in systemic vasculitis and is an index of outcome. *Q J Med* 1997a; **90**: 391–9.

Exley A, Bacon PA, Luqmani RA *et al*. Development and initial validation of the vasculitis damage index (VDI) for the standardised clinical assessment of damage in systemic necrotising vasculitis. *Arthritis Rheum* 1997b; **40**: 371–80.

Falk RC, Jeanette JC. Anti-neutrophil cytoplasmic antibodies with specificity for myeloperoxidase in patients with systemic vasculitis and idiopathic necrotising and crescentic glomerulonephritis. *N Eng J Med* 1988; **318**: 1651–7.

Fauci AS, Haynes BF, Katz P *et al*. Wegener's granulomatosis: prospective clinical and therapeutic experience with 85 patients for 21 years. *Ann Intern Med* 1983; **98**: 76–85.

Frankel AH, Singer DR, Winnearls CG *et al*. Type II essential mixed cryoglobulinaemia; presentation, treatment and outcome in 13 patients. *Q J Med* 1992; **82**: 101–24.

Fries JF, Hunder GG, Bloch DA *et al*. The American College of Rheumatology 1990 criteria for the classification of vasculitis: summary. *Arthritis Rheum* 1990; **33**: 1135–6.

Frohnert PP, Sheps SG. Long term follow up of periarteritis nodosa. *Am J Med* 1967; **43**: 8–14.

Godman GC, Churg J. Wegener's granulomatosis: pathology and review of the literature. *Arch Pathol* 1954; **58**: 533–53.

Gordon M, Luqmani RA, Adu D *et al*. Relapses in patients with systemic vasculitis. *Q J Med* 1993; **86**: 779–89.

Grau GE, Roux-Lombard P, Gysler C *et al*. serum cytokine changes in systemic vasculitis. *Immunology* 1989; **68**: 196–8.

Gross WL, Csernok E. Immunodiagnostic and pathophysiologic aspects of ANCA in vasculitis. *Curr Opin Rheumatol* 1995; **7**: 11–19.

Gross WL. Systemic necrotizing vasculitis. *Ballière's Clinical Rheumatology* 1997; **11**: 259–84.

Guillevin L, Lhote F, Jarrousse B *et al*. Treatment of polyarteritis nodosa and Churg Strauss syndrome. A meta analysis of 3 propsective controlled trials including 182 patients over 12 years. *Ann Intern Med* 1992; **143**: 405–16.

Guillevin L, Lhote F, Leon A *et al*. Treatment of polyarteritis nodosa related to hepatitis B with shortterm therapy with anti-viral agents and plasma exchanges. A prospective trial in 33 patients. *J Rheumatol* 1993; **30**: 289–98.

Guillevin L, Lhote F, Leon A *et al*. Treatment of polyarteritis nodosa related to hepatitis B with interferon alpha and plasma exchanges. *Ann Rheum Dis* 1994; **53**: 334–7.

Guillevin L, Lhote F, Cohen P *et al*, Corticosteroids and pulse cyclophosphamide and plasma exchanges versus corticosteroids and pulse cyclophosphamide alone in the treatment of polyarteritis nodosa and Churg Strauss syndrome with factors predicting poor prognosis. *Arthritis Rheum* 1995; **38**: 1638–45.

Guillevin L, Lhote F, Gayraud M *et al*. Prognostic factors in polyarteritis nodosa and Churg Strauss syndrome: a prospective study in 342 patients. *Medicine* 1996; **75**: 17–28.

Hagan EC, Stegeman CA, D'Amaro J *et al*. Decreased frequency of HLA-DR13DR6 in Wegener's granulomatosis. *Kidney Int* 1995; **48**: 801–5.

Hagan EC, Andrassy K, Csernok E *et al*. Development and standardisation of solid phase assays for the detection of antineutrophil cytoplasmic antibodies. *J Immunol Meth* 1996; **196**: 1–15.

Hall S, Barr W, Lie J *et al*. Takayasu arteritis: a study of 32 North American patients. *Medicine* 1985; **64**: 89–99.

Heeringa P, Brouwer E, Cohen Tervaert JW, Weening JJ, Kallenberg CGM. Animal models of anti-neutrophil cytoplasmic antibody associated vasculitis. *Kidney Int* 1998; **53**: 253–63.

Hillarby MC, Hopkins J, Greenan DM. A re-analysis of the association between rheumatoid arthritis with and without extra-articular features, HLA-DR4, and DR4 subtypes. *Tissue Antigens* 1991; **37**: 39–41.

Hillarby MC, Ollier WER, Davis M *et al*. Unusual DQA-DR haplotypes in rheumatoid vasculitis. *Br J Rheumatol* 1993; **32**: 93–6.

Hirsch F, Couderc J, Sapin C *et al*. Polyclonal effect of HgCL2 in the rat, its possible role in an experimental autoimmune disease. *Eur J Immunol* 1982; **12**: 620–5.

Hoffman GS, Kerr GS, Leavitt RY *et al*. Wegener's granulomatosis: an analysis of 158 patients. *Ann Intern Med* 1992a; **116**: 488–98.

Hoffman GS, Leavitt RY, Kerr GS *et al*. The treatment of Wegener's granulomatosis with glucocorticoids and methotrexate. *Arthritis Rheum* 1992b; **35**: 1322–9.

Hoffman GS, Leavitt RY, Kerr GS *et al*. Treatment of glucocorticoid resistant or relapsing Takayasu arteritis with methotrexate. *Arthritis Rheum* 1994; **37**: 578–82.

Hoffman GS, Spechs K. Anti-neutrophil cytoplasmic antibodies. *Arthritis Rheum* 1998; **41**: 1521–37.

Hunder GG, Arend WP, Bloch DA *et al*. The American College of Rheumatology 1990 criteria for the classification of vasculitis: introduction. *Arthritis Rheum* 1990; **33**: 1065–7.

Hutchings CJ, Hillarby MC, McMahon MJ *et al*. HLA-DPA1 and HLA-DPB1 in rheumatoid arthritis and its subsets. *Disease Markers* 1993; **11**: 37–44.

International Study Group of Behçet's Disease. *Lancet* 1990; **335**: 1078–80.

Ishikawa K, Maetani S. Long term outcome for 120 Japanese patients with Takayasu's disease. Clinical and statistical analyses of related prognostic factors. *Circulation* 1994; **90**: 1855–60.

Jayne DRW, Lockwood CM. Pooled intravenous immunoglobulin in the management of systemic vasculitis. *Adv Exp Med Biol* 1993; **336**: 469–72.

Jayne DRW, Lockwood CM. Intravenous immunoglobulin as sole therapy for systemic vasculitis. *Br J Rheumatol* 1996; **35**: 1150–3.

Jeanette JC, Falk RJ, Andrassy K *et al*. Nomenclature of systemic vasculitides. Proposal of an international consensus conference. *Arthritis Rheum* 1994; **37**: 187–92.

Jin DK, Kohsaka T, Koo JW *et al*. Complement 4 locus II gene deletion and DQA1*0301 gene: genetic risk factors for IgA nephropathy and Henoch-Schonlein nephritis. *Nephron* 1996; **73**: 390–5.

Kaslow RA, Bailowitz A, Lin FY *et al*. Association of epidemic Kawasaki syndrome with the HLA-A2, B44, Cw5 antigen combination. *Arthritis Rheum* 1985; **28**: 938–40.

Kato S, Kimura M, Tsjui K *et al*. HLA antigens in Kawasaki disease. *Pediatrics* 1978; **61**: 252–5.

Kawasaki T. Acute febrile mucocutaneous syndrome with lymphoid involvement with specific desquamation of the fingers and toes in children: clinical observations in 50 cases. *Jap J Allergol* 1967; **16**: 178–222.

Keren G, Danon YL, Orgad S *et al*. HLA Bw51 is increased in mucocutaneous lymph node syndrome in Israeli patients. *Tissue Antigens* 1982; **20**: 144–6.

Kerr GS, Hallahan CW, Giodano J *et al*. Takayasu's arteritis. *Ann Intern Med* 1994; **120**: 919–29.

Khraishi MM, Gladman DD, Dagenais P *et al*. HLA antigens in North American patients with Takayasu arteritis. *Arthritis Rheum* 1992; **35**: 573–9.

Klein RG, Hunder GG, Stanson AW *et al*. Large artery involvement in giant cell (Temporal) arteritis. *Ann Intern Med* 1975; **83**: 806–12.

Krensky AM, Grady S, Shanley KM *et al*. Epidemic and endemic HLA-B and DR associations in mucocutaneous lymph node syndrome. *Hum Immunol* 1983; **6**: 75–7.

Kussmaul A, Maier R. Uber eine bisher nicht beschriebene eigenthümliche Arterienerkrankung (Periarteritis nodosa), die mit Morbus Brightü und rapid fortschreitender allgemeiner Muskellähmung einhergeht. *Deutsche Archive Klinical Medizin* 1866; **1**: 484–514.

Lamb AR. Periarteritis nodosa — a clinical and pathological review of the diseases. *Arch Intern Med* 1914; **14**: 481–516.

Lanham JG, Elkon KB, Pusey CD *et al*. Systemic vasculitis in asthma and eosinophilia: a clinical approach to the Churg Strauss syndrome. *Medicine* 1984; **63**: 65–81.

Leavitt RY, Fauci AS, Bloch DA *et al*. The American College of Rheumatology 1990 criteria for the classification of Wegener's granulomatosis. *Arthritis Rheum* 1990; **33**: 1101–7.

Leung DYM, Schlievert PM, Meissner HC. The immunopathogenesis and management of Kawasaki syndrome. *Arthritis Rheum* 1998; **41**: 1538–47.

Lie JT. Vascular involvment in Behçet's disease: arterial, venous and vessels of all sizes. *J Rheumatol* 1992; **19**: 341–3.

Lockwood CM, Thiru S, Isaacs JD *et al*. Humanised monoclonal antibody therapy for intractable systemic vasculitis. *Lancet* 1993; **341**: 1620–2.

Lockwood CM, Thiru S, Stewart S *et al*. Treatment of refractory Wegener's granulomatosis with humanised monoclonal antibodies. *Q J Med* 1996; **89**: 903–12.

Lospalutto J, Dorvand B, Miller W *et al*. Cryoglobulinaemia based on interaction between a gamma macroglobulin and S gamma globulin. *Am J Med* 1962; **32**: 142–7.

Lüdemann J, Utecht B, Gross WL. Anti-neutrophil cytoplasmic antibodies (ANCA) in Wegener's granulomatosis recognize an elastinolytic enzyme. *J Exp Med* 1990; **171**: 357–62.

Lupi-Herrera E, Sanchez-Torres G, Marcushamer J *et al*. Takayasu's arteritis. Clinical study of 107 cases. *American Heart Journal*, 1977; **93**: 94–103.

Luqmani RA, Bacon PA, Beaman M *et al*. Classical versus nonrenal Wegener's granulomatosis. *Q J Med* 1994a; **87**: 161–7.

Luqmani RA, Bacon PA, Moots RJ *et al*. Birmingham Vasculitis Activity Score (BVAS) in systemic necrotising vasculitis. *Q J Med* 1994b; **87**: 671–8.

Mathieson PW, Thiru S, Oliviera DBG. Mercuric chloride treated Brown Norway rats develop widespread tissue injury including necrotising vasculitis. *Lab Invest* 1992; **67**: 121–9.

Mayet WJ, Csernok E, Szymkowiak C *et al*. Human endothelial cells express PR3, the target antigen of anticytoplasmic antibodies in Wegener's granulomatosis. *Blood* 1993; **82**: 1221–9.

Mayet W-J, Schwarting A, Orth T *et al*. Antibodies to proteinase 3 mediate expression of vascular cell adhesion molecule-1 (VCAM-1). *Clin Exp Immunol* 1996; **103**: 259–67.

Mazodier P, Elzouki A-NY, Segelmark M *et al*. Systemic necrotizing vasculitides in sever alpha 1-antitrypsin deficiency. *Q J Med* 1996; **89**: 599–611.

McDuffie FC, Sams WM, Maldonaldo JE *et al*. Hypocomplementaemia with cutaneous vasculitis and arthritis. Possible immune complex syndrome. *Mayo Clin Proc* 1973; **48**: 340–8.

McLean RH, Wyatt RJ, Julian BA. Complement phenotypes in glomerulonepthritis: increased frequency of homozygous null C4 phoentypes in IgA nephropathy and Henoch–Schonlein purpura. *Kidney Int* 1984; **26**: 855–60.

Mehregan DR, Hall MJ, Gibson CE. Urticarial vasculitis: a histopathological and clinical review of 72 cases. *J Am Acad Dermatol* 1992; **26**: 441–8.

Meltzer M, Elias K, McCluskey RT *et al*. Cryoglobulinaemia — a clinical and laboratory study. *Am J Med* 1966; **40**: 828–36.

Meroni PL, Youinou P. Endothelial cell antibodies. In: *Autoantibodies*, eds Peter JD, Shoenfeld Y. Elsevier Science BV, Amsterdam, 1996; 245–51.

Miescher PA, Huang YP, Izui S. Type II cryoglobulinaemia. *Sem Haematol* 1995; **32**: 80–5.

Mineshita S, Tian D, Wang LM *et al*. Histocompatibility antigens associated with Behcet's disease in northern Han Chinese. *Int Med* 1992; **31**: 1073–75.

Mizoguchi M, Matsuki K, Mochizuki M *et al*. Human leukocyte antigen in Sweet's syndrome and its relationship to Behçet's disease. *Arch Dermatol* 1988; **124**: 1069–73.

Mizuki N, Inoko H, Mizuki N *et al*. Human leukocyte antigen serologic and DNA typing of Behcet's disease and it primary association with B51. *Invest Opthal Vis Sci* 1992; **33**: 3332–40.

Nakamaru Y, Maguchi S, Takizawa M *et al*. The association between human leukocyte antigens (HLA) and cytoplasmic antineutrophil cytoplasmic antibody (cANCA)-positive Wegener's granulomatosis in a Japanese population. *Rhinology* 1996; **34**: 163–5.

Newburger JW, Takashi M, Burns JC. Treatment of Kawasaki disease with intravenous immunoglobulins. *N Eng J Med* 1986; **315**: 341–6.

Ninet JP, Bachet P, Dumontet CM, *et al*. Subclavian and axillary involvement in temporal arteritis and polymyalgia rheumatica. *Am J Med* 1990; **88**: 13–20.

Noronha IL, Kruger C, Andrassy K *et al*. In situ production of TNF-α, IL-1β, and IL-2R in ANCA positive glomerulonephritis. *Kidney Int* 1993; **43**: 682–92.

Novak SN, Pearson CM. Cycophosphamide therapy in of Wegener's granulomatosis. *N Eng J Med* 1971; **284**: 938–42.

Ostergaard JR, Storm K, Lamm Lu. Lack of association between HLA and Schoenlein–Henoch purpura. *Tissue Antigens* 1990; **35**: 234–5.

Pall AA, Howie AJ, Adu D *et al*. Glomerular VCAM-1 expression in renal vasculitis. *J Clin Pathol* 1996; **49**: 238–42.

Papiha SS, Murty GE, Ad'Hia A *et al*. Association of Wegener's granulomatosis with HLA antigens and other genetic markers. *Ann Rheum Dis* 1992; **51**: 246–8.

Piesch P, Vohr HW, Degitz K *et al*. Immunological alterations induced by mercuric compounds II. Mercuric chloride and gold sodium thiomalate enhance serum IgE and IgG in susceptable mouse strains. *Int Arch Allergy Appl Immunol* 1989; **90**: 47–53.

Qasim FJ, Thiru S, Gillespie K. Gold and D-penicillamine induce vasculitis and up-regulate mRNA for IL-4 in the Brown Norway rat: support for a role for Th2 cell activity. *Clin Exp Immunol* 1997; **108**: 438–45.

Rao JK, Weinberger M, Oddone EZ *et al*. The role of anti-neutrophil antibody (cANCA) testing in the diagnosis of Wegener's granulomatosis. *Ann Intern Med* 1995; **123**: 925–32.

Reid AJC, Harrison BDW, Watts RA *et al*. Churg Strauss syndrome in a district hospital. *Q J Med* 1998; **91**: 219–29.

Reuter H, Wraight EP, Qasim FJ. Management of systemic vasculitis: contributions of scintigraphic imaging to evaluation of disease activity and classification. *Q J Med* 1995; **88**: 509–16.

Salvarani C, Gabriel SE, O'Fallon WM *et al*. The incidence of giant cell arteritis in Olmstead County, Minnesota: apparent fluctuations in cyclic pattern. *Ann Intern Med* 1995; **123**: 192–4.

Savage COS, Winearls CG, Evans DJ *et al*. Microscopic polyarteritis: presentation, pathology and prognosis. *Q J Med* 1985; **56**: 467–82.

Savage COS, Pottinger BE, Gaskin G *et al*. Vascular damage in Wegener's granulomatosis and microscopic polyarteritis: presence of anti-endothelial cell antibodies and their relation to anti-neutrophil cytoplasm antibodies. *Clin Exp Immunol* 1991; **85**: 14–19.

Scott DGI, Bacon PA, Elliott PJ *et al*. Systemic vasculitis in district general hospital 1972–80: clinical and laboratory features, classification and prognosis of 80 cases. *Q J Med* 1982; **203**: 292–311.

Somer T, Finegold SM. Vasculitides associated with infections, immunization, and antimicrobial drugs. *Clin Infect Dis* 1995; **20**: 1010–36.

Spencer SJW, Burns A, Gaskin G *et al*. HLA class II specificities in vasculitis with antibodies to neutrophil cytoplasmic antigens. *Kidney Int* 1992; **41**: 1059–63.

Spertini F, Donati Y, Welle I *et al*. Prevention of murine cryoglobulinaemia and associated pathology by monoclonal anti-idiotype antibody. *J Immunol* 1989; **143**: 2508–13.

Springer TA. Traffic signals for lymphocyte recirculation and leucocyte emigration: the multistep paradigm. *Cell* 1994; **76**: 301–14.

Stegeman CA, Cohen Tervaert JW, Huitema MG *et al*. Serum levels of soluble adhesion molecules: ICMA-1, VCAM-1 and E-selection in patients with Wegener's granulomatosis: relationship to disease activity and relevance during follow up. *Arthritis Rheum* 1994; **37**: 1228–35.

Stegeman CA, Cohen Tervaert JW, de Jong PE *et al*. Trimethoprim-sulphamethoxazole (co-trimoxazole) for the prevention of relapses in Wegener's granulomatosis. *N Eng J Med* 1996; **335**: 16–20.

Sutcliffe N, Morris V, Gomperts B *et al*. Relationship between the development of blindness in Churg–Strauss syndrome and anti-myeloperoxidase antibodies. *Br J Rheumatol* 1997; **36**: 273–5.

Takayasu M. Cases with unusual changes of the central vessels in the retina. *Acta Societas Ophthalmol Jap* 1908; **12**: 554.

Thomson JB, Hulse D, Galbraith I *et al*. Autoantibody associations with MHC class II antigens in scleroderma and autoimmune vasculitis. *Autoimmunity* 1994; **19**: 265–9.

van der Woude FJ, Rasmussen N, Lobatto S *et al*. Auto-antibodies against neutrophils and monocytes: tool for diagnosis and marker of disease activity in Wegener's granulomatosis. *Lancet* 1985; i: 425–9.

Varagunam M, Nwosu Z, Adu D *et al*. Little evidence for anti-endothelial cell antibodies in microscopic polyarteritis and Wegener's granulomatosis. *Nephrol Dialysis Transplant* 1993; **8**: 113–17.

Volkman DJ, Mann DL, Fauci AS. Association between Takayasu's arteritis and a B-cell alloantigen in North Americans. *N Eng J Med* 1982; **306**: 464–5.

Voskuyl AE, Hazes MJW, Schreuder GMT *et al*. HLA-DRB1, DQA1, and DQB1 genotypes and risk of vasculitis in patients with rheumatoid arthritis. *J Rheumatol* 1997; **24**: 852–5.

Wainwright J, Davson J. The renal appearances in micro-scopic form of polyarteritis nodosa. *J Pathol Bacteriol* 1950; **62**: 189–96.

Watts RA, Scott DGI. Classification and epidemiology of the vasculitides. *Bailliere's Clin Rheum* 1997; **11**: 191–217.

Westedt ML, Breedveld FC, Schreuder GM *et al*. Immuno-genetic heterogeneity of rheumatoid arthritis. *Ann Rheum Dis* 1986; **45**: 534–8.

Weyand CM, Xie C, Goronzy JJ. Homozygosity for the HLA-DRB1 allele selects for extraarticular manifesta-tions of rheumatoid arthritis. *J Clin Invest* 1992a; **89**: 2033–9.

Weyand CM, Kicok KC, Hunder GG *et al*. The HLA-DRB1 locus as a genetic component in giant cell arteritis. Mapping of a disease-linked sequence motif to the antigen binding site of the HLA-DR molecule. *J Clin Invest* 1992b; **90**: 2355–61.

Weyand CM, Hicok, KC, Hunder GG *et al*. Tissue cytokine patterns in polymyalgia and giant cell arteritis. *Ann Intern Med* 1994, **121**: 2184–91.

Weyand CM, Tetzlaff N, Björnsson J *et al*. Disease patterns and tissue cytokine profiles in giant cell arteritis. *Arthritis Rheum* 1997; **40**: 19–26.

Wilkinson IMS, Russell RWR. Arteritis of the head and neck in giant cell arteritis. *Arch Neurol* 1972; **27**: 378–91.

Wintrobe MM, Beuell MV. Hypoproteinaemia associated with multiple myeloma. *Bull Johns Hopkins Hosp* 1933; **52**: 156–65.

Yajima M, Numano F, Park YB *et al*. Comparative studies of patients with Takayasu arteritis in Japan, Korea and India. *Jap Circulation J* 1994; **58**: 9–14.

Yang JJ, Tuttle R, Falk RJ *et al*. Frequency of anti-bactericidal/ permeability-increasing protein (BPI) and anti-azurocidin in patients with renal disease. *Clin Exp Immunol* 1996; **105**: 125–31.

Yoshida M, Kimura A, Katsuragi K *et al*. DNA typing of HLA-B gene in Takayasu's arteritis. *Tissue Antigens* 1993; **42**: 87–90.

Zanelli E, Gonzalez-Gay MA, David CS. Could HLA-DRB1 be the protective locus for rheumatoid arthritis? *Immunol Today* 1995; **16**: 274–8.

Zeek PM. Periarteritis nodosa — a critical review. *Am J Clin Pathol* 1952; **22**: 777–90.

Zhao MH, Lockwood CM. Azurocidin is a novel antigen for anti-neutrophil cytoplasmic autoantibodies (ANCA) in systemic vasculitis. *Clin Exp Immunol* 1996; **103**: 397–402.

Zhao MH, Jones SH, Lockwood CM. Bactericidal/permeability-increasing protein (BPI) is an important antigen for anti-neutrophil cytoplasmic autoantibodies (ANCA) in vasculitis. *Clin Exp Immunol* 1995; **99**: 49–56.

Index